Blood Stem Cell Transplantation

Blood Stem Cell Transplantation

Edited by

JOSY REIFFERS, MD
Laboratoire de Greffe de Moëlle
Université Victor Segalen Bordeaux 2
33076 Bordeaux Cedex
FRANCE

JOHN M GOLDMAN, DM, FRCP, FRCPath
Chairman, Department of Haematology
Imperial College School of Medicine
Hammersmith Hospital
London W12 0NN
UK

JAMES O ARMITAGE, MD
Professor and Chairman
Department of Internal Medicine
University of Nebraska Medical Center
Omaha NE 68198-3332
USA

MARTIN DUNITZ

© Martin Dunitz Ltd 1998

First published in the United Kingdom in 1998 by
Martin Dunitz Ltd
The Livery House
7–9 Pratt Street
London NW1 0AE

A CIP catalogue record for this book is available from the British Library

ISBN 1-85317-291-X

Composition by Wearset, Boldon, Tyne and Wear
Printed and bound in Great Britain by
Biddles Ltd, Guildford and King's Lynn

Contents

Contributors

Douglas Adkins, MD
Division of Bone Marrow Transplantation and
Stem Cell Biology
Washington University School of Medicine
660 S. Euclid Avenue
St. Louis MO 63110
USA

James O Armitage, MD
Professor and Chairman
Department of Internal Medicine
University of Nebraska Medical Center
600 South 42nd Street
Omaha NE 68198-3332
USA

Bart Barlogie, MD, PhD
Division Director
Department of Medicine
Division of Hematology/Oncology
University of Arkansas for Medical Sciences
4301 West Markham
Little Rock AR 72205
USA

James Bender, PhD
Scientific Director
Baxter Healthcare Corporation
Biotech Group
Immunotherapy Division
9 Parker
Irvine CA 92618
USA

Philip J Bierman, MD
Associate Professor
Department of Internal Medicine
University of Nebraska Medical Center
600 South 42nd Street
Omaha NE 68198-3332
USA

Jean-Michel Boiron, MD
Hôpital Haut-Lévêque
CHU Bordeaux
33604 Pessac
FRANCE

Hal E Broxmeyer, PhD
Walther Oncology Center
1044 West Walnut Street
Indianapolis IN 46202
USA

John M Cunningham, MD
Division of Experimental Hematology
Department of Hematology/Oncology
St Jude Children's Research Hospital
332 North Lauderale
Memphis TN 38103
USA

Peter Dreger, MD
Second Department of Medicine
University of Kiel
Chemnitzstrasse 33
D-24116 Kiel
GERMANY

Adrian P Gee, MIBiol, PhD
Director, Stem Cell Processing Laboratory
Section of Bone and Marrow Transplantation
Department of Hematology
MD Anderson Cancer Center
1515 Holcombe Boulevard
Houston TX 77030
USA

George E Georges, MD
Fred Hutchinson Cancer Research Center
Clinical Research Division
1124 Columbia Street
Seattle WA 98104
USA

John M Goldman, DM, FRCP, FRCPath
Chairman, Department of Haematology
Imperial College School of Medicine
Hammersmith Hospital
Du Cane Road
London W12 0NN
UK

Rainer Haas, MD
Professor
Department of Internal Medicine V
University of Heidelberg
Hospitalstrasse 3
69115 Heidelberg
GERMANY

Helen E Heslop, MD
Division of Bone Marrow Transplantation
Department of Hematology/Oncology
St Jude Children's Research Hospital
332 North Lauderale
Memphis TN 38103
USA

Stefan Hohaus, MD
Department of Internal Medicine V
University of Heidelberg
Hospitalstrasse 3
69115 Heidelberg
GERMANY

Sundar Jagannath, MD
Chief, Bone Marrow Transplant
Department of Medicine
Division of Hematology/Oncology
University of Arkansas for Medical Sciences
4301 West Markham
Little Rock AR 72205
USA

Stephen M Jane, MD, PhD
Bone Marrow Unit
Royal Melbourne Hospital
Melbourne
Victoria 3050
AUSTRALIA

Gunnar Kvalheim, MD, PhD
Department of Medical
Oncology/Radiotherapy
Clinical Stemcell Laboratory
The Norwegian Radium Hospital
Montebello
N-0310 Oslo
NORWAY

Robert CF Leonard, FRCP, FRCPE
Department of Clinical Oncology
Western General Hospital
Crewe Road
Edinburgh EH4 2XU
UK

Gérald Marit, MD
Hôpital Haut-Lévêque
CHU Bordeaux
33604 Pessac
FRANCE

Nikhil C Munshi, MD
Chief, Molecular Oncology
Department of Medicine
Division of Hematology/Oncology
University of Arkansas for Medical Sciences
4301 West Markham
Little Rock AR 72205
USA

Yago Nieto, MD
Bone Marrow Transplant Program
University of Colorado Health Sciences Center
4200 East 9th Avenue
Denver CO 80262
USA

Stephen G O'Brien, MRCP, MRCPath
Department of Haematology
University of Wales College of Medicine
Heath Park
Cardiff CF4 4XN
UK

Ruth Pettengell, MB ChB, FRACP
Department of Oncology and Haematology
St George's Hospital
Blackshaw Road
London SW17 0RE
UK

Josy Reiffers, MD
Laboratoire de Greffe de Moëlle
Université Victor Segalen Bordeaux 2
146 rue Léo Saignat
33076 Bordeaux Cedex
FRANCE

Brenda M Sandmaier, MD
Fred Hutchinson Cancer Research Center
Clinical Research Division
1124 Columbia Street
Seattle WA 98104
USA

Norbert Schmitz, MD
Bone Marrow Transplantation Unit and
Department of Hematopathology
University of Kiel
Schwarenweg 20
D-24105 Kiel
GERMANY

Elizabeth J Shpall, MD
Associate Director
Bone Marrow Transplant Program
University of Colorado Health Sciences Center
4200 East 9th Avenue
Denver CO 80262
USA

Erlend B Smeland, MD, PhD
Department of Medical Immunology
Clinical Stemcell Laboratory
The Norwegian Radium Hospital
Montebello
N-0310 Oslo
NORWAY

Gary Spitzer, MD
Bone Marrow Transplantation Program
Lombardi Cancer Center
Georgetown University Hospital
3800 Reservoir Road NW
Washington DC 20007
USA

Rainer Storb, MD
Professor of Medicine
Fred Hutchinson Cancer Research Center
Clinical Research Division
1124 Columbia Street
Seattle WA 98104
USA

Guido Tricot, MD
Department of Medicine
Division of Hematology/Oncology
University of Arkansas for Medical Sciences
4301 West Markham
Little Rock AR 72205
USA

Maria Teresa Voso, MD
Department of Internal Medicine V
University of Heidelberg
Hospitalstrasse 3
69115 Heidelberg
GERMANY

1

Animal models

George E Georges, Brenda M Sandmaier and Rainer Storb

CONTENTS • **Introduction** • **Stem cells circulate in peripheral blood** • **Stem cell characterization** • **In vitro assays for stem cells** • **Stem cell phenotype** • **Mobilization of stem cells** • **Cytokine-mobilized stem cells** • **Murine stem cell mobilization** • **Large animals** • **Graft-versus-host disease and blood stem cell transplantation** • **Summary**

INTRODUCTION

Significant progress has been made in the past few years in the development of blood stem cell transplantation as a method for treatment of patients with hematologic and non-hematologic malignancies. Work using animal models has helped set the stage for these developments. This chapter will highlight the background history and recent progress of that work.

The primary animal models include inbred mice and rats and random-bred dogs, rabbits and non-human primates. The need for animal models is clear: there are unacceptable risks to patients when clinically untested modifications are made to transplant protocols. Animal models serve as the means with which to reliably assess the biology and the likely outcome of new approaches to stem cell transplantation. In general, the inbred mouse has been a very useful model for studying the basic biology of hematopoiesis, as well as for providing rapid readouts for studying basic principles of transplantation. The major caveat with the murine

Species	RBC per ml ($\times 10^9$)	Weight (kg)	Blood volume (ml)	RBC life span (days)	RBC per day	Life expectancy (years)	RBC per life of animal
Mouse	9.0	0.025	1.8	50	3.2×10^8	2	2.4×10^{11}
Human	6.0	70	4900	120	2.5×10^{11}	80	7.3×10^{15}
Cat	7.5	4	280	70	3.0×10^{10}	15	1.6×10^{14}
Dog	7.2	18	1550	115	9.7×10^{10}	13	4.6×10^{14}

Table 1.1 Red blood cell demands of different species[a]

[a]Adapted from Abkowitz et al.[57]

model is that the demands on stem cells are radically different and extrapolation of transplantation results from mice to humans for clinical use is questionable. These differences in demand are best illustrated by the fact that the mouse makes as many red blood cells in a lifetime as a human makes in one day or as a dog makes in 2.5 days (Table 1.1).

The outbred dog is a useful large animal model with consistently relevant outcomes that are similar to the clinical experience in human marrow transplantation. In addition, the large litters provide a model for sibling transplants, which are not easily done in non-human primates. The non-human primate model bears the closest resemblance to clinical transplantation, although monkeys and apes are more difficult to maintain as study subjects, and therefore discourage the development of truly novel transplantation approaches.

STEM CELLS CIRCULATE IN PERIPHERAL BLOOD

That blood stem cells circulate at a low frequency in the peripheral blood has been known for over 30 years. In 1962, Goodman et al[1] demonstrated that pooled blood isolated from normal F_1 hybrid donor mice could successfully restore hematopoiesis in supralethally irradiated and myeloablated homozygous parent mice. They specifically postulated the existence of a blood stem cell population with marrow repopulation potential that was present in the donor mouse's peripheral blood. Similar findings were reported by other investigators in guinea pigs[2] and dogs.[3] To determine the cell dose necessary for allogeneic engraftment in large animals, Storb et al[4] infused large doses of leukapheresed donor mononuclear cells (a total of 20×10^9 mononuclear cells collected daily over 7 days from peripheral blood) into lethally irradiated unrelated dogs, which resulted in restoration of marrow function (engraftment). The incidence of graft-versus-host disease (GVHD) was high. Sufficient hematopoietic progenitor cells were not obtained from the thoracic ducts of donors to enable autologous

engraftment.[5] This suggested that stem cells did not circulate in the lymphatics. Cross-circulation experiments in baboons indicated that hematopoietic progenitor cells were present in the peripheral blood of non-human primates as well.[6,7]

While these studies proved that peripheral blood stem cells (PBSC) existed and were a potential source of cells for transplantation, marrow cells provided a more clinically reliable and easily accessible source of hematopoietic repopulation cells. In steady state, the best estimate of the ratio of hematopoietic progenitor cells in the blood to those in the marrow is approximately 1:100.[8] Due to the low frequency of PBSC, attempts to generalize the use of PBSC in lieu of marrow was not pursued. If, however, marrow harvest resulted in an insufficient number of cells needed for transplant, blood-derived stem cells could be used as a supplemental source to ensure engraftment. For example, in patients with aplastic anemia, where there is a higher risk of graft failure associated with low numbers of transplanted marrow cells, supplemental buffy coat infusion from donors have been successfully used to increase the number of stem cells infused.[9]

Although there had been some concern that PBSC had limited proliferation capacity and did not include the requisite pluripotent stem cell population necessary for long-term hematopoiesis,[10] canine models have convincingly demonstrated long-term repopulation by allogeneic cells.[11,12] As early as 1981, both Goldman et al[13] and Korbling et al[14] demonstrated that leukapheresed autologous cryopreserved PBSC could restore hematopoiesis after myeloablative chemotherapy in patients with chronic myelogenous leukemia. While this did not prove long-term repopulation, it supported the principle, since patients transplanted in blast crisis were converted into chronic phase after infusion of PBSC that had been collected in chronic phase.

In comparison with marrow, the unmanipulated leukapheresis product containing PBSC has an order of magnitude greater number of mature T cells. In the allogeneic mouse and dog transplant models, higher T-cell doses at time of transplant have been correlated with increased severity of acute GVHD.[4,15,16] Since GVHD remains one of the major causes of morbidity and mortality, there has, up until the recent advent of mobilization strategies, been a significant disincentive for the use of PBSC as an alternative source for allogeneic grafts. High numbers of T cells in the PBSC leukapheresis product have not been relevant to the autologous transplant setting.

STEM CELL CHARACTERIZATION

Historically, a major obstacle to studying circulating hematopoietic progenitor cells was that the phenotype of the cells responsible for pluripotent reconstitution of hematopoiesis was unknown. Over the past decade there have been advances in the phenotypic characterization of hematopoietic progenitor cells, including identification of specific cell-surface markers (CD34 or c-kit) and cell metabolism-specific dyes. Despite this progress, stem cells remain best defined functionally as having the capacity to restore complete long-term hematopoietic cell differentiation and production in the lethally irradiated host.

Based on animal models and clinical data thus far, successful allogeneic PBSC engraftment requires the equivalent intensity of conditioning that is necessary for marrow transplantation. Similarly, a minimum threshold cell dose of PBSC is necessary to ensure successful allogeneic transplants. In the allogeneic dog model, a minimum of 0.6×10^8 mononuclear marrow cells per kilogram is necessary for successful engraftment after myeloablative conditioning (9.2 Gy total-body irradiation). In contrast, at least one order of magnitude higher number of non-cytokine-mobilized peripheral blood cells (2×10^9 mononuclear cells/kg) are necessary for allogeneic engraftment.[5,17] This is due to the lower frequency of stem cells in the blood compared with marrow, and does not appear to be due to functional differences in stem cells derived from peripheral blood versus marrow.

Several investigators have developed assays to quantify the number of stem cells necessary for successful transplantation. The colony-forming unit spleen (CFU-S), colony-forming unit granulocyte–macrophage (CFU-GM) and other derivative assays, initially developed in the mouse model, are indirect measures of primitive precursor cells present in the marrow or blood. More recently, these assays have been used to determine optimal stem cell mobilization regimens, which will be discussed in subsequent sections of this chapter.

IN VITRO ASSAYS FOR STEM CELLS

Till and McCulloch described the CFU-S in 1961.[18] In this assay, normal mouse marrow cells are injected into lethally irradiated syngeneic mice. Macroscopically visible multilineage (myeloid and lymphoid) colonies of cells in the spleens of the irradiated recipients were identified at either 8 or 14 days after injection. Neither the 8- nor the 14-day CFU-S cells were true stem cells, however, since they were incapable of long-term hematopoiesis.[19,20] A subpopulation of these CFU-S were capable of generating multilineage colonies in spleens of secondary irradiated recipient mice.[21]

This assay has been subsequently refined into the pre-CFU-S assay, which is a double transplantation technique.[20] It defines a population of primitive hematopoietic progenitor cells as being capable of reconstituting hematopoiesis (14 days after primary transplantation) and then differentiating into CFU-S in secondary irradiated recipients. While the pre-CFU-S assay does not definitively identify true clonal hematopoietic stem cells, it provides a quantitative means of comparing primitive hematopoietic stem cell activity in various cell populations.

Another approach to identifying cells with long-term repopulating capacity in the mouse is the competitive repopulating unit (CRU) assay (also referred to as competitive repopulating index (CRI)).[22,23] This is an in vivo limiting dilution assay, which quantifies genetically marked cells that are individually capable of regenerating at least 5% of the entire hematopoietic system, including both myeloid and lymphoid cells and maintaining production of these cells for at least 6 months. These relatively long-term pluripotent cells are infused simultaneously with short-term myeloprotective cells (or unmanipulated, distinctly marked marrow cells) into irradiated recipient mice. Thus, CRU cells must compete with committed progenitors for long-term repopulation.

A similar but more quantitative in vitro approximation of stem cell number is the long-term-culture initiating cells (LTC-IC) assay.[24] LTC-IC are immature, multipotent progenitor cells, which are quantitated by limited dilution analysis. Another commonly used in vitro assay to describe more committed progenitor cells measures CFU-GM. This quantifies the number of precursor cells that develop characteristics of granulocytes after a shorter duration of culture (typically 10–14 days).

These in vitro assays have been developed to assess the number of progenitor cells in peripheral blood and marrow. They serve only as surrogate markers for truly primitive pluripotent stem cells in a given animal model. It remains unproven whether or not increased frequencies of in vitro progenitor cells correlate with increased numbers of long-term marrow repopulating stem cells.

STEM CELL PHENOTYPE

Much work has been devoted to identifying the specific cellular phenotype of stem cells. A more detailed discussion of the characteristics of stem cells can be found in later chapters. While a unique cell surface antigen has not been identified in stem cells, multistep selective depletion of differentiated hematopoietic cells results in a subpopulation of 'lineage-negative' cells that include stem cells. CD34, a stem cell marker, has been identified and characterized in humans, dogs and mice. In non-human primates, monoclonal antibodies to human CD34 are cross-reactive, and identify a population of stem cells.[25] Additionally, c-kit and Ly-6A/E (or Sca-1) have been identified as stem cell markers in mice.[26] These cell

surface proteins distinguish more primitive hematopoietic cells from lineage-specific cells.[27] Not all CD34+ or c-kit+ cells have self-renewal potential; most are multipotent for lymphoid and myeloid lineages.[28]

During steady-state conditions, the subset of primitive cells that have evidence of self-renewal potential are resistant to 5-fluorouracil (5-FU) or other active cell-cycle toxic agents.[29] Because stem cells replicate infrequently and are quiescent, they would be expected to have low numbers of active mitochondria. Rhodamine-123 (Rh-123) is a dye that binds to cells high in mitochondrial content. Several investigators have shown that primitive hematopoietic cells (lineage-negative, c-kit+) with low Rh-123 staining maintain long-term repopulating capacity.[30,31] A second metabolic agent, Hoechst 33342 (Ho) (a DNA-affiliating dye), can identify cells not in cell cycle. Thus, a combination of the two metabolic dyes and monoclonal antibodies have been used to identify a primitive, pluripotent progenitor cell that is Ho-low, Rh-123-low, lineage-negative, c-kit+ and capable of long-term hematopoiesis.[32] Wolf[33] has shown that injection of single Ho-low, Rh-123-low, cells into lethally irradiated mice results in donor hematopoietic reconstitution in 15% of cases.

Thus, significant progress in the isolation and characterization of stem cells has been made over the past few years. Despite the in vitro assays to characterize stem cells, the ability of progenitor cells to repopulate ablated marrow for long-term hematopoiesis remains the key functional definition of stem cells.

In larger animals it has not been possible to isolate in vitro a homogeneous population of pluripotent primitive stem cells. However, immunoaffinity selection of a stem-cell-containing population using anti-CD34 monoclonal antibodies has been possible in baboons.[25] While the CD34 antigen does not define stem cells, it permits 100- to 1000-fold enrichment of the population of stem cells isolated from blood or marrow. With the cloning of the canine *CD34* gene[34] and the development of monoclonal antibodies to the recombinant CD34 antigen, more sophisticated in vitro blood stem cell manipulation will be possible in that model (McSweeney et al, personal communication). It will be possible to investigate the long-term engraftment potential of allogeneic purified CD34$^+$ cells and the specific role of T cells or natural killer cells in the dog. Since cellular manipulation of PBSC (such as subtraction or addition of T cells) for non-malignant or currently treatable malignant diseases in humans can be ethically questionable, especially in the allogeneic transplant setting, animal models are necessary for these studies.

MOBILIZATION OF STEM CELLS

Along with the development of improved assays to identify progenitor cells from marrow or blood, one of the critical advances in blood stem cell transplantation has been the observation that stem cells can be mobilized from marrow into the peripheral blood. In 1977, Cline and Golde[35] and Richman et al[36] reported that the number of CFU-GM were markedly increased in humans given endotoxin, dextran sulfate or chemotherapy.

Animal models have been useful in studying new strategies for stem cell mobilization, since they have responses similar to stem cell mobilization in humans. Although the use of chemotherapy-mobilized stem cells is now clinically widespread in the autologous clinical transplant setting, animal models were necessary to define the kinetics and show clinical feasibility.

In the autologous dog model, Abrams et al[37] demonstrated that infusion of cryopreserved PBSC mobilized after chemotherapy was able to restore hematopoiesis after myeloablative total-body irradiation (TBI). Peripheral blood mononuclear cells (PBMC) were collected 14–16 days after myelosuppressive cyclophosphamide (CY) treatment – during the rapid leukocyte recovery phase following the CY-induced leukocyte nadir. Following collection and cryopreservation, as few as 0.5×10^8 PBMC/kg could protect dogs from otherwise lethal TBI (9.0 Gy). In comparison with non-mobilized peripheral blood, chemotherapy-mobilized leukapheresed cells provided 11 times more CFU-GM and were 12.5 times more potent in reconstituting hematopoiesis. Potency was defined in terms of the total number of nucleated cells needed for successful engraftment. Thus, the collection and infusion of PBSC had become significantly more efficient.

In a similar manner, Appelbaum et al[38] demonstrated successful autologous transplantation of dogs with lymphoma using leukapheresed PBSC obtained after combination chemotherapy. The leukapheresis of chemotherapy-mobilized stem cells has rapidly developed into a clinically widespread technique for autologous transplantation of patients with a variety of malignancies, including lymphoma, acute myeloid leukemia, breast and ovarian cancer.

One of the most compelling reasons for the rapid widespread clinical application of autologous PBSC transplantation has been the more rapid engraftment seen with mobilized PBSC compared with marrow. This results in a reduction in the amount of supportive care and inpatient hospital days. It has contributed to the improved clinical safety of autologous transplants.[39] The accelerated recovery of hematopoiesis is due to the infusion of large numbers of mature, proliferating committed progenitor cells in addition to sufficient long-term marrow-repopulating stem cells with the leukapheresis cell product. This is reflected in the marked increase in the number of committed precursor cells in assays of CFU-S (mice) and CFU-GM (canine and primate) in animal models of chemotherapy-mobilized stem cells.

In autologous clinical transplants, there has been concern that the risk of relapse of the underlying malignancy is significantly increased when there is infusion of contaminating malignant cells with cryopreserved stem cells following high-dose chemotherapy.[40] Clinical studies are currently underway involving purging of PBSC via CD34$^+$ immunoaffinity selection, thereby reducing the relapse rate following autotransplants.[41] There have been no published reports of blood stem cell tumor purging in animal models.

CYTOKINE-MOBILIZED STEM CELLS

The discovery and cloning of the many cytokines involved in hematopoiesis have been key factors in the tremendous advances in the understanding of cell growth regulation. Many of the cytokines have the additional property of stimulating marked increases in hematopoietic progenitor cells circulating in the peripheral blood. Cytokines are thought to act on primitive or precursor cells at different stages of differentiation. Thus, recent efforts have been focused on combining different cytokines to maximize the number of stem cells in circulation. If the efforts were successful, the number of apheresis procedures necessary to achieve a sufficient collection of PBSC could be reduced to one brief session. (Refer to Table 1.2 for a summary of cytokines studied for mobilization.)

The first cytokines shown to mobilize stem cells into the peripheral blood were granulocyte colony-stimulating factor (G-CSF) and granulocyte–macrophage colony-stimulating factor (GM-CSF). During Phase I clinical trials, increases of up to 100-fold in the number of CFU-GM were observed with both cytokines.[42,43] These observations led to speculation that cytokines could be used to mobilize transplantable stem cells into the peripheral blood.

The following section summarizes results from murine, canine and non-human primate models of stem cell mobilization and transplantation. Many of the cytokines have cross-species reactivity, which has permitted rapid assessment of biological effects in several animal models. Other cytokines appear to have suboptimal biologic activity in unrelated species and have required the cloning of that species' homologous cytokine.

MURINE STEM CELL MOBILIZATION

Molineux et al[44] published the first study demonstrating the transplantation potential of G-CSF-mobilized PBSC in the mouse. Donor mice were subcutaneously administered G-CSF (250 µg/kg/ day × 4 days) until maximal progenitor cell circulation was achieved. As little as 10 µl of blood (2.5×10^5 cells) from male B6D2F$_1$ mice restored complete hematopoiesis in 15.2 Gy (^{60}Co γ over 16 hours) lethally irradiated female syngeneic recipients. Donor chimerism of 100% was shown for up to 10 months after transplant, and there were no discernible differences in hematopoiesis between the G-CSF-mobilized PBSC and marrow control chimeras.

Neben et al[45] compared the marrow and peripheral blood compartments for the presence of stem cells after mobilization. C57B1/6J (B6) mice were treated with CY 200 mg/kg, followed by or in lieu of rhG-CSF 250 mg/kg/day × 4 days. At day +6 after onset of mobilization, limited numbers of Ficoll-Hypaque gradient separation mononuclear cells – obtained from either marrow, spleen or peripheral blood – were transplanted into syngeneic lethally irradiated recipients (12.5 Gy, split course 3 hours apart at 1.11 Gy/min).

Compared with non-mobilized controls, the committed progenitor CFU-S content in peripheral blood increased 11-fold following G-CSF mobilization, 15-fold following CY and 36-fold following CY plus G-CSF. The primitive stem cell content of mobilized peripheral blood approached that of normal marrow in the donors treated with CY, with G-CSF and with CY plus G-CSF (competitive repopulating index, CRI, of normal marrow and normal peripheral blood was 0.43 and 0.006 respectively, while CRI of blood mobilized with CY, with G-CSF and with CY plus G-CSF was 0.21, 0.41 and 0.28 respectively). In addition, the stem cell content reversibly decreased in the marrow of mice treated with a combination of CY plus G-CSF, but remained unchanged following G-CSF alone.

These studies demonstrated that the hematopoietic stem cells can be temporarily and reversibly mobilized into the peripheral blood and nearly approach marrow levels. The differences in the repopulating ability following specific techniques used for mobilization suggested that different subpopulations of stem cells may have been mobilized. This has led to attempts to identify other cytokines that may

Table 1.2 Summary of cytokines used to mobilize PBSC

Stimulus	Timing of mobilization	Mouse	Dog	Primate	Rescue of lethally irradiated recipient
G-CSF	4–7 days	5–20-fold ↑ CFU-GM[46] 11–18-fold ↑ CFU-S[45,55]	3–7 fold ↑[62] CFU-GM	10–50 fold ↑ CFU-GM[64,65]	Mouse, allogeneic dog, baboon, allogeneic rabbit
GM-CSF	5–14 days				
SCF	7–10 days	1.5–3.7-fold ↑ CFU-GM[46] 14-fold ↑ CFU-S[53]	1.4–12-fold ↑[62] CFU-GM	12-fold ↑ CFU-GM[70] 0–10-fold ↑ CFU-GM[64]	Mouse, autologous dog
SCF + G-CSF	5–10 days	13–20-fold ↑ CFU-GM[46] 7–10-fold ↑ CFU-S[48]	12–45-fold ↑[62] CFU-GM	50–300-fold ↑ CFU-GM[64,65]	Mouse, allogeneic dog, baboon
IL-1β	Single dose	10-fold ↑ CFU-S[77]		100-fold ↑ CFU-GM[68]	Mouse, autologous monkey
IL-3	11–14 days	30-fold ↑ CFU-GM[77]		14-fold ↑ CFU-GM[70]	
IL-3 + GM-CSF	11–14 days IL-3 followed by 5 days GM-CSF			65-fold ↑ CFU-GM[70]	
IL-6	14 days	8.7-fold ↑ CFU-S[50]			Mouse
IL-6 + G-CSF	14 days	132-fold ↑ CFU-S[50]			
IL-7	7 days	6-fold ↑ CFU-S[51]			Mouse
IL-8	Single dose	20-fold ↑ CFU-GM[52]		10–100-fold ↑ CFU-GEMM[66]	Mouse
IL-11	7 days	1.9-fold ↑ CFU-S[53]		60–140-fold ↑ CFU-GM[67]	
IL-11 + SCF	7 days				Mouse
IL-11 + G-CSF	4 days IL-11 followed by 4 days G-CSF	10.6-fold ↑ CFU-S[53]		90–350-fold ↑ CFU-GM[67]	
FLT-3 + G-CSF	5 days	384-fold ↑ CFU-S[55]			
MIP-1α	Single dose	2-fold ↑ CFU-S[56]			
MIP-1α + G-CSF	2 days G-CSF followed by single-dose MIP-1α	25-fold ↑ CFU-S[56]			
Anti-VLA-4	4 days			10–100-fold ↑ CFU-GM[71]	
Anti-VLA-4 + G-CSF	5 days followed by 2 days anti-VLA-4			200–1300-fold ↑ CFU-GM[71]	

even further enhance the ability to mobilize PBSC efficiently.

Accordingly, Briddell et al[46] administered low-dose recombinant rat stem cell factor (rrSCF) and recombinant human (rh)G-CSF in combination, which resulted in even higher concentrations of both primitive and mature progenitor cells in the peripheral blood than if either cytokine was used singly. Splenectomized male (C57BL/6J × DBA/2J)F$_1$ mice were mobilized with rrSCF (pegylated form, 25 µg/kg/day), rhG-CSF (200 µg/kg/ day) for 7 days alone or in combination. Mobilized PBSC obtained as fractionated low-density peripheral blood cells were infused in a cell dose escalation study into syngeneic lethally irradiated (11.5 Gy, equal split dose, 4 hours apart) female mice. PBSC mobilized by SCF plus G-CSF resulted in greater survival at 90 days compared with mice receiving an equal number of mononuclear cells mobilized with G-CSF. The synergistic effect of the two cytokines may be explained by the SCF expanding both primitive and mature hematopoietic progenitor cells and the G-CSF mobilizing progenitor cells into the periphery.

Yan et al[47] have shown that PBSC mobilized with a combination of SCF and G-CSF could be sequentially transplanted to tertiary recipients and reconstitute hematopoiesis for more than 26 months. At 12–24 months after transplant, the female recipients had donor engraftment greater than 90%, as documented by Y-chromosome specific polymerase chain reaction (PCR) probe in spleen, thymus and lymph node cells. Marrow cells from these recipients were further transplanted to syngeneic secondary female recipients (myeloablated with 12.0 Gy, split dose, 4 hours apart). At 6 months, 98% of the secondary recipients had male-derived hematopoiesis by whole-blood PCR analysis, with single-colony marrow culture PCR analysis confirming greater than 90% male-derived hematopoiesis. Marrow cells from the secondary recipients were further passaged to tertiary recipients, with 90% of mice exhibiting male-derived hematopoiesis 6 months after transplant. In contrast, fewer than 50% of secondary recipients of PBSC mobilized with G-CSF alone showed sustained male-derived hematopoiesis by single-colony marrow culture PCR analysis. This indicated that PBSC mobilized with SCF plus G-CSF provided increased numbers of long-term reconstituting stem cells compared with PBSC mobilized with G-CSF alone.

These studies have been further supported by the findings of Bodine et al,[48] who used a quantitative competitive repopulation assay to assess the ability of combined SCF and G-CSF to mobilize repopulating stem cells. Comparing results in C57BL/6J splenectomized mice receiving SCF plus G-CSF for 3–7 days with those given an equal number of marrow cells from unstimulated HW80 mice (genetically identical to C57BL/6J except at the β-globin locus), there was a dramatic shift in hematopoiesis in favor of the mice treated with SCF plus G-CSF. Specifically, 80–90% of the hemoglobin was derived from C57BL/6J (donor) mice 4 months post-transplant in the histocompatible recipient WBB6F$_1$ mice irradiated with 9.0 Gy from a ^{137}Cs source. In addition, the efficiency of recombinant retroviral human multidrug-resistance gene (*MDR-1*) transfer into PBSC mobilized with SCF plus G-CSF was 2–5-fold greater than into PBSC mobilized with standard (5-FU) chemotherapy.

Based on quantitative models of hematopoiesis that were originally described by Chervenick,[49] these studies indicate that splenectomized mice treated with SCF plus G-CSF undergo a threefold expansion in total absolute number of stem cells, from a baseline of 3000 to an increase of 9000 per mouse. In addition, the cytokine combination mobilized 70% of stem cells from the marrow compartment to the peripheral blood compared with <0.1% of stem cells in the blood of nonmobilized controls.

Several of the interleukin (IL) cytokines have been studied to determine their effect on mobilization of stem cells in mice. There have been recent reports on the use of these cytokines as single agents or in combination with G-CSF to rapidly mobilize PBSC and reconstitute hematopoiesis in myeloablated recipients. IL-6 is a cytokine previously reported to stimulate primitive hematopoietic stem cells. IL-6 has been used to support and expand progenitor cells in vitro. Suzuki et al[50] have shown that rhIL-6 (10 µg/day × 14 days) combined with rhG-CSF (0.35 µg/day × 14 days) resulted in a 132-fold increase in CFU-S compared with control mice. IL-6 or G-CSF alone resulted in 8-fold and 11-fold increases respectively in CFU-S. Survival of lethally irradiated (10 Gy) syngeneic C57BL/6 mice at day 100 after infusion of 100 µl of blood from animals mobilized with combined IL-6 and G-CSF was 92%. Mice rescued with IL-6 or G-CSF single-cytokine-mobilized blood had survival rates of 31% and 46% respectively. This compared with 0% survival of mice rescued with non-mobilized blood. The relatively poor survival of mice rescued with G-CSF-mobilized PBSC in that study is most likely related to differences in G-CSF administration compared with other investigators. Specifically, G-CSF dose (0.35 µg vs 4 µg per day) and method of administration (continuous infusion for 14 days vs subcutaneous daily injection for 5–7 days) were different. Possible synergy between the three cytokines SCF, IL-6 and G-CSF awaits further investigation.

Grzegorzewski et al[51] have reported that rhIL-7 at 5 µg twice daily for 7 days in mice stimulated a sixfold increase in CFU-S in peripheral blood. As few as 10^6 peripheral blood leukocytes (PBL) from IL-7-treated C57BL/6 (Ly 5.1) donors rescued 90% of lethally irradiated (11 Gy, equal split dose 3 hours apart) recipient C57BL/6 (Ly 5.2) mice compared with no survivors from the same number of PBL from control donors. In recipients transplanted with IL-7-mobilized PBSC, >90% donor hematopoiesis (Ly 5.1 antigen) was documented at 6 months post-transplant in marrow, spleen and thymus. These studies suggest that IL-7 can efficiently mobilize PBSC; whether or not the IL-7-mobilized stem cells are capable of the long-term hematopoiesis necessary in larger animals is unknown. Potential synergies between IL-7 and other cytokines to mobilize stem cells remain to be examined.

IL-8 is a cytokine that is involved in chemotaxis and activation of neutrophils. In large animals, injection of IL-8 results in immediate neutropenia, followed by granulocytosis, neutrophil margination and infiltration, plasma exudation, and angiogenesis. Laterveer et al[52] have reported that mice given 30 µg of rhIL-8 as a single intraperitoneal dose showed a 20-fold increase in CFU-GM in peripheral blood within 15 minutes of injection. As few as 1.5×10^6 PBMC isolated from IL-8-treated Balb/c male mice reconstituted hematopoiesis in 100% of myeloablated (8.5 Gy) female recipients (studied ⩽60 days post-transplant). This compared with no survivors among controls. The rapid mobilization followed by rapid reversal of PBSC following IL-8 may provide synergy with G-CSF or SCF for more efficient stem cell mobilization.

Mauch et al[53] showed that either twice daily subcutaneous or continuous infusion of 250 µg/day rhIL-11 for 7 days in mice resulted in an increase in the progenitor cell (CFU-S) content but not the primitive cell content (measured by CRI) of blood and spleen. Six-month repopulating ability of PBSC, spleen or marrow cells from B6-Hbb^s-treated mice mixed 1:1 with B6-Hbb^d marrow cells was assessed in lethally irradiated (12.5 Gy, split dose) B6-Hbb^s. The combination of IL-11 and SCF synergistically increased the capacity of PBSC and spleen cells to provide 6-month hematopoiesis. However, as single agents in splenectomized donor mice, SCF increased the long-term competitive repopulating ability of blood (CRI = 1.63) while IL-11 did not (CRI = 0). IL-11 enhanced SCF mobilization of stem cells from marrow to blood, since CRI of marrow from splenectomized donor mice after combination IL-11 and SCF decreased to 0.3 while CRI of marrow after SCF treatment was 0.8 (control = 1.0). Although IL-11 may not be useful as a single-agent cytokine for PBSC mobilization, its synergistic effect with SCF was clearly demonstrated.

The recently cloned rhflt-3 ligand[54] had a synergistic effect in combination with rhG-CSF in increasing peripheral blood mobilization of CFU-S.[55] Mice injected with both flt-3 ligand 20 µg/kg and G-CSF 250 µg/kg for 5 days yielded a 384-fold increase in CFU-S compared with an 18-fold increase in CFU-S with G-CSF alone. It is not yet known if these findings translate into the ability of flt-3 ligand to mobilize stem cells that are capable of long-term hematopoiesis in lethally irradiated recipients.

Lord et al[56] reported that BB-10010, a variant of human macrophage inflammatory protein-1 (MIP-1α), mobilized mouse PBSC in synergy with G-CSF. Thirty minutes after a single subcutaneous dose of MIP-1α (2.5 µg/kg of BB-10010), there was a twofold increase in circulating CFU-S and progenitors with marrow repopulating ability (MRA, similar in design to the pre-CFU-S assay). Following 2 days of G-CSF treatment (twice daily injections of 100 µg/kg), circulating CFU-S and MRA increased by 25- and 27-fold respectively. A single administration of MIP-1α after 2 days of G-CSF treatment increased circulating CFU-S and MRA even further to 38- and 100-fold. Splenectomized mice had even greater increases in CFU-S and MRA, with similar pattern of mobilization. The long-term engraftment potential of rapidly mobilized primitive progenitor cells using the combination of cytokines awaits future study.

The important conclusions from these studies are that PBSC transplants in the mouse are feasible, and that the technology for assessing long-term hematopoiesis makes the mouse a useful tool for quickly comparing mobilization strategies. It is important to stress that 6-month hematopoiesis in the mouse does not translate into long-term hematopoiesis in humans, however. The various cytokines assayed indicate that there are multiple agents capable of mobilizing stem cells. The synergistic effect of combined or sequential cytokine administration may promote higher yields of mobilized stem cells. Further progress in this area awaits the elucidation of the specific molecular and cellular mechanisms by which cytokines influence stem cell mobilization. That so many cytokines have been shown to mobilize stem cells suggests that complex signalling within the hematopoietic cell differentiation can be strongly influenced at several points to enhance the peripheralization of progenitor cells. Elucidation of the cellular mechanisms of mobilization will lead to better understanding of the control of hematopoiesis.

LARGE ANIMALS

While mouse studies have shown the enormous potential for using cytokine-mobilized blood stem cells as a source of stem cells for hematopoietic transplantation, large-animal studies are necessary to determine the PBSC's efficacy to maintain long-term hematopoiesis after transplant. Compared with large animals, mice have much more limited hematopoietic demands over the lifespan of the animal. For example, Abkowitz et al[57] have estimated that the cat has at least 3750 times more red blood cells produced per lifetime compared with the mouse. Humans have over 30 000 times the number of blood cells produced per lifespan compared to the mouse (Table 1.1). Thus, questions of stem cell self-renewal potential and long-term hematopoiesis can really be convincingly studied only in larger animals in order to draw meaningful clinical comparisons.

In addition to the questions of long-term hematopoiesis, the large-animal models are more accurate at predicting the incidence and severity of GVHD in humans. For example, with most mouse strain combinations, GVHD is not observed after crossing non-major histocompatibility complex (MHC) H-2 class barriers.[15,16,58] In many cases, even MHC H-2 disparity may not result in fatal GVHD. In contrast, acute GVHD is uniformly seen in MHC-incompatible canine, simian or human marrow stem cell graft recipients.[59,60] Canine studies were the first to show fatal GVHD in recipients of marrow from DLA-identical littermates when transplants were done without postgrafting immunosuppression, a finding that was subsequently confirmed in humans.[61] Thus, the large-animal models have been more accurate and more relevant to predicting clinical outcome in humans. For this reason, large-animal models will continue to be necessary to assess new treatment/mobilization regimens and hematopoietic stem cell manipulation procedures prior to use in humans.

Canine stem cell mobilization

Studies in outbred dogs showed recombinant canine (rc)G-CSF and rcSCF to be synergistic with regard to mobilizing transplantable progenitor cells into the peripheral blood.[62] rcG-CSF (10 µg/kg/day) for 7 days led to a 5.4-fold increase in CFU-GM/ml of blood, compared with 7 days of high-dose rcSCF (200 µg/kg/day), which gave an 8.2-fold increase. Low-dose SCF (25 µg/kg/day) administered for 7 days had no effect on CFU-GM. However, rcG-CSF plus low-dose SCF resulted in a 21.6-fold increase in CFU-GM, a significant difference compared with low-dose SCF alone ($p = 0.03$). The 25 µg/kg/day dose level for low-dose SCF was based on the observation that this may approximate the maximum tolerated dose in humans.[63]

To assess the ability of G-CSF and SCF to increase the circulation of cells capable of rescuing dogs after lethal TBI, 1×10^8 mononuclear cells/kg were collected and cryopreserved from dogs after 7 days of treatment with G-CSF, SCF or a combination of the two. One month later, dogs were exposed to 9.2 Gy TBI and transplanted with the previously collected cells. All three control animals transplanted with 1×10^8 non-mobilized PBMC/kg died with marrow aplasia 11–29 days after TBI. Similarly, dogs give PBSC mobilized with low-dose SCF only failed to recover. In contrast, all 15 dogs given PBSC collected after G-CSF, high-dose SCF, or low-dose SCF plus G-CSF recovered granulocyte function. The mean period to obtain 500 PMN/µl was 17 days (G-CSF), 18.8 days (SCF) and 13.6 days (low-dose SCF plus G-CSF). The mean period to reach 20 000 platelets/µl was 42 days (G-CSF), 46 days (SCF) and 37 days (low-dose SCF plus G-CSF). In the combination group, all five dogs survived with stable trilineage engraftment to >180 days. This study was not designed to study long-term repopulation, since PBSC may have provided only short-term repopulation until reconstitution of autologous hematopoiesis from radiation-resistant stem cells occurred. The study showed that both SCF and G-CSF dramatically increased the level of PBSC and that these growth factors act synergistically to mobilize stem cells from the marrow into the blood.

Non-human primate stem cell mobilization

Andrews et al[64,65] have shown that rhSCF in combination with rhG-CSF mobilized greater numbers of progenitor cells that could be collected by a single 2-hour leukapheresis than did rhG-CSF alone. One group of baboons was administered SCF (25 µg/kg/day) plus G-CSF (100 µg/kg/day), while a second group received G-CSF alone (100 µg/kg/day). Each animal underwent a single 2-hour leukapheresis on the day that the number of progenitor cells per volume of blood was maximal (day 10 for SCF plus G-CSF and day 5 for G-CSF-treated animals). For baboons administered SCF plus G-CSF, the leukapheresis products contained eightfold more progenitor cells (CFU-GM) compared with animals treated with G-CSF alone.

In baboons that were exposed to a lethal dose of 10.7 Gy TBI followed by administration of cryopreserved leukapheresed cells, more rapid autologous trilineage engraftment was observed using PBSC mobilized by SCF plus G-CSF compared with G-CSF alone. In animals transplanted with PBSC mobilized by SCF plus G-CSF, the times to engraftment of neutrophils (ANC > 500) and platelets (>20 000) were 12 and 8 days respectively, compared with 24 and 42 days using PBSC mobilized by G-CSF alone. These results demonstrate enhanced mobilization of progenitor cells with long-term engraftment potential using SCF plus G-CSF in non-human primates, which is similar to findings in dogs and splenectomized mice and in preliminary results from phase I/II studies in humans.

In findings similar to those described in mice, Laterveer et al[66] reported that IL-8 led to a dose-dependent 10–100-fold increase in CFU-GEMM in peripheral blood of rhesus monkeys, within 30 minutes of injection. By 4 hours after injection, CFU-GEMM had returned to pretreatment levels. Hastings et al[67] reported that concomitant administration of rhIL-11 (100 µg/kg/day) and rhG-CSF (10 µg/kg/day) subcutaneously for 7 days in *Cynomolgus* monkeys resulted in a 61–141-fold increase in CFU-GM above baseline. This was not significantly different than G-CSF administration alone. However, monkeys receiving IL-11 $\times$ 4 days followed by G-

CSF × 4 days showed a 90–350-fold increase in CFU-GM above baseline. This suggested that IL-11 followed by G-CSF enhances stem cell mobilization, and that IL-11 acted via a distinct hematopoietic cell differentiation mechanism.

Gasparetto et al[68] showed in *Cynomolgus* monkeys that rhIL-1β (1 μg/kg, single intravenous dose) resulted in a 100-fold increase in CFU-GM 4 days after injection and a 10–15-fold increase in secondary CFU-GM (similar to LTC-IC assays) for 2–7 days after injection. Autologous PBSC (1×10^7 mononuclear cells) collected either 24 or 72 hours after IL-1β was able to rescue all four monkeys following 10 Gy TBI, but only two of the four survived with normal neutrophil counts beyond 60 days. One of two non-mobilized control monkeys survived long-term following PBSC autotransplant. In addition, Gasparetto et al reported that neither a single injection of IL-3 (20 μg/kg), G-CSF (50 μg/kg) nor GM-CSF (50 μg/kg) resulted in significant CFU-GM or secondary CFU-GM increases. It is not clear if humans could tolerate the dose of IL-1β needed to mobilize PBSC in this study; dose-limiting toxicity including fever and hypotension was reported in patients receiving 0.1 μg/kg IL-1β following 5-FU administration.[69]

In rhesus monkeys, Geissler et al[70] compared IL-3 (33 μg/kg/day subcutaneously for 11–14 days) followed by GM-CSF (5.5 μg/kg/day for 5–14 days) with either GM-CSF or IL-3 alone. There was a 65-fold increase in peripheral blood CFU-GM in the sequential protocol compared with 12- and 14-fold respectively in the others. This study contrasts with the findings of Gasparetto et al, emphasizing the point that optimal PBSC mobilization depends upon dose, duration and method of administration of specific cytokines.

It is unknown what specific molecular signals cause mobilization of hematopoietic progenitor cells from marrow to peripheral blood. However, it appears that cellular interactions between hematopoietic cells and their microenvironment (such as marrow stromal cells) are important for development and function, and several adhesion molecules may be critical for these interactions.

Investigating the role of the cytoadhesion molecule VLA-4 on hematopoietic cells, Papayannopoulou and Nakamoto[71] have shown that systemic treatment of primate with antibody to the VLA-4 integrin molecule (HP1/2 administered intravenously for 4 days at a dose of 1 mg/kg) resulted in a 10–100-fold increase in circulating CFU-GM. There was a synergistic effect observed with G-CSF (30 mg/kg/day for 5 days) followed by anti-VLA-4 antibody administration (HP1/2, 1 mg/kg/day for 2 days), with a significant increase in CFU noted compared with G-CSF alone. The total CFU/ml increased from 2500 (G-CSF) to 13 000 (G-CSF plus anti-VLA-4 antibody). This suggests independent mechanisms by which G-CSF and anti-VLA-4 antibody can mobilize stem cells. Based on studies in mice and humans, VLA-4 is an adhesion molecule on hematopoietic cells. The anti-VLA-4 antibody appears to block the interaction between hematopoietic stem cells and marrow stroma, resulting in increased stem cell mobilization. The anti-VLA-4 antibody may be clinically useful to increase the yield of PBSC for transplantation. The identification of additional cell-surface/adhesion molecules that are involved in stem cell mobilization may reveal additional mechanisms with which to improve blood stem cell yield for clinical use.

The optimal time to harvest PBSC mobilized by either chemotherapy, cytokines or antibodies to adhesion molecules has been identified as the day(s) of peak CFU after mobilization. For clinical purposes, this is a cumbersome assay since there is significant interlaboratory variation in the measurement of CFU, and since progenitor assays take 10–14 days to read. Thus, there has been interest in using CD34 antigen flow cytometric analysis as a rapid and reliable clinical marker for measuring peak PBSC. Based on recent evidence in human studies, it appears that the day(s) of peak $CD34^+$ cells in the peripheral blood after cytokine mobilization correlates with the optimal time for leukapheresis of transplantable PBSC.[72]

GRAFT-VERSUS-HOST DISEASE AND BLOOD STEM CELL TRANSPLANTATION

There have been no published reports describing the use of non-syngeneic donors in the mouse model to evaluate graft rejection or GVHD. However, the potential clinical application of allogeneic PBSC makes it vital to study the parameters influencing graft rejection and GVHD in large animals. This is particularly important in view of the larger numbers of T cells in unfractionated leukapheresed PBSC.[73] Previous studies in both small and large animals have shown high T-cell (10^7 cells/kg) doses to result in increased acute GVHD.[4,15,16] In humans given buffy coat infusion post-transplant (which has a 1- to 2-log increase in T-cell content compared with marrow), there is an increased incidence of chronic GVHD.[74]

The dog has been a very useful model for studying clinically relevant problems of GVHD in allogeneic marrow transplantation. The question of whether or not PBSC are more likely to cause acute or chronic GVHD remains an important issue. While preliminary clinical evidence suggests that there is no increased incidence of acute GVHD in allogeneic human PBSC transplants, the incidence of chronic GVHD remains unknown. Thus, it was important to determine the feasibility of the dog model to assess GVHD in this setting.

Sandmaier et al[75] used mobilized PBSC obtained via leukapheresis for allogeneic transplantation in dogs. PBSC were obtained after either 7 days of low-dose rcSCF (25 μg/kg/day) plus rcG-CSF (10 μg/kg/day), or after G-CSF alone. Donors showed up to 25-fold increases in peripheral blood CFU-GM after growth factor treatment. Eighteen dogs were given a median of 17.1×10^8 mononuclear cells/kg (median number of CFU-GM infused was 27×10^4 kg) from littermate donors after 9.2 Gy of TBI. No postgrafting immunosuppression was given. In DLA-haploidentical littermate recipients given PBSC mobilized with SCF plus G-CSF or G-CSF, the rate of engraftment was higher (100%) than observed with marrow alone, where 75% of dogs failed to engraft. All haploidentical recipients developed fatal hyperacute GVHD. Recipients of DLA-identical transplants all developed GVHD, which was fatal in 30% and transient in 70%. The incidence and severity of acute GVHD was similar to that expected after marrow grafts. This model will allow for further treatment, including

T-cell depletion to minimize GVHD without increasing graft rejection.

The only other reported animal model of allogeneic G-CSF-mobilized PBSC used rabbits.[76] Adult outbred red Burgundy rabbits served as donors of histoincompatible New Zealand White recipients of the opposite sex. Three different schedules of PBSC collection and infusion were tested, none of which showed significant differences in engraftment rate or incidence of GVHD. PBSC were mobilized with rhG-CSF (10 μg/kg/day administered subcutaneously for 14 or 18 days), collected during either three or six apheresis sessions, and infused at a single time or 4 or 5 days after recipients were given a single dose of 10 Gy TBI delivered at 0.2 Gy/min from a ^{60}Co source. This dose of TBI was not lethal, and resulted in 50% recovery of autologous hematopoiesis. Recipients were administered cyclosporin as GVHD prophylaxis. Repetitive collections and infusions of PBSC decreased the period of aplasia compared with historical controls receiving unmanipulated marrow. Two of the 15 animals died of TBI toxicity, while all others engrafted. Two animals became long-term complete chimeras, 8 died of acute GVHD and 3 died of infection. These results indicated that PBSC mobilized with G-CSF could engraft across MHC barriers with an incidence of GVHD that was no different from unmanipulated marrow.

These large-animal studies suggest that allogeneic mobilized PBSC have a higher rate of sustained engraftment than marrow and cause no higher incidence of GVHD despite the infusion of increased numbers of lymphocytes. The improved rate of engraftment in mismatched transplants could be due to increased numbers of transplanted hematopoietic progenitor cells or T cells in the graft. It remains to be determined if there is any immunologic difference between growth-factor-mobilized PBSC compared with marrow.

SUMMARY

Animal models have been developed that are very useful for the study of PBSC in both autologous and allogeneic transplantation. Although the existence of stem cells in the peripheral blood has been known for over 30 years, clinical use of PBSC has become feasible only recently with the advent of mobilization of these cells from marrow to blood with the help of hematopoietic growth factors. This chapter has reviewed studies that have been critical in identifying cytokines capable of enhancing PBSC mobilization. Large-animal models such as dogs and non-human primates, which have been historically instrumental for the development of clinical marrow transplantation, represent ideal settings for evaluating clinically relevant issues in allogeneic PBSC transplantation.

Animals such as the mouse and rat with limited hematopoietic demands lend themselves to the study of stem cell mobilization and the basic molecular biology of hematopoiesis. However, large-animal models will continue to be crucial for studying long-term hematopoiesis with its increased stem cell demands. Attempts to improve the safety and effectiveness of PBSC for allogeneic transplantation with in vitro manipulation of hematopoietic cells using molecular biology and immunologic techniques will continue to require the use of large-animal models.

ACKNOWLEDGEMENTS

The authors are indebted to Bonnie Larson, Harriet Childs and Sue Carbonneau for their assistance in the preparation of the manuscript. This work was supported in part by Grants CA18221, CA31787, DK42716 and HL36444 awarded by the National Institutes of Health, DHHS, Bethesda, MD. Support was also received from the Josef Steiner Krebsstiftung, Bern, Switzerland, awarded to one of the investigators (R Storb).

REFERENCES

1. Goodman JW, Hodgson GS, Evidence for stem cells in the peripheral blood of mice. *Blood* 1962; **19:** 702–14.
2. Malinin TI, Perry VP, Kerby CC, Dolan MF, Peripheral leukocyte infusion into lethally irradiated guinea pigs. *Blood* 1965; **25:** 693–702.
3. Epstein RB, Graham TC, Buckner CD et al, Allogeneic marrow engraftment by cross circulation in lethally irradiated dogs. *Blood* 1966; **28:** 692–707.
4. Storb R, Epstein RB, Ragde H, Thomas ED, Marrow engraftment by allogeneic leukocytes in lethally irradiated dogs. *Blood* 1967; **30:** 805–11.
5. Storb R, Epstein RB, Thomas ED, Marrow repopulating ability of peripheral blood cells compared to thoracic duct cells. *Blood* 1968; **32:** 662–7.
6. Storb R, Graham TC, Epstein RB et al, Demonstration of hematopoietic stem cells in the peripheral blood of baboons by cross circulation. *Blood* 1977; **50:** 537–42.
7. Storb R, Buckner CD, Epstein RB et al, Clinical and hematologic effects of cross circulation in baboons. *Transfusion* 1969; **9:** 23–31.
8. Trobaugh FE, Jr, Lewis JP, Repopulating potential of blood and marrow. *J Clin Invest* 1964; **43:** 1306.
9. Storb R, Doney KC, Thomas ED et al, Marrow transplantation with or without donor buffy coat cells for 65 transfused aplastic anemia patients. *Blood* 1982; **59:** 236–46.
10. Micklem HS, Anderson N, Ross E, Limited potential of circulating haemopoietic stem cells. *Nature* 1975; **256:** 41–3.
11. Carbonell F, Calvo W, Fliedner TM et al, Cytogenetic studies in dogs after total body irradiation and allogeneic transfusion with cryopreserved blood mononuclear cells: Observations in long-term chimeras. *Int J Cell Cloning* 1984; **2:** 81–8.
12. Korbling M, Fliedner TM, Cavalo W, Albumin density gradient purification of canine hemopoietic blood stem cells (HBSC): Long-term allogeneic engraftment without GVH reaction. *Exp Hematol* 1979; **7:** 277–88.
13. Goldman JM, Catovsky D, Goolden AWG et al, Buffy coat autografts for patients with chronic granulocytic leukaemia in transformation. *Blut* 1981; **42:** 149.
14. Korbling M, Burke P, Braine H et al, Successful engraftment of blood-derived normal hemopoietic stem cells in chronic myelogenous leukemia. *Exp Hematol* 1981; **9:** 684–90.

15. van Bekkum DW, de Vries MJ, *Radiation Chimaeras.* Radiobiological Institute of the Organisation for Health Research TNO, Rijswijk Z.H. Netherlands. New York: Academic Press, 1967.

16. van Bekkum DW, Löwenberg B, *Bone Marrow Transplantation. Biological Mechanisms and Clinical Practice.* New York: Marcel Dekker, 1985.

17. Storb R, Epstein RB, Ragde H, Thomas ED, Marrow grafts by combined marrow and leukocyte infusions in unrelated dogs selected by histocompatibility typing. *Transplantation* 1968; **6:** 587–93.

18. Till JE, McCulloch EA, A direct measurement of the radiation sensitivity of normal mouse bone marrow cells. *Radiat Res* 1961; **14:** 213–22.

19. Ploemacher RE, van der Sluijs JP, van Beurden CA et al, Use of limiting-dilution type long-term marrow cultures in frequency analysis of marrow-repopulating and spleen colony-forming hematopoietic stem cells in the mouse. *Blood* 1991; **78:** 2527–33.

20. Jones RJ, Wagner JE, Celano P et al, Separataion of pluripotent haematopoietic stem cells from spleen colony-forming cells. *Nature* 1990; **347:** 188–9.

21. Siminovitch L, Till JE, McCulloch EA, Decline in colony-forming ability of marrow cells subjected to serial transplantation into irradiated mice. *J Cell Comp Physiol* 1964; **64:** 23–31.

22. Fraser CC, Szilvassy SJ, Eaves CJ, Humphries RK, Proliferation of totipotent hematopoietic stem cells in vitro with retention of long-term competitive in vivo reconstituting ability. *Proc Natl Acad Sci USA* 1992; **89:** 1968–72.

23. Harrison DE, Jordan CT, Zhong RK, Astle CM, Primitive hemopoietic stem cells: direct assay of most productive populations by competitive repopulation with simple binomial, correlation and covariance calculations. *Exp Hematol* 1993; **21:** 206–19.

24. Sutherland HJ, Lansdorp PM, Henkelman DH et al, Functional characterization of individual hematopoietic stem cells cultured at limiting dilution on supportive marrow stromal layers. *Proc Natl Acad Sci USA* 1990; **87:** 3584–8.

25. Berenson RJ, Andrews RG, Bensinger WI et al, Antigen CD34$^+$ marrow cells engraft lethally irradiated baboons. *J Clin Invest* 1988; **81:** 951–5.

26. Spangrude GJ, Biological and clinical aspects of hematopoietic stem cells. *Annu Rev Med* 1994; **45:** 93–104.

27. Li CL, Johnson GR, Long-term hemopoietic repopulation by Thy-11^0, Lin$^-$, Ly6A/E$^+$ cells. *Exp Hematol* 1992; **20:** 1309–15.

28. Spangrude GJ, Johnson GR, Resting and activated subsets of mouse multipotent hematopoietic stem cells. *Proc Natl Acad Sci USA* 1990; **87:** 7433–7.

29. Hodgson GS, Bradley TR, Properties of haematopoietic stem cells surviving 5-fluorouracil treatment: evidence for a pre-CFU-S cell? *Nature* 1979; **281:** 381–2.

30. Bertoncello I, Hodgson GS, Bradley TR, Multiparameter analysis of transplantable hemopoietic cells: I. The separation and enrichment of stem cells homing to marrow and spleen on the basis of rhodamine-123 fluorescence. *Exp Hematol* 1985; **13:** 999–1006.

31. Li CL, Johnson GR, Murine hematopoietic stem and progenitor cells: I. Enrichment and biologic characterization. *Blood* 1995; **85:** 1472–9.

32. Wolf NS, Kone A, Priestley GV, Bartelmez SH, In vivo and in vitro characterization of long-term repopulating primitive hematopoietic cells isolated by sequential Hoechst 33342-rhodamine 123 FACS selection. *Exp Hematol* 1993; **21:** 614–22.

33. Wolf NS, Hematopoietic repopulation with a single injected stem cell [abstract]. *Blood* 1995; **86**(Suppl 1): 111a.

34. McSweeney PA, Rouleau KA, Storb R et al, Canine CD34: Cloning of the cDNA and evaluation of an antiserum to recombinant protein *Blood* 1996; **88:** 1992–2003.

35. Cline MJ, Golde DW, Mobilisation of hematopoietic stem cells (CFU-C) into the peripheral blood of man by endotoxin. *Exp Hematol* 1977; **5:** 186.

36. Richman CM, Weiner RS, Yankee RA, Increase in circulating stem cells following chemotherapy in man. *Blood* 1976; **47:** 1031–9.

37. Abrams RA, McCormack K, Bowles C, Deisseroth AB, Cyclophosphamide treatment expands the circulating hematopoietic stem cell pool in dogs. *J Clin Invest* 1981; **67:** 1392–9.

38. Appelbaum FR, Deeg HJ, Storb R et al, Cure of malignant lymphoma in dogs with peripheral blood stem cell transplantation. *Transplantation* 1986; **42:** 19–22.

39. To LB, Roberts MM, Haylock DN et al, Comparison of hematological recovery times and supportive care requirements of autologous recovery phase peripheral blood stem cell transplants, autologous bone marrow transplants and allogeneic bone marrow transplants. *Bone Marrow Transplant* 1992; **9:** 277–84.

40. Brugger W, Bross KJ, Glatt M et al, Mobilization

of tumor cells and hematopoietic progenitor cells into peripheral blood of patients with solid tumors. *Blood* 1994; **83:** 636–40.

41. Gale RP, Reiffers J, Juttner CA, What's new in blood progenitor cell autotransplants? *Bone Marrow Transplant* 1994; **14:** 343–6.

42. Dührsen U, Villeval J, Boyd J et al, Effects of recombinant human granulocyte colony-stimulating factor on hematopoietic progenitor cells in cancer patients. *Blood* 1988; **72:** 2074–81.

43. Socinski MA, Cannistra SA, Elias A et al, Granulocyte–macrophage colony stimulating factor expands the circulating haemopoietic progenitor cell compartment in man. *Lancet* 1988; **i:** 1194–8.

44. Molineux G, Pojda Z, Hampson IN et al, Transplantation potential of peripheral blood stem cells induced by granulocyte colony-stimulating factor. *Blood* 1990; **76:** 2153–8.

45. Neben S, Marcus K, Mauch P, Mobilization of hematopoietic stem and progenitor cell subpopulations from the marrow to the blood of mice following cyclophosphamide and/or granulocyte colony-stimulating factor. *Blood* 1993; **81:** 1960–7.

46. Briddell RA, Hartley CA, Smith KA, McNiece IK. Recombinant rat stem cell factor synergizes with recombinant human granulocyte colony-stimulating factor in vivo in mice to mobilize peripheral blood progenitor cells that have enhanced repopulating potential. *Blood* 1993; **82:** 1720–3.

47. Yan XQ, Hartley C, McElroy P et al, Peripheral blood progenitor cells mobilized by recombinant human granulocyte colony-stimulating factor plus recombinant rat stem cell factor contain long-term engrafting cells capable of cellular proliferation for more than two years as shown by serial transplantation in mice. *Blood* 1995; **85:** 2303–7.

48. Bodine DM, Seidel NE, Zsebo KM, Orlic D, In vivo administration of stem cell factor to mice increases the absolute number of pluripotent hematopoietic stem cells. *Blood* 1993; **82:** 445–55.

49. Chervenick PA, Boggs DR, Marsh JC et al, Quantitative studies of blood and bone marrow neutrophils in normal mice. *Am J Physiol* 1968; **215:** 353–60.

50. Suzuki H, Okano A, Suzuki C et al, A synergistic increase in transplantable peripheral blood stem cells in mice by co-administration of recombinant human interleukin 6 and recombinant human granulocyte colony-stimulating factor. *Transplantation* 1995; **59:** 1596–1600.

51. Grzegorzewski KJ, Komschlies KL, Jacobsen SEW et al, Mobilization of long-term reconstituting hematopoietic stem cells in mice by recombinant human interleukin 7. *J Exp Med* 1995; **181:** 369–74.

52. Laterveer L, Lindley IJD, Hamilton MS et al, Interleukin-8 induces rapid mobilization of hematopoietic stem cells with radioprotective capacity and long-term myelolymphoid repopulating ability. *Blood* 1995; **85:** 2269–75.

53. Mauch P, Lamont C, Neben TY et al, Hematopoietic stem cells in the blood after stem cell factor and interleukin-11 administration: evidence for different mechanisms of mobilization. *Blood* 1995; **86:** 4674–80.

54. Lyman SD, James L, Johnson L et al, Cloning of the human homologue of the murine flt3 ligand: a growth factor for early hematopoietic progenitor cells. *Blood* 1994; **83:** 2795–801.

55. Shimazaki C, Beckendorf J, Kikuta T et al, FLT-3 ligand synergistically enhances the in vivo response to G-CSF for mobilizing hematopoietic stem/progenitor cells into blood in mice [abstract]. *Blood* 1995; **86**(Suppl 1): 111a.

56. Lord BI, Woolford LB, Wood LM et al, Mobilization of early hematopoietic progenitor cells with BB-10010 – a genetically engineered variant of human macrophage inflammatory protein-1-alpha. *Blood* 1995; **85:** 3412–15.

57. Abkowitz JL, Persik MT, Shelton GH et al, Behavior of hematopoietic stem cells in a large animal. *Proc Natl Acad Sci USA* 1995; **92:** 2031–5.

58. Dicke KA, van Hooft JI, van Bekkum DW, The selective elimination of immunologically competent cells from bone marrow and lymphatic cell mixtures. II. Mouse spleen cell fractionating on a discontinuous albumin gradient. *Transplantation* 1968; **6:** 562–70.

59. Storb R, Graham TC, Shiurba R, Thomas ED, Treatment of canine graft-versus-host disease with methotrexate and cyclophosphamide following bone marrow transplantation from histoincompatible donors. *Transplantation* 1970; **10:** 165–72.

60. Thomas ED, Buckner CD, Rudolph RH et al, Allogeneic marrow grafting for hematologic malignancy using HL-A matched donor–recipient sibling pairs. *Blood* 1971; **38:** 267–87.

61. Storb R, Rudolph RH, Thomas ED, Marrow grafts between canine siblings matched by serotyping and mixed leukocyte culture. *J Clin Invest* 1971; **50:** 1272–5.

62. de Revel T, Appelbaum FR, Storb R et al, Effects of granulocyte colony stimulating factor and stem cell factor, alone and in combination, on the mobilization of peripheral blood cells that engraft lethally irradiated dogs. *Blood* 1994; **83:** 3795–9.

63. Crawford L, Lau D, Erwin R et al, A phase I trial of recombinant methionyl human stem cell factor (SCF) in patients with advanced non-small cell lung carcinoma (NSCLC) [abstract]. *Proc Am Soc Clin Oncol* 1993; **12:** 135a.

64. Andrews RG, Briddell RA, Knitter GH et al, In vivo synergy between recombinant human stem cell factor and recombinant human granulocyte colony-stimulating factor in baboons: Enhanced circulation of progenitor cells. *Blood* 1994; **84:** 800–10.

65. Andrews RG, Briddell RA, Knitter GH et al, Rapid engraftment by peripheral blood progenitor cells mobilized by recombinant human stem cell factor and recombinant human granulocyte colony-stimulating factor in nonhuman primates. *Blood* 1995; **85:** 15–20.

66. Laterveer L, Lindley IJD, Heemskerk DPM et al, Rapid mobilization of hematopoietic progenitor cells in rhesus monkeys by a single intravenous injection of interleukin-8. *Blood* 1996; **87:** 781–8.

67. Hastings R, Kaviani MD, Schlerman F et al, Mobilization of hematopoietic progenitors by rhIL-11 and rhG-CSF in non-human primates [abstract]. *Blood* 1994; **84**(Suppl 1): 23a.

68. Gasparetto C, Smith C, Gillio A et al, Enrichment of peripheral blood stem cells in a primate model following administration of a single dose of rh-IL-1 beta. *Bone Marrow Transplant* 1994; **14:** 717–23.

69. Crown J, Jakubowski A, Kemeny N et al, A phase I trial of recombinant human interleukin-1β alone and in combination with myelosup-pressive doses of 5-fluorouracil in patients with gastrointestinal cancer. *Blood* 1991; **78:** 1420–7.

70. Geissler K, Valent P, Mayer P et al, Recombinant human interleukin-3 expands the pool of circulating hematopoietic progenitor cells in primates – synergism with recombinant human granulocyte–macrophage colony-stimulating factor. *Blood* 1990; **75:** 2305–10.

71. Papayannopoulou T, Nakamoto B, Peripheralization of hemopoietic progenitors in primates treated with anti-VLA-4 integrin. *Proc Natl Acad Sci USA* 1993; **90:** 9374–8.

72. Schots R, Van Riet I, Damiaens S et al, The absolute number of circulating $CD34^+$ cells predicts the number of hematopoietic stem cells that can be collected by apheresis. *Bone Marrow Transplant* 1996; **17:** 509–15.

73. Noga SJ, Davis JM, Vogelsang GB et al, The combined use of elutriation and CD8/magnetic bead separation to engineer the bone marrow allograft. In: *Advances in Bone Marrow Purging and Processing*. New York: Wiley–Liss, 1992.

74. Storb R, Prentice RL, Sullivan KM et al, Predictive factors in chronic graft-versus-host disease in patients with aplastic anemia treated by marrow transplantation from HLA-identical siblings. *Ann Intern Med* 1983; **98:** 461–6.

75. Sandmaier BM, Storb R, Santos EB et al, Allogeneic transplants of canine peripheral blood stem cells mobilized by recombinant canine hematopoietic growth factors. *Blood* 1996; **87:** 3508–13.

76. Gratwohl A, Baldomero H, John L et al, Transplantation of G-CSF mobilized allogeneic peripheral blood stem cells in rabbits. *Bone Marrow Transplant* 1995; **16:** 63–8.

77. Fibbe WE, Hamilton MS, Laterveer LL et al, Sustained engraftment of mice transplanted with IL-1 primed blood-derived stem cells. *J Immunol* 1992; **148:** 417–21.

2

Characterization of blood stem cells

Gunnar Kvalheim and Erlend B Smeland

CONTENTS • **Introduction** • **Mobilization of stem cells to peripheral blood** • **Phenotypic characterization of peripheral blood progenitor cells** • **Functional characterization of peripheral blood progenitor cells** • **Mobilization of tumour cells into blood** • **Further perspectives**

INTRODUCTION

Normal haematopoiesis occurs in bone marrow in humans, and is characterized by the generation of mature cells of all haematopoietic lineages from pluripotent stem cells. The bone marrow consists of haematopoietic progenitor and precursor cells at various differentiation stages closely associated with the bone-marrow stromal elements. The pluripotent stem cells are characterized by their capability of self-renewal and the capacity to generate long-term, multi-lineage reconstitution of haematopoiesis after marrow ablation.[1–5] Pluripotent stem cells are very rare, and represent only about 1 in 100 000 bone-marrow mononuclear cells. Small numbers of primitive haematopoietic progenitor cells are also found in the circulation, as first demonstrated in studies in mice, and later confirmed in other species, including humans.[6–12] However, the numbers of progenitor cells in blood can be drastically increased after mobilization with chemotherapy and/or cytokines,[13–21] thus making mobilized peripheral blood an attractive stem cell source for clinical use. There are several advantages of using peripheral blood progenitor cells (PBPC) instead of bone marrow in clinical transplanta-

tion protocols.[11,12,22] Reinfusion of PBPC after high-dose therapy has produced significant shortening in the time of cytopenia, particularly thrombocytopenia. This has led to reductions in the number of platelet transfusions required and the number of days in hospital following high-dose therapy. The haematopoietic graft can be collected without general anaesthesia, and also allows harvesting of stem cells in patients with bone-marrow fibrosis. Clinical data from patients given ablative high-dose therapy including total body irradiation following re-infusion of autologous PBPC show that the quality of human PBPC is at least equivalent to that corresponding to bone-marrow grafts. Based on these observations, there is strong evidence that PBPC contain the true lymphohaematopoietic stem cells. Although the observation time after transplant is short and the long-term reconstitution of haematopoieses is not known, the successful use of allogeneic PBPC transplantation confirms this hypothesis. Furthermore, the development of modern leukapheresis technology has made mobilized peripheral blood an attractive source of progenitor cells for clinical use.

MOBILIZATION OF STEM CELLS TO PERIPHERAL BLOOD

Several decades ago it was shown in various species, using cross-circulation experiments or by infusion of autologous or allogeneic leukocytes, that peripheral blood contains marrow-regenerating cells that are able to engraft the ablated marrow of irradiated recipients.[6–9] This led to the demonstration of haematopoietic progenitor cells in normal human peripheral blood as well,[10–12] and subsequently to the first clinical use of peripheral blood stem cell transplantations.[23–26] Primitive haematopoietic cells are normally present in very low numbers in peripheral blood.[11,12] However, it was noted that there was a dramatic increase in the numbers of circulating early haematopoietic cells during recovery from cytotoxic chemotherapy and thus that chemotherapeutic agents were able to mobilize stem cells.[13–17] Later it was found that certain haematopoietic growth factors can augment the mobilization of circulating progenitor cells when given after chemotherapy.[11,12,18,19] More recently, growth factors alone have also been found to produce a marked increase in the percentage of progenitor cells in blood.[12,27–29] Several growth factors, including granulocyte colony-stimulating factor (G-CSF), granulocyte–macrophage (GM)-CSF, interleukin (IL)-1, IL-3, IL-8, IL-11 and stem cell factor (SCF), have been shown to mobilize progenitor cells into the circulation.[12,19–21,30–44] G-CSF is the most widely used cytokine for mobilization of stem cells. Daily administration of G-CSF permits the harvest of PBPC at days 6 and 7 after initiation of the G-CSF treatment. The use of chemotherapy and G-CSF to mobilize PBPC permits the harvest of PBPC in the haematopoietic regeneration phase occurring usually at days 10–15 after initiation of chemotherapy. Recently, combinations of cytokines have been tried out in animal studies, and early studies in humans demonstrate that combinations of certain cytokines, like G-CSF + SCF, G-CSF + GM-CSF or IL-11 + SCF, may be superior to single cytokines with regard to mobilization of haematopoietic progenitor cells.[39,43,44]

The mechanism by which the progenitor cells mobilize from bone marrow into the peripheral blood is not known. As pointed out by previous investigators, the capability to mobilize PBPC is directly related to previous chemotherapy and irradiation. This type of treatment has a toxic effect not only on haematopoietic progenitor cells but also on stromal cells. The imbalance between the interaction of haematopoietic progenitor cells and stromal cells in the bone marrow is most likely the reason why extensively chemotherapy-treated or irradiated patients mobilized poorly compared with those mobilized with little or no previous chemoradiotherapy. Therefore studies on stromal cell function are becoming an increasing area of investigation.

Phenotypic characterization of peripheral blood progenitor cells

During the past few decades, major achievements have been made in our understanding of haematopoiesis, in part due to the revolution in molecular cell biology. The development of monoclonal antibodies against leukocyte differentiation antigens, the identification of assay systems for haematopoietic progenitor cells, and the identification and production of numerous recombinant cytokines with effects on haematopoietic cells have provided important tools for the study of early haematopoiesis. Furthermore, these discoveries have facilitated the characterization, enrichment and functional study of the most primitive haematopoietic cells, in particular in mice, but also in humans.

Expression of CD34 on peripheral blood progenitor cells

The use of monoclonal antibodies against CD (cluster of differentiation) antigens has greatly facilitated the precise characterization of different haematopoietic lineages and allowed the precise delinement of distinct maturation steps within different cell lineages.[45] Monoclonal antibodies against the same antigens are grouped together based on the reactivity and biochemical and/or genetic characterization of the corresponding antigen.[45] So far, more than 160 different antigens expressed on leukocytes have been described, and these are termed 'CD antigens'.

CD34, a transmembrane cell surface glycoprotein, was initially identified by the My10 monoclonal antibody, which was raised against the immature myeloid cell line KG-1a.[46] Subsequently, it has been shown that CD34 expression is restricted, with the exception of capillary endothelium, to human haematopoietic progenitor cells as well as stromal cell precursors in bone marrow.[46–51] In humans, most committed progenitor cells capable of forming colonies in semi-solid culture assays have been found to reside in the CD34+ population of bone-marrow mononuclear cells.[51–55] CD34+ cells, which represent the most immature 1–4% of bone-marrow mononuclear cells, also include more primitive haematopoietic progenitor cells.[51,56–59] Recent data have shown that enriched CD34+ marrow cells can reconstitute haematopoiesis in vivo in humans and non-human primates,[60,61] and although murine studies suggest that at least some long-term reconstituting cells express low or negligible levels of CD34,[62] available data in humans strongly suggest that the CD34+ population in human bone marrow includes most pluripotent stem cells. The existence of CD34− stem cells in humans cannot be excluded, however.

Enumeration of CD34+ cells is difficult, but development of excellent monoclonal antibodies and standardization of the flow cytometric procedure have made it possible to use determinations of the percentage or number of CD34+ cells in routine clinical use.[63–65] The levels of CD34+ cells are very low in unmobilized blood, representing approximately 0.1% of blood mononuclear cells.[12] Such values lie around the detection limit for determination of small populations by flow cytometry.

The levels of CD34+ cells in blood increase markedly after mobilization, and the percentage of CD34+ cells in the apheresis products may approach the percentages in bone-marrow grafts.[12,28,66,67] The rise in CD34 numbers in peripheral blood can be used to determine the optimal time for apheresis, and monitoring of CD34+ cells is now widely used for this purpose.[12,28,66,67] Several studies have demonstrated that the peak concentrations of circulating CD34+ cells as well as the kinetics of mobilization vary with the mobilizing regimen and/or the pretreatment of the patient.[68–71] The combination of chemotherapy and growth factor usually act synergistically with regard to mobilization of PBPC. In the allogeneic setting, using mobilized blood from normal donors, cytotoxic drugs naturally cannot be used. Therefore cytokines alone have been used for mobilization of normal donors. Still, sufficient progenitor cells are currently often obtained by just one apheresis, even with the use of a single cytokine for mobilization. However, the numbers of circulating CD34+ cells vary significantly between donors, even with identical mobilizing regimens.[68] Moreover, recent data suggest that combinations of cytokines such as G/GM-CSF and G-CSF/SCF may be better than the use of single cytokines.[39,43,44,68] For instance, it is noted that some subjects who mobilize poorly with G-CSF alone may show a normal mobilization after the combination of G-CSF/GM-CSF.[68]

Identification of subsets of CD34+ cells in mobilized blood

The CD34+ population is heterogeneous and pluripotent stem cells constitute only a minor fraction of the whole CD34+ population. Therefore several attempts have been made to further enrich for the most immature human haematopoietic cells by determination of subsets of CD34+ cells. In particular, available data suggest that the most primitive cells are enriched in the CD34+CD38−, CD34+HLA-DR− or CD34+Thy-1+ subpopulations.[58,59,72–77] Both the CD34+CD38− and CD34+HLA-DR− cells represent only a few percent of the CD34+ population, and have been found to be enriched for the most immature cells capable of in vitro growth, as well as cells giving rise to multilineage reconstitution in in vivo models of human haematopoiesis in chimaeric animals.[72]

There is actually little overlap between the CD34$^+$CD38$^-$ and CD34$^+$HLA-DR$^-$ populations in fetal and adult bone marrow, and studies comparing these populations suggest that the CD34$^+$CD38$^-$ cells are more homogeneous and are relatively more enriched for the most primitive haematopoietic cells detectable by in vitro assays than CD34$^+$HLA-DR$^-$ cells.[59,73] The CD34$^+$Thy-1$^+$ population represents a larger fraction of the CD34$^+$ population (approximately 10–25%), and also contains primitive progenitor cells.[74-77] It should be emphasized that although CD34$^+$CD38$^-$, CD34$^+$HLA-DR$^-$ and CD34$^+$Thy-1$^+$ cells contain primitive progenitors, all of these populations are still heterogeneous, and putative pluripotent stem cells represent only a small fraction of these populations (Figure 2.1). A problem with the use of antibodies against the CD38, HLA-DR and Thy-1 antigens to characterize stem cells is the gradual overlap between positive and negative cells. This makes it difficult to precisely compare the results from different laboratories with regard to the content of these populations, since small variations in sensitivity and thus the detection limit can greatly influence the percentages obtained.

Several groups have compared the levels of immature CD34$^+$ subsets in mobilized peripheral blood versus bone marrow and/or cord blood. The data suggest that the CD34$^+$CD38$^-$ and the CD34$^+$HLA-DR$^-$ subsets are present in similar proportions in mobilized peripheral blood versus bone marrow, while cord blood may express a relatively higher proportion of the CD34$^+$CD38$^-$ subset.[68,78-81] Interestingly, Ho et al recently demonstrated that the percentage of CD34$^+$CD38$^-$ cells varied with the mobilizing regimen, in that blood mobilized with G-CSF contained a lower percentage of such cells than blood mobilized either with GM-SCF or with G-CSF plus GM-CSF.[68,82] In addition, the total number of CD34$^+$CD38$^-$ cells were found to be lower in G-CSF-mobilized samples.

Mobilized peripheral blood has been reported to contain similar or higher percentages of CD34$^+$Thy-1$^+$ cells among CD34$^+$ cells, as compared with adult bone marrow.[83-86]

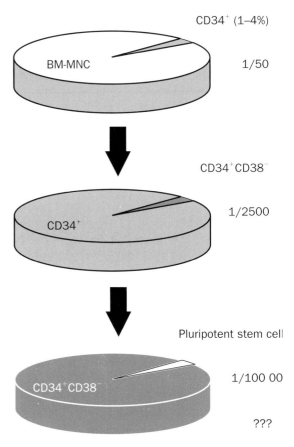

CD34$^+$ (1–4%)

BM-MNC

1/50

CD34$^+$CD38$^-$

1/2500

CD34$^+$

Pluripotent stem cell

1/100 00

CD34$^+$CD38$^-$

???

Figure 2.1 Phenotypical heterogeneity of human haematopoietic progenitor cells. CD34$^+$ cells represent the most immature 1–4% of bone-marrow mononuclear cells and up to similar percentages of mononuclear cells from mobilized peripheral blood. CD34$^+$ cells are heterogeneous, and contain most committed progenitor cells capable of in vitro colony formation in semi-solid medium in addition to more primitive cells. The CD34$^+$CD38$^-$ subset represents a few percent of the CD34$^+$ population (approximately 1/2500 bone-marrow mononuclear cells), and is markedly enriched for the most immature haematopoietic cells detectable by currently available assays. However, although CD34$^+$CD38$^-$ cells are rather homogeneous with regard to size and morphology, pluripotent stem cells represent only a small fraction of the CD34$^+$CD38$^-$ cells (estimated frequency 1/100 000 bone-marrow mononuclear cells).

Moreover, the high levels of CD34$^+$Thy-1$^+$ cells were only temporarily present in sequential apheresis samples, despite the continuous presence of CD34$^+$ cells.[83,86] Donahue and co-workers, using non-human primates, also demonstrated a difference between bone-marrow-derived CD34$^+$ cells and CD34$^+$ cells from mobilized peripheral blood with regard to cell cycle state, since CD34$^+$ cells from peripheral blood had a lower percentage of cells in the S + G2/M phases.[86]

Several studies have compared the levels of other subsets of CD34$^+$ cells in mobilized blood and in bone marrow. Thus it has been shown that peripheral blood and cord blood CD34$^+$ cells contain relatively lower percentages of early B-lineage cells expressing CD10 and CD19, and relatively more cells co-expressing myeloid markers than bone-marrow CD34$^+$ cells.[68,78–80] Moreover, circulating CD34$^+$ cells have been found to express lower levels of leukocyte function antigen-1 (LFA-1) and very late antigen-4 (VLA-4) compared with CD34$^+$ cells from bone marrow.[87]

Taken together, available data demonstrate that there are clear differences between CD34$^+$ cells in mobilized blood and bone marrow with regard to the immunophenotype. However, the data strongly suggest that mobilized peripheral blood contain levels of CD34$^+$ cells with an immature phenotype that are comparable to the levels in bone marrow.

Phenotyping of progenitor cells in PBPC products and engraftment

Several studies have shown that there is a direct relation between the number of CD34$^+$ cells in the PBPC product reinfused and time to engraftment of neutrophils and platelets after high-dose therapy, at least for doses below $(2–3) \times 10^6$ CD34$^+$ cells/kg body weight.[71,88,89] However, the dose relationship is steep, and most studies indicate that more than 2×10^6 CD34$^+$ cells/kg are needed for timely multilineage engraftment.[88–91] Moreover, in autologous transplantations using mobilized peripheral blood, it has been found that doses of CD34$^+$ cells higher than 5×10^6 cells/kg are associated with early trilineage engraftment.[92] When fewer CD34$^+$ cells per kg are used, recovery of neutrophils can still be fast, but very often a delay in platelet recovery occurs. Recently, Mavroudis et al[89] presented data suggesting that the dose of CD34$^+$ cells predicted post-transplantation survival as well as speed of engraftment. Thus patients given doses of CD34$^+$ cells below 1×10^6 cells/kg had a higher transplantation-related mortality than patients given more than 1×10^6 cells/kg.[94] Moreover, doses of CD34$^+$ cells above 2×10^6 cells/kg led to faster rates of recovery than doses below 2×10^6 cells/kg. Our own experiences and others have shown that the use of enriched CD34$^+$ cells to reconstitute haematopoiesis after high-dose therapy in autografts and recently in allografts gives a similar pattern of engraftment to that with unseparated PBPC. This clinical observation confirms that CD34$^+$ cells in the PBPC products contain both early progenitor cells and more mature progenitor cells contributing to both early and late reconstitution of haematopoiesis.

Körbling et al found that the cytokine-mobilized CD34$^+$ and CD34$^+$Thy-1$^+$ concentrations in blood before apheresis predicted apheresis-derived stem cell yield.[84] In spite of this, there is still uncertainty regarding the clinical usefulness of CD34$^+$ subset analysis in relation to predictions of short- and long-term engraftment. At present, there are no data showing a correlation between CD34$^+$CD38$^-$ or CD34$^+$Thy-1$^+$ cells, and haematopoietic reconstitution. However, data by Dercksen et al suggested that the numbers of CD34$^+$CD41$^+$ cells and CD34$^+$CD33$^-$ cells correlated significantly better with time to platelet and neutrophil engraftment respectively than did the total number of CD34$^+$ cells.[88]

The low numbers of CD34$^+$CD19$^+$CD10$^+$ early B-lineage cells in mobilized blood have raised concerns with regard to the potential of these cells to generate lymphocytes after transplantation. However, available data suggest that mobilized peripheral blood CD34$^+$ cells have both B- and T-cell potential.[85]

FUNCTIONAL CHARACTERIZATION OF PERIPHERAL BLOOD PROGENITOR CELLS

Colony assays in semi-solid medium

During the development from pluripotent stem cells to the mature progeny, the cells gradually become more and more lineage-restricted and lose their capability of self-renewal. Colony assays in semi-solid medium have been extremely useful for studies of haematopoietic progenitor cells. Each colony represent the result of proliferation and differentiation of a single progenitor cell, and the phenotype of the mature colony reflects the potential of this cell to develop into cells of the various lineages,

depending on the growth factors added.[93,94] In such assays, committed cells, which can give rise to cells of single lineages, can be detected. These are named after the cell type of the colonies obtained (for instance colony-forming unit–granulocyte (CFU-G), CFU-M, CFU-E/BFU-E or CFU-Meg). In addition, bi- or multipotent cells giving rise to colonies with cells of different lineages can be detected (GFU-GM, CFU-GEMM and CFU-mix). A schematic drawing of haematopoietic differentiation in relation to the various in vitro assay systems is shown in Figure 2.2. As the determination of different types of colonies requires more close morphological evaluation, and because granulocyte–macrophage colonies often dominate, many

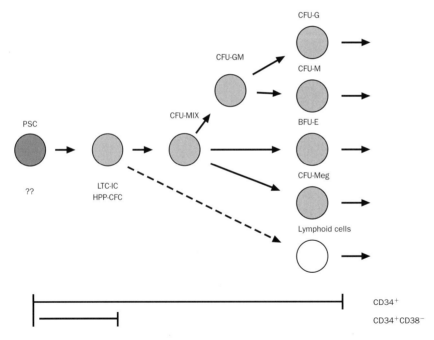

Figure 2.2 Functional in vitro assays detecting haematopoietic progenitor cells. Colony assays in semi-solid medium detect committed progenitor cells giving rise to colonies consisting of morphologically mature cells of various lineages. Such colonies are termed colony-forming units (CFUs) or burst-forming units (BFUs), and are named after the cell type present in the colony: CFU-G (CFU-granulocyte), CFU-M (CFU-monocyte/macrophage), CFU-Meg (CFU-megakaryocyte), BFU-E (BFU-erythrocyte), CFU-GM (CFU-granulocyte–macrophage); CFU-mix/CFU-GEMM (colonies consisting of granulocytes, macrophages, erythrocytes and megakaryocytes). Such colonies are thus derived from unipotent progenitors (like CFU-G), bipotent progenitors (like CFU-GM) or multipotent progenitors (like CFU-mix/CFU-GEMM). Even more immature cells can also be detected by in vitro cultures (long-term culture-initiating cells (LTC-IC) or high-proliferative-potential colony-forming cells (HPP-CFC).

investigators often use the total number of colonies formed (total colony-forming cells, CFC). Colony assays are critically dependent on the culture conditions used, including the type of serum and the cytokines used for stimulation. Therefore such assays are difficult to standardize, and may vary considerably between different laboratories. Recently, however, the availability of commercially available standardized regents has led to increased reproducibility of such assays.

As for CD34[+] cells, there is a marked increase in CFC after mobilization, and several studies suggest that CD34[+] cells from mobilized blood have a higher cloning efficiency in standard colony assays than CD34[+] cells from adult bone marrow.[79–81,95] The numbers of CFU-GM or total CFC have frequently been used to assess the quality of apheresis products, and there is a close correlation between CD34[+] numbers and CFU-GM/CFC numbers.[82] As for CD34[+] cells, variations in CFC content and cloning efficiency of PBPC have been described.[68] CFU assays are not standardized, and large differences in the plating efficacy of CFU can be observed among laboratories. Therefore the minimal number of CFU required to obtain haematopoietic reconstitution after high-dose therapy is not known. Furthermore, it has been suggested that CFU assays do not correlate well with long-term repopulating ability of stem cells, and it therefore seems important also to employ other assays capable of detecting and enumerating more primitive progenitor stem cells.

Assays detecting immature cells

In vitro assays

The most immature progenitor cells do not grow in standard colony assays, and often require a stromal support for growth in vitro. During the past few decades, several in vitro assays have been described that allow growth of immature cells, including assays for LTC-IC (long-term culture-initiating cells) and HPP-CFCs (high-proliferative-potential colony-forming cells).[96,97] Of these, the LTC-IC assay especially has been used in several studies in order to characterize the immature cells in peripheral blood. The assay is based on the ability of immature cells to generate progenitor cells in standard colony assays after preculture for 5–8 weeks on a stromal cell layer. The cells giving rise to secondary colonies are immature, and more mature cells present at onset will die or mature during the preculture period.[96] In mice, a close overlap has been demonstrated between LTC-ICs and cells giving rise to long-term haematopoietic reconstitution. Thus the LTC-IC assay is currently the best functional assay in vitro in humans for identification of primitive cells that closely approximate the pluripotent stem cell.[98] The CD34[+]CD38[−], CD34[+]Thy-1[+] and CD34[+]HLA-DR[−] populations have all been shown to be enriched in LTC-IC, although none of these populations contain all LTC-IC.[59,81] In fact, a modification of the LTC-IC assay by extended preculture has recently been described.[99] The extended LTC-IC (ELTC-IC) assay detects even more primitive cells than week-5 or week-8 LTC-IC.[99] Unfortunately, the LTC-IC and the ELTC-IC assays are time-consuming and cumbersome to perform, and are therefore impractical for routine identification and enumeration of circulating stem cells.

In vivo assays

The ultimate assays for stem cell function are in vivo assays, and such assays have been widely used in mice. Till and McCulloch developed in 1961 the first functional quantitative in vivo assay for the enumeration of candidate stem cells in mice.[100] After injection of marrow into lethally irradiated mice, they observed colonies developing on the surface of the spleen. When these were further investigated, it was found that each colony contained precursor cells from granulocyte, erythroid and megakaryocyte lineages. Furthermore, when cells from the spleen colonies were collected and reinjected, they were capable of forming new spleen colonies. The spleen colony assay (CFU-S) became very useful for the identification of primitive haematopoietic cells in mice, but later data have shown that the pluripotent stem cells are distinct from CFU-S.[101] In vivo assays of human stem cells require the use of chimaeric animals. Multilineage reconstitution of human haematopoiesis has been demonstrated in immune-deficient animals, especially after addition of human cytokines, and in a sheep in utero model.[72,102] However, these in vivo assays are not suitable for clinical use.

Normal peripheral blood contain very small amounts of LTC-IC (approximately 1/100 of the relative content of LTC-IC present in bone-marrow mononuclear cells).[103] By analogy with the phenotypical characterization of mobilized peripheral blood, it has been demonstrated that the content of LTC-IC in blood also increase markedly after mobilization, although the relative increases vary.[81,98,104–106] Recently, Prosper et al found that G-CSF mobilizes LTC-IC in normal donors to a greater extent than committed progenitors or CD34$^+$ cells.[81] Although a fraction of these had functional characteristics of primitive LTC-IC similar to those in bone marrow, the majority represented more mature LTC-IC.

Studies primarily in mice suggest that different cells are responsible for early and late engraftment. While the most primitive pluripotent stem cells are most likely responsible for long-term reconstitution, more intermediate multipotent cells are involved in early engraftment.[98] In humans, it is generally believed that increased clonogenicity or other functional changes in committed cells are responsible for the earlier engraftment observed after transplantation with peripheral blood stem cells versus bone marrow.[98] In contrast, LTC-IC are reported not to be involved in early engraftment, but instead may be responsible for long-term reconstitution.[98] Recently, this notion has been challenged in mice, where it was found that highly enriched populations of primitive cells were able to give rise to early as well as late engraftment.[107] It is interesting to note that in humans autografts consisting of highly purified CD34$^+$Thy-1$^+$Lin$^-$ cells also give engraftment after high-dose therapy.[108] The time to engraftment in such patients tends to be slightly delayed in comparison with what has been observed when CD34$^+$ cells are used. The most likely explanation for this difference in

time to reconstitution between CD34$^+$ cells and CD34$^+$Thy-1$^+$Lin$^-$ cells is that CD34$^+$ cells contain a higher number of mature progenitor cells giving rise to the early engraftment.

Taken together, experimental data on human progenitor cells and clinical data using peripheral blood stem cells strongly suggest that mobilized blood contains long-term reconstituting cells. This is supported by animal studies, which demonstrate that long-term repopulating cells are found in peripheral blood after mobilization.[109–112] Recently, Varas et al, employing genetically labelled mice, found that G-CSF mobilizes into peripheral blood the complete clonal repertoire of haematopoietic precursors that reside in the bone marrow of mice.[113] Moreover, gene-marking studies in humans have demonstrated that CD34$^+$-enriched peripheral blood cells contribute to long-term, multilineage engraftment after autologous transplantation for more than 18 months.[114] Murray et al have also demonstrated multilineage growth of human peripheral blood CD34$^+$Thy-1$^+$Lin$^-$ cells using in vivo assays in chimaeric severe combined immunodeficiency (SCID)-hu mice, supporting this conclusion.[85] This is in agreement with clinical experiences, since there are no available data to suggest the development of late graft failures after transplantations using peripheral blood autografts. However, the final proof with regard to the content of cells with long-term repopulating ability in mobilized blood, will require long-term follow up in patients treated with high-dose therapy and allogeneic PBPC support.

Functional assays – predictive value with regard to rate of engraftment?

Studies that have compared haematopoietic recovery following the use of bone marrow with that following PBPC as stem cell support after high-dose therapy have shown that PBPC reduce the time to reconstitute neutrophils and especially platelets to 8–10 days. It has been generally assumed that the rapid engraftment obtained with PBPC grafts is caused either by their high content of clonogenic cells or by some other change in their function that accompanies their ability to be mobilized.

Data have been published related to the correlation between the speed of engraftment and the progenitor content of the PBPC graft. Some investigators have found that patients given more than 1×10^5 colony-forming cells (CFC) per kilogram body weight have faster recovery of haematopoiesis compared with those given less than 1×10^5 CFC/kg, while other studies show no significant relation between the speed of engraftment and the number of CFC reinfused.[115–118] Clonogenic in vitro assays are difficult to standardize, and the most likely explanation for these conflicting data is the large variation in the number of CFC present in PBPC grafts.

Murine studies suggest that the majority of committed cells capable of forming colonies in progenitor cell assays are not responsible for long-term lymphohaematopoietic reconstitution. Bone marrow autografts purged with 4-hydroperoxycyclophosphamide (4-HC) have been depleted to undetectable levels of progenitor stem cell colonies. In spite of this, most patients autotransplanted with these grafts have been found to recover their blood counts, although delayed engraftment, especially of platelets, has frequently been observed.[119] This emphasizes that also in humans, CFC/CFU-GM assays cannot be used as a reliable predictor for long-term reconstitution of haematopoiesis after high-dose therapy. Moreover, there are so far no data to support a predictive role for assays of primitive progenitor cells like LTC-IC with regard to early or late engraftment potential. Sutherland and co-workers found that the LTC-IC content did not correlate with the content of total clonogenic cells or the total CD34[+] cell content of leukapheresis products.[98] However, a limited number of LTC-IC studies have been published, and more patients should be evaluated before a firm conclusion can be drawn as to whether or not levels of primitive progenitor cells at various stages contribute to early or late haematopoietic recovery. Several studies are under way.

MOBILIZATION OF TUMOUR CELLS INTO BLOOD

Autologous stem cell transplantation as rescue therapy after high-dose therapy is a safe procedure. However, death after such treatment is mostly due to relapse of the disease.[120] Applying sensitive techniques to detect tumour cells, contamination can be observed in histologically normal bone-marrow autografts in 20–70% of patients undergoing high-dose treatment.[121] PBPC autografts are increasingly used also in the belief that these products will have a low probability of containing tumour cells. However, recent findings demonstrate that tumour cell involvement is also frequent in peripheral blood stem cell autografts.[121–124]

Previous reports in metastatic breast cancer patients have demonstrated that malignant cells, like haematopoietic progenitor stem cells, migrate or egress from the bone marrow in response to chemotherapy and growth factors such as G-CSF and GM-CSF.[125] Since the tumour cells appear simultaneously with CD34[+] cells in the blood, collected PBPC will, under these circumstances, also contain contaminating tumour cells. In our own work with high-risk stage II breast cancer patients entering an adjuvant Scandinavian study, randomized between dose-escalating chemotherapy plus G-CSF versus high-dose therapy with PBPC support, micrometastatic detection was performed on bone marrow and blood at diagnosis and on the PBPC product. At diagnosis, 40% had tumour cells present in bone marrow and 19% in the blood. After two cycles of chemotherapy, patients were mobilized with chemotherapy and G-CSF. Since 30% of the PBPC products were contaminated with tumour cells, these data show that the regimen used to mobilize PBPC also mobilized tumour cells simultaneously into the blood (Figure 2.3).

Our results also indicate that tumour cells remaining in the PBPC product may be chemoresistant, since three cycles of chemotherapy were not capable of eradicating these cells. Similar findings have been observed in patients with other diseases such as myelomas, follicular lymphomas and Hodgkin's disease

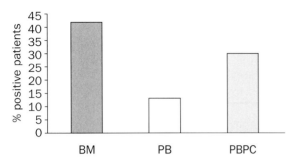

Figure 2.3 The presence of micrometastases in bone marrow and blood at diagnosis and in the PBPC product was tested in 38 high-risk stage II breast cancer patients employing immunocytochemistry with anticytokeratin antibodies. Although the patients were treated with two cycles of chemotherapy prior to mobilization with chemotherapy and G-CSF, 30% of the PBPC products had contaminating tumour cells. In contrast, 13% presented with tumour cells in the blood at diagnosis. This indicates that tumour cells are mobilized into the blood by the use of chemotherapy and G-CSF. BM = bone marrow; PB = peripheral blood; PBPC = peripheral blood progenitor cells.

(our own experiences). The work by Brenner et al and others,[126,127] provides strong evidence that re-entry of contaminating tumour cells to the bone marrow occurs when grafts containing tumour cells are reinfused after high-dose therapy. This observation indicates that tumour cells, like haematopoietic progenitor cells, might have similar molecular mechanisms of homing and release from bone marrow.

The possible contribution of purging of malignant cells to the efficacy of autologous progenitor stem cell transplantation is not known, since prospective clinical studies have not been performed. However, gene-marking studies of autografted cells to trace the origin of relapse after ABMT have indicated that tumour cells remaining in the reinfused marrow contribute to recurrence of the disease.[126,127] This conclusion is further supported by results in patients with follicular lymphomas, indicating

that efficient bone-marrow purging improves disease-free survival.[128]

Several methods have been developed for purging of malignant cells from autografts.[129] Our own experiences with immunomagnetic beads to purge malignant lymphoma cells from bone marrow and PBPC have shown that available methods are efficient and safe, resulting in rapid and sustained engraftment when re-infusion is performed after high-dose therapy.[130–137] Experimental and clinical experiences have demonstrated that autografts can be purged with immunomagnetic beads and an anti-HLA-DR antibody without any adverse effect on reconstitution of haematopoiesis.[130,134] This clinical observation supports the hypothesis that HLA-DR-expressing progenitor cells might not be required to reconstitute haematopoiesis after high-dose therapy.

Since the CD34 antigen is generally not expressed on cancer cells from tumours such as lymphomas, myelomas and breast cancers, positive enrichment of CD34$^+$ cells containing the repopulating haematopoietic progenitor cells might also be a method to deplete contaminating malignant cells from autografts.[138–140] Our experiences with the use of immunobeads in combination with Isolex 300 for the enrichment of CD34$^+$ cells from leukapheresis products in lymphoma patients and breast cancer patients show high purity (97.8%) and yield (62%) of CD34$^+$ cells (Figure 2.4). In spite of this, and in keeping with previous reports employing other methods of CD34$^+$ enrichment, most patients who presented tumour cells in the PBPC prior to CD34 enrichment still had persistent tumour cells after the CD34 selection, although the total numbers of tumour cells were considerably reduced.

Our own preclinical experiences show that when CD34$^+$ cell enrichment is followed by immunomagnetic purging using the B-cell or T-cell mixture of monoclonal antibodies as described earlier, lymphoma cells can be efficiently eradicated. In breast cancer patients, CD34$^+$ cell enrichment followed by one cycle of immunomagnetic purging, employing the anti-breast cancer monoclonal antibodies directly attached to the beads, eradicates the breast

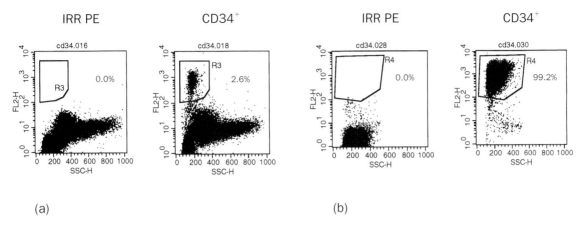

(a) (b)

Figure 2.4 Flow cytometry determination of (a) CD34$^+$ cells in mobilized peripheral blood and (b) positively selected CD34$^+$ cells. PBPC were collected from a breast cancer patient mobilized with chemotherapy and G-CSF. Enrichment of CD34$^+$ cells was performed with Isolex 300. Flow cytometry was performed after staining of the starting PBPC product and the enriched CD34$^+$ cell product with the (PE)-labelled anti-CD34 monoclonal antibody HPAC-2. Control cells were stained with an isotype-matched PE-labelled irrelevant monoclonal antibody. FL2 = relative phycoerythrin fluorescence; SSC = side light scatter; IRR PE = phycoerythrin-labelled irrelevant, isotype-matched monoclonal antibody.

cancer cells, with an insignificant loss of CD34$^+$ cells.

Several clinical studies confirm that CD34$^+$ enriched cells give a fast and sustained engraftment. The use of purged CD34$^+$ cell products as autotransplants opens up the possibility of harvesting progenitor stem cells with only growth factors and prior to any cancer treatment, without the risk of tumour cell contamination. Since such purified CD34$^+$ cells have not been influenced by chemoradiotherapy, this also might minimize the risk of developing secondary haematopoietic malignancies.

FURTHER PERSPECTIVES

There is still a need for better characterization of the cells that are responsible for the various phases of haematological reconstitution after peripheral blood transplantations. Pluripotent stem cells are not characterized as well in humans as in the murine system. Therefore it is

important to obtain a better and more reproducible phenotypical detection of the most primitive subset of haematopoietic cells, preferably by the use of novel antigens that are strongly expressed on such cells. Assays for the most primitive haematopoietic cells are cumbersome, time-consuming and difficult to standardize. Several groups are therefore exploiting molecular biology to characterize gene expression in early haematopoietic cells, and it is hoped that the use of RT-PCR analyses of gene expression will in the future give an important supplement to the characterization of such cells.

Little is understood about the molecular signals that mediate the release of haematopoietic progenitor cells from haematopoietic stroma or about the surface characteristics of the cells that allow their ingress, or re-entry, into the marrow compartment.[141] Since it appears that malignant cells mobilize to the blood together with progenitor cells, it is not unlikely that similar mechanisms for tumour cells and progenitor cells exist. Furthermore, some leukaemic cells, with the exception of chronic myeloid leukaemias, have recently been demonstrated to home to marrow stroma and proliferate in a similar way as normal progenitor cells do. Therefore further knowledge of the regulation of migration and trafficking of normal haematopoietic progenitor cells may also give a better understanding of the metastatic activity of cancer cells.

Clinically, it has been shown that expansion in vitro of a small number of CD34[+] cells stimulated by combinations of multiple cytokines appears to give haematopoietic reconstitution when reinfused after high-dose therapy.[142]

Since in this study the conditioning of the patients prior to reinfusion was not totally ablative, it has been suggested that the use of such expanded cells has not proved that they contain enough primitive progenitor cells to give a long and sustained engraftment. The final confirmation that a small number of expanded CD34[+] cells will contain a sufficient number of stem cells to reconstitute patients after high-dose therapy can be obtained only when such cells are used in allotransplantation. For ethical reasons, such a study is difficult to perform in humans until more knowledge of haematopoietic stem cells exists.

REFERENCES

1. Ogawa M, Differentiation and proliferation of hematopoietic stem cells. *Blood* 1993; **81:** 2844–53.

2. Metcalf D, Hematopoietic regulators: redundancy or subtlety? *Blood* 1993; **82:** 3515–23.

3. Till JE, McCulloch EA, Siminovitch L, A stochastic model of stem cell proliferation, based on the growth of spleen colony-forming cells. *Proc Natl Acad Sci USA* 1964; **51:** 29–36.

4. Nakahata T, Gross AJ, Cornetta K, A stochastic model of self-renewal and commitment to differentiation of the primitive hematopoietic stem cells in culture. *J Cell Physiol* 1982; **113:** 455–88.

5. Spangrude GJ, Heimfeld SH, Weissman IL, Purification and characterization of mouse hematopoietic stem cells. *Science* 1988; **241:** 58–62.

6. Brecher G, Cronkite EP, Post-radiation parabiosis and survival in rats. *Proc Soc Exp Biol Med* 1951; **77:** 292–9.

7. Storb R, Graham TC, Epstein RB et al, Demonstration of hematopoietic stem cells in the peripheral blood of baboons by cross circulation. *Blood* 1977; **50:** 537–42.

8. Kiem HP, Davorovsky B, von Kalle C et al, Retrovirusmediated gene transduction into canine peripheral blood repopulating cells. *Blood* 1994; **83:** 1467–73.

9. Demetri GD, Elias AD, Current understanding of PBPCs and hematopoietic growth factors. *Adv Oncol* 1994; **10:** 11–28.

10. Barr RD, Wang-Peng J, Hematopoietic stem cells in human peripheral blood. *Science* 1975; **190:** 284–5.

11. Hong D-S, Deeg HJ, Hematopoietic stem cells: sources and applications. *Med Oncol* 1994; **11:** 63–8.

12. Stadmauer EA, Schneider CJ, Silberstein LE, Peripheral blood progenitor cell generation and harvesting. *Semin Oncol* 1995; **22:** 291–300.

13. To DN, Haylock RJ, Kimber RJ et al, High levels of circulating hematopoietic stem cells in very early remission from acute non-lymphoblastic leukemia and their collection and cryopreservation. *Br J Haematol* 1984; **58:** 399–410.

14. Richman CM, Weiner RS, Yankee RA, Increase in circulating stem cells following chemotherapy in man. *Blood* 1996; **47:** 1031–9.

15. Reiffers J, Bernard P, David B et al, A successful autologous transplantation with peripheral blood hematopoietic cells in patient with acute leukemia. *Exp Hematol* 1986; **14:** 312–15.

16. Gianni AM, Sierra S, Bregni M et al, Rapid and complete hematopoietic reconstruction following combined transplantation of autologous blood and bone marrow cells. A changing role for high dose chemo-radiotherapy? *Hematol Oncol* 1989; **7:** 139–48.

17. Tavassoli M, The role of conditioning regimens in homing of transplanted hematopoietic cells. *Bone Marrow Transplant* 1992; **10:** 15–17.

18. Duhrsen U, Villeval JL, Boyd J et al, Effects of

recombinant granulocyte colony-stimulating factor on hematopoietic progenitor cells in cancer patients. *Blood* 1988; **72:** 2074–81.

19. Sheridan WP, Bergley CG, Juttner CA, Effect of peripheral-blood progenitor cells mobilised by filgrastim (G.CSF) on platelet recovery after high-dose chemotherapy. *Lancet* 1992; **339:** 640–4.

20. Stadtmauer E, Biggs D, Sickles C, G-CSF mobilized peripheral blood stem cells with high dose therapy for responding patients with metastatic breast cancer. *J Cell Biochem* 1994; **18B:** 102.

21. Bolwell BJ, Fishleder SW, Andresen AE et al, G-CSF primed peripheral blood progenitor cells in autologous bone marrow transplantation: Parameters affecting bone marrow enfragment. *Bone Marrow Transplant* 1993; **12:** 609–14.

22. Tanaka J, Kasai M, Imamura M, Asaka M, Clinical application of allogenic peripheral blood stem cells transplantation. *Ann Hematol* 1995; **71:** 265–9.

23. Haines ME, Goldman JM, Worsley AM et al, Chemotherapy and autografting for patients with chronic granulocytic leukemia in transformation: probable prolongation of life for some patients. *Br J Haematol* 1984; **58:** 711–22.

24. Kessinger A, Armitage JO, Landmark JD et al, Autologous peripheral hematopoietic stem cell transplantation restores hematopoietic function following marrow ablative therapy. *Blood* 1988; **77:** 723–7.

25. Körbling M, Dorken B, Ho AD et al, Autologous transplantation of blood-derived hematopoietic stem cells after myeloblative therapy in a patient with Burkitt's lymphoma. *Blood* 1986; **67:** 529–32.

26. Williams SF, Bitran JD, Richards JM et al, Peripheral blood-derived stem cell collections for use in autologous transplantation after high dose chemotherapy: an alternative approach. *Bone Marrow Transplant* 1990; **5:** 129–33.

27. Eaves C, Peripheral blood stem cells reach new heights. *Blood* 1993; **82:** 1957–9.

28. Smith AM, Peripheral blood progenitor cell transplantation: Clinical, practical, and economic considerations. *J Hematol* 1994; **3:** 331–48.

29. Reisner Y, Segall H, Hematopoietic stem cell transplantation for cancer therapy. *Curr Opin Immunol* 1995; **7:** 687–93.

30. Sheridan WP, Begley CG, To LB, Phase II study of autologous filgrastim (G.CSF)-mobilized peripheral blood progenitor cells to restore hematopoiesis after high dose chemotherapy

for lymphoid malignancies. *Bone Marrow Transplant* 1994; **14:** 105–11.

31. Chao NJ, Schriber JR, Grimes K et al, Granulocyte colony-stimulating factor 'mobilized' peripheral blood progenitor cells accelerate granulocyte and platelet recovery after high dose chemotherapy. *Blood* 1993; **81:** 2031–5.

32. Bensinger W, Singer J, Appelbaum F et al, Autologous transplantation with peripheral blood mononuclear cells collected after administration of recombinant granulocyte stimulating factor. *Blood* 1993; **81:** 3158–63.

33. Ahmed T, Preti RA, Raziz E et al, Peripheral blood mononuclear mobilization with sargramostim (GM-CSF). In: *Advances in Bone Marrow Purging and Processing: Fourth International Symposium* (Gee AP, Gross S, Worthington-White DA, eds). New York: Wiley, 1994: 457–62.

34. Peters WP, Rosner G, Ross M et al, Comparative effects of granulocyte–macrophage colony-stimulating factor (GM-CSF) and granulocyte colony-stimulating factor (G-CSF) on priming peripheral blood progenitor cells for use with autologous bone marrow after high-dose chemotherapy. *Blood* 1993; **81:** 1709–19.

35. Fibbe W, Hamilton M, Laterveer L et al, Sustained engraftment of mice transplanted with IL-1 primed blood-derived stem cells. *J Immunol* 1992; **148:** 417–21.

36. Andrews RG, Bensinger W, Knitter G et al, The ligand for c-kit, stem cell factor, stimulates the circulation of cells that engraft lethally irradiated baboons. *Blood* 1992; **80:** 2715–20.

37. Andrews RG, Bartelmez S, Knitter G et al, A c-kit ligand, recombinant stem cell factor, mediates reversible expansion of multiple CD34[+] colony-forming cell types in blood and marrow of baboons. *Blood* 1992; **80:** 920–7.

38. Guillaume T, d'Hodt V, Symann M, IL-3 and peripheral blood stem cell harvesting. *Stem Cells* 1993; **11:** 173–81.

39. Briddell RA, Hartley CA, Smidt KA, McNiece IK, Recombinant rat stem cell factor synergizes with recombinant human granulocyte colony-stimulating factor in vivo in mice to mobilize peripheral blood and progenitor cells that have enhanced repopulating potential. *Blood* 1993; **82:** 1720–3.

40. Sutherland H, Eaves C, Lansdorp P et al, Kinetics of committed and primitive blood progenitor mobilization after chemotherapy and growth factor treatment and their use in autotransplants. *Blood* 1993; **82:** 1720.

41. Bodine D, Seidel N, Orlic D, In vivo administration of stem cell factor to mice increases the absolute number of pluripotent stem cells. *Blood* 1993; **82**: 3808.

42. Laterveer L, Lindley I, Hamilton M et al, Interleukin-8 induces rapid mobilization of hematopoietic stem cells with radioactive capacity and long-term myelophoid repopulating ability. *Blood* 1995; **85**: 2269–75.

43. deRevel T, Appelbaum F, Storb R et al, Effects of granulocyte colony-stimulating factor and stem cell factor, alone and in combination, on the mobilization of peripheral blood cells that engraft lethally irradiated dogs. *Blood* 1994; **83**: 3795–9.

44. Mauch P, Lamont C, Neben T-Y et al, Hematopoietic stem cells in the blood after stem cell factor and interleukin-11 administration: Evidence for different mechanisms of mobilization. *Blood* 1995; **86**: 4674–80.

45. Schlossman SE, Boumsell L, Gilks W et al (eds), *Leucocyte Typing V. White Cell Differentiation Antigens.* Volume 2. *Proceedings of 5th International Workshop and Conference, Boston, 1993.* Oxford: Oxford University Press, 1995.

46. Civin CI, Strauss LC, Brovall C et al, Antigenic analysis of hematopoiesis. III. A hematopoietic progenitor cell surface antigen defined by a monoclonal antibody raised against KG-la cells. *J Immunol* 1984; **133**: 157–65.

47. Andrews RG, Singer JW, Bernstein ID, Monoclonal antibody 12-8 recognizes a 115-kd molecule present on both unipotent and multipotent hematopoietic colony-forming cells and their precursors. *Blood* 1986; **67**: 842–5.

48. Fina L, Molgaard HV, Robertson D et al, Expression of the CD34 gene in vascular endothelial cells. *Blood* 1990; **75**: 2417–26.

49. Tindle RW, Nichols RAB, Chan L et al, A novel monoclonal antibody BI-3C5 recognizes myeloblasts and non-B non-T lymphoblasts in acute leukemias and CGL blast crises, and reacts with immature cells in normal bone marrow. *Leuk Res* 1985; **9**: 1–9.

50. Simmons PJ, Torok-Storb B, CD34 expression by stromal precursors in normal human adult bone marrow. *Blood* 1991; **78**: 2848–53.

51. Smeland EB, Funderud S, Kvalheim G et al, Isolation and characterization of human hematopoietic progenitor cells: An effective method for positive selection of CD34$^+$ cells. *Leukemia* 1992; **6**: 845–52.

52. Andrews RG, Singer JW, Bernstein ID, Precursors of colony-forming cells in human can be distinguished from colony-forming cells by expression of the CD33 and CD34 antigens and light scatter properties. *J Exp Med* 1989; **169**: 1721–31.

53. Civin CL, Trischmann TM, Fackler MJ et al, Report of the CD34 cluster workshop. In: *Leukocyte Typing IV. White Cell Differentiation Antigens* (Knapp W, Dorken B, Gilks WR et al, eds). Oxford: Oxford University Press, 1990: 818–25.

54. Gabbianelli M, Sargiacomo M, Pelosi E et al, Pure human hematopoietic progenitors: permissive action of basic fibroblast growth factor. *Science* 1990; **2**: 1561–4.

55. Katz FE, Tindle R, Sutherland DR, Greaves MF, Identification of a membrane glycoprotein associated with haematopoietic progenitor cells. *Leuk Res* 1985; **9**: 191–8.

56. Verfaillie C, Blakolmer K, McGlave P, Purified primitive human hematopoietic progenitor cells with long-term in vitro repopulating capacity adhere selectively to irradiated bone marrow stroma. *J Exp Med* 1990; **172**: 509–19.

57. Andrews RG, Singer JW, Bernstein ID, Human hematopoietic precursors in long-term culture: single CD34$^+$ cells that lack detectable T cell, B cell, and myeloid cell antigens with marrow stromal cells. *J Exp Med* 1990; **172**: 355–8.

58. Terstappen LWMM, Huang S, Safford M et al, Sequential generations of hematopoietic colonies derived from single nonlineage-committed CD34$^+$CD38$^-$ progenitor cells. *Blood* 1991; **77**: 1218–27.

59. Rusten L, Jacobsen SEW, Kaalhus O et al, Functional differences between CD38$^-$ and DR$^-$ subfractions of CD34$^+$ bone marrow cells. *Blood* 1994; **84**: 1473–81.

60. Berenson RJ, Andrews RG, Bensinger WI et al, Antigen CD34$^+$ marrow cells engraft lethally irradiated baboons. *J Clin Invest* 1988; **81**: 951–5.

61. Berenson RJ, Bensinger WI, Hill RS et al, Engraftment after infusion of CD34$^+$ marrow cells in patients with breast cancer or neuroblastoma. *Blood* 1991; **77**: 1717–22.

62. Osawa M, Hanada K-i, Hamada H, Nakauchi H, Long-term lymphohematopoietic reconstitution by a single CD34-low/negative hematopoietic stem cell. *Science* 1996; **273**: 242–5.

63. Kreissig C, Kirsch A, Serke S, Characterization and measurement of CD34-expressing hematopoietic cells. *J Hematother* 1994; **3**: 263–89.

64. Sutherland HJ, Eaves AC, Eaves CJ, Quantitative assays of human hemopoietic

progenitor cells. In: *Bone Marrow Processing and Purging: A Practical Guide* (Gee AP, ed). Boca Raton, FL: CRC Press, 1991: 155–71.

65. Johnsen HE, Knudsen LM, Nordic flow cytometry standards for CD34$^+$ cell enumeration in blood and leukaphereis products: report from the Second Nordic Workshop. *J Hematother* 1996; **5:** 237–45.

66. Fielding AK, Watts MJ, Goldstone AH, Peripheral blood progenitor cells versus bone marrow. *J Hematother* 1994; **3:** 203–11.

67. Siena S, Bregni M, Gianni MA, Estimation of peripheral blood CD34$^+$ cells for autologous transplantation in cancer patients. *Exp Hematol* 1993; **21:** 203–5.

68. Ho AD, Young D, Maruyama M et al, Pluripotent and lineage-committed CD34$^+$ subsets in leukapheresis products mobilized by G-CSF, GM-CSF vs. a combination of both. *Exp Hematol* 1996; **24:** 1460–8.

69. Bender JG, Unverzagt KL, Walker DE et al, Identification and comparison of CD34-positive cells and their subpopulations from normal peripheral blood and bone marrow using multicolor flow cytometry. *Blood* 1991; **77:** 2591–6.

70. Bender JG, Unverzagt K, Walker DE et al, Phenotypic analysis and characterization of CD34$^+$ cells from normal human bone marrow, cord blood, peripheral blood and mobilized peripheral blood from patients undergoing autologous stem cell transplantation. *Clin Immunol Immunopathol* 1994; **70:** 10–18.

71. Bender JG, Lum LK, Unverzagt KL et al, Correlation of colony-forming cells, long-term culture initiating cells and CD34$^+$ cells in apheresis products from patients mobilized for peripheral blood progenitors with different regimens. *Bone Marrow Transplant* 1994; **13:** 479–85.

72. Srour EF, Zanjani ED, Cornetta K et al, Persistence of human multilineage, self-renewing lymphohematopoietic stem cells in chimeric sheep. *Blood* 1993; **82:** 3333–42.

73. Huang S, Terstappen LWMM, Lymphoid and myeloid differentiation of single human CD34$^+$, CD38$^-$ hematopoietic stem cells. *Blood* 1994; **83:** 1515–26.

74. Humeau L, Bardin F, Maroc C et al, Phenotypic, molecular, and functional characterization of human peripheral blood CD34$^+$/THY1$^+$ cells. *Blood* 1996; **87:** 949–55.

75. Craig W, Kay R, Cutler RL, Landsdorp PM, Expression of Thy-1 on human hematopoietic progenitor cells. *J Exp Med* 1993; **177:** 1331–42.

76. Mayani H, Lansdorp PM, Thy-1 expression is linked to functional properties of primitive hematopoietic progenitor cells from human umbilical cord blood. *Blood* 1994; **83:** 2410–17.

77. Péault B, Weissman IL, Buckle AM et al, Thy-1 expressing CD34$^+$ human cells express multiple hematopoietic potentialities in vitro and in SCID-hu mice. *Nouv Rev Fr Hematol* 1993; **35:** 91–3.

78. Inaba T, Shimazaki C, Hirati T et al, Phenotypic differences of CD34-positive stem cells harvested from peripheral blood and bone marrow obtained before and after peripheral blood stem cell collection. *Bone Marrow Transplant* 1994; **13:** 527–32.

79. Steen R, Tjønnefjord GE, Egeland T, Comparison of the phenotype and clonogenicity of normal CD34$^+$ cells from umbilical cord blood, granulocyte colony-stimulating factor-mobilized peripheral blood, and adult human bone marrow. *J Hematother* 1994; **3:** 253–62.

80. Van Epps DE, Bender J, Lee W et al, Harvesting, characterization, and culture of CD34$^+$ cells from human bone marrow, peripheral blood and cord blood. *Blood Cells* 1994; **20:** 411–23.

81. Prosper F, Stroncek D, Verfaillie CM, Phenotypic and functional characterization of long-term culture-initiating cells present in peripheral blood progenitor collections of normal donors treated with granulocyte colony-stimulating factor. *Blood* 1996; **88:** 2033–42.

82. Lane TA, Law P, Maruyama M et al, Harvesting and enrichment of hematopoietic progenitor cells mobilized into the peripheral blood of normal donors by granulocyte–macrophage colony-stimulating factor (GM-CSF) or G-CSF: Potential role in allogenic marrow transplantation. *Blood* 1995; **85:** 275–82.

83. Haas R, Möhle R, Murea S et al, Characterization of peripheral blood progenitor cells mobilized by cytotoxic chemotherapy and recombinant human granulocyte colony-stimulating factor. *J Hematother* 1994; **3:** 323–30.

84. Körbling M, Huh YO, Durett A et al, Allogenic blood stem cell transplantation: Peripheralization and yield of donor-derived primitive hematopoietic progenitor cells (CD34$^+$Thy-1^{dim}) and lymphoid subsets, and possible predictors of engraftment and graft-versus-host disease. *Blood* 1995; **86:** 2842–8.

85. Murray L, Chen B, Galy A et al, Enrichment of human hematopoietic stem cell activity in the CD34$^+$Thy-1$^+$Lin$^-$ subpopulation from mobilized peripheral blood. *Blood* 1995; **85:** 368–78.

86. Donahue RE, Kirby MR, Metzger ME et al, Peripheral blood CD34$^+$ cells differ from bone marrow CD34$^+$ cells in Thy-1 expression and cell cycle status in nonhuman primates mobilized or not mobilized with granulocyte colony-stimulating factor and/or stem cell factor. *Blood* 1996; **87:** 1644–53.

87. Möhle R, Haas R, Hunstein W, Expression of adhesion molecules and c-kit on CD34$^+$ hematopoietic progenitor cells: Comparison of cytokine-mobilized blood stem cells with normal bone marrow and peripheral blood. *J Hematother* 1993; **2:** 483–9.

88. Dercksen MW, Rodenhuis S, Dirkson MKA et al, Subsets of CD34$^+$ cells and rapid hematopoietic recovery after peripheral-blood stem-cell transplantation. *J Clin Oncol* 1995; **13:** 1922–32.

89. Mavroudis D, Read E, Cottler-Fox M et al, CD34$^+$ cell dose predicts survival, posttransplant morbidity, and rate of hematologic recovery after allogenic marrow transplants for hematologic malignancies. *Blood* 1996; **88:** 3223–9.

90. Weaver C, Hazelton B, Birch R et al, An analysis of engraftment kinetics as a function of the CD34 content of peripheral blood progenitor cell collections in 692 patients after administration of myeloablative chemotherapy. *Blood* 1995; **86:** 3961–9.

91. Bensinger W, Appelbaum F, Rowley S et al, Factors that influence collection of and engraftment of autologous peripheral blood stem cells. *J Clin Oncol* 1995; **13:** 2547–55.

92. Bender JG, To LB, Williams S, Schwartzberg LS, Defining a therapeutic dose of peripheral blood stem cells. *J Hematother* 1992; **1:** 329–41.

93. Metcalf D, The molecular control of cell division, differentiation commitment and maturation of haematopoietic cells. *Nature* 1989; **339:** 27–30.

94. Moore MA, Clinical implications of positive and negative hematopoietic stem cell regulators. *Blood* 1991; **78:** 1–19.

95. Pettengell R, Testa NG, Swindell R et al, Transplantation potential of hematopoietic cells released into the circulation during routine chemotherapy for non-Hodgkin's lymphoma. *Blood* 1993; **82:** 39–48.

96. Sutherland HJ, Eaves CJ, Eaves AC et al, Characterization and partial purification of human marrow cells capable of initiating long-term hematopoiesis in vitro. *Blood* 1989; **74:** 1563–70.

97. Bradley TR, Hodgson GS, Detection of primitive macrophage progenitor cells in mouse bone marrow. *Blood* 1979; **54:** 1446–50.

98. Sutherland HJ, Hogge DE, Lansdorp PM et al, Quantitation, mobilization, and clinical use of long-term culture-initiating cells in blood cell autografts. *J Hematother* 1995; **4:** 3–10.

99. Hao Q-L, Thiemann T, Åpetersen D et al, Extended long-term culture reveals a highly quiescent and primitive human hematopoietic progenitor population. *Blood* 1996; **88:** 3306–13.

100. Till JE, McCulloch EA, A direct measurement of the radiation sensitivity of normal mouse bone marrow cells. *Radiat Res* 1961; **14:** 213–17.

101. Lord BI, Dexter TM, Which are the hematopoietic stem cells? *Exp Hematol* 1995; **23:** 1237–41.

102. Civin CI, Almeida-Porada G, Lee M-J et al, Sustained, retransplantable, multilineage engraftment of highly purified adult human bone marrow stem cells in vitro. *Blood* 1996; **88:** 4102–9.

103. Udomsakti C, Landsdorp PM, Hogge DE et al, Characterization of primitive hematopoietic cells in normal human peripheral blood. *Blood* 1992; **80:** 2513–21.

104. Sutherland HJ, Eaves CJ, Lansdorp PM et al, Kinetics of committed and primitive blood progenitor mobilization after chemotherapy and growth factor treatment and their use in autotransplants. *Blood* 1994; **83:** 3808–14.

105. Pettengell R, Luft T, Henschler R et al, Direct comparison by limiting dilution analysis of long-term culture-initiating cells in human bone marrow, umbilical cord blood and blood stem cells. *Blood* 1994; **84:** 3653–9.

106. Weaver A, Ryder D, Crother D et al, Increased numbers of long-term culture-initiating cells in apheresis product of patients randomized to receive increasing doses of stem cell factor administered in combination with chemotherapy and a standard dose of granulocyte colony-stimulating factor. *Blood* 1996; **88:** 3323–8.

107. Uchida N, Aguila HL, Fleming WH et al, Rapid and sustained hematopoietic recovery in lethally irradiated mice transplanted with purified Thy-1,1^{10}Lin$^-$Sca-1$^+$ hematopoietic stem cells. *Blood* 1994; **83:** 3758–79.

108. Archimbaud E, Philip I, Coiffier B et al, CD34^{++}Thy1$^+$Lin$^-$ peripheral blood stem cells (PBSC) transplantation after high dose therapy for patients with multiple myeloma. *Blood* 1996; **88**(Suppl 1): 2370.

109. Molineux G, Pojda Z, Hampson IN et al, Transplantation potential of peripheral blood stem cells induced by granulocyte colony-stimulating factor. *Blood* 1990; **76:** 2153–8.

110. Briddell RA, Hartley CA, Smith KA, McNiece IK, Recombinant rat stem cell factor synergizes with recombinant human granulocyte colony-stimulating factor in vivo in mice to mobilize peripheral blood progenitor cells that have enhanced repopulating potential. *Blood* 1993; **82:** 1720–3.

111. Carbonell F, Calvo W, Fliedner TM et al, Cytogenetic studies in dogs after total irradiation and allogenic transfusion with cytopreserved blood mononuclear cells. *Int J Cell Cloning* 1984; **2:** 81–8.

112. Yan X-Q, Hartley C, McElroy P et al, Peripheral blood progenitor cells mobilized by recombinant human granulocyte colony-stimulating factor plus recombinant rat stem cell factor containing long-term engrafting cells capable of cellular proliferation for more than two years as shown by serial transplantation in mice. *Blood* 1995; **85:** 2303–7.

113. Varas F, Bernad A, Bueren JA, Granulocyte colony-stimulating factor mobilizes into peripheral blood the complete clonal repertoire of hematopoietic precursors residing in the bone marrow of mice. *Blood* 1996; **88:** 2495–501.

114. Dunbar CE, Cottler-Fox M, O'Shaughnessy JA et al, Retrovirally marked CD34-enriched peripheral blood and bone marrow cells contribute to long-term engraftment after autologous transplantation. *Blood* 1995; **85:** 3048–57.

115. Arnold R, Schmeiser T, Heit W et al, Hematopoietic reconstitution after bone marrow transplantation. *Exp Hematol* 1986; **14:** 271–7.

116. To LB, Roberts MM, Haylock DN et al, Comparison of hematopoietic recovery times and supportive care requirements of autologous recovery phase peripheral blood stem cell transplants, autologous bone marrow transplants and allogenic bone marrow transplants. *Bone Marrow Transplant* 1992; **9:** 277–84.

117. Torres A, Alonso MC, Gomez-Villagran JL et al, No influence of number of donor CFU-GM on granulocyte recovery in bone marrow transplantation for acute leukemia. *Blut* 1992; **50:** 89.

118. Atkinson K, Norrie S, Chan P et al. Lack of correlation between nucleated bone marrow cell dose, marrow CFU-GM dose or marrow CFU-E and the rate of HLA-identical sibling marrow engraftment. *Br J Hematol* 1985; **60:** 245–51.

119. Kaizer H, Stuart RK, Brookmeyer R et al, Autologous bone marrow transplantation in acute leukemia: a phase I study of in vitro treatment with 4-hydroperoxycyclophosphamide to purge tumour cells. *Blood* 1985; **65:** 1504–10.

120. International Consensus Conference on Intensive Chemotherapy Plus Hematopoietic Stem Cell Transplantation in Malignancies, Lyon, 1993. Conclusions from the Jury. *Ann Oncol* 1993; **4**(Suppl 1): 1–81.

121. Shpall EJ, Jones RB, Release of tumor cells from bone marrow. *Blood* 1994; **83:** 623–5.

122. Ross AA, Cooper BW, Lazarus HM et al, Detection and viability of tumor cells in peripheral blood stem cell collections from breast cancer patients using immunocytochemical and clonogenic assay techniques. *Blood* 1993; **82:** 2605–10.

123. Negrin RS, Pesando J, Detection of tumor cells in purged bone marrow and peripheral-blood mononuclear cells by polymerase chain reaction amplification of bcl-2 translocations. *J Clin Oncol* 1994; **12:** 1021–7.

124. Corradini P, Voena C, Astolfi M et al, High dose sequential chemotherapy in multiple myeloma: Residual tumor cells are detectable in bone marrow and peripheral blood cell harvest and after autografting. *Blood* 1995; **85:** 1596–602.

125. Brugger W, Bross KJ, Glatt M et al, Mobilization of tumor cells and hematopoietic progenitor cells into peripheral blood of patients with solid tumors. *Blood* 1994; **83:** 636–40.

126. Brenner MK, Rill DR, Moen RC et al, Gene-marking to trace origin of relapse after autologous bone-marrow transplantation. *Lancet* 1993; **341:** 85–6.

127. Deisseroth A, Zu Z, Claxton D et al, Genetic marking shows that Ph$^+$ cells present in autologous transplants of chronic myelogenous leukemia (CML) contribute to relapse after autologous bone marrow in CML. *Blood* 1994; **83:** 3068–76.

128. Gribben JG, Freedman AS, Neuberg D et al, Immunological purging of marrow assessed by PCR before autologous bone marrow transplantation for B-cell lymphoma. *N Engl J Med* 1991; **28:** 1525–33.

129. Kvalheim G, Purging of autografts: Methods and clinical significance. *Ann Med* 1996; **28:** 167–73.

130. Kvalheim G, Fodstad Ø, Pihl A et al, Elimination of B-lymphoma cells from human bone marrow: Model experiments using

monodisperse magnetic particles coated with primary monoclonal antibodies. *Cancer Res* 1987; **47:** 846–51.

131. Wang MY, Fodstad Ø, Luwig WD et al, An effective, direct immunomagnetic procedure for purging acute lymphoblastic leukemia cells from human bone marrow. *Pathol Oncol Res* 1995; **1:** 32–7.

132. Kvalheim G, Sørensen O, Fodstad Ø et al, Immunomagnetic removal of B-lymphoma cells from human bone marrow: a procedure for clinical use. *Bone Marrow Transplant* 1988; **3:** 31–41.

133. Wang MY, Kvalheim G, Kvaløy S et al, An effective immuno-magnetic method for bone marrow purging in T cell malignancies. *Bone Marrow Transplant* 1992; **9:** 319–23.

134. Kvalheim G, Funderud S, Kvaløy S et al, Successful clinical use of an anti-HLA-DR monoclonal antibody for autologous bone marrow transplantation. *J Natl Cancer Inst* 1988; **80:** 1322–5.

135. Kvalheim G, Jakobsen E, Holte H et al, Autologous bone marrow transplantation of non-Hodgkin's lymphoma patients with marrow purged with immunomagnetic beads. *Prog Clin-Biol-Res* 1994; **389:** 133–8.

136. Kvalheim G, Wang MY, Pharo A et al, Purging of tumor cells from leukopheresis products: Experimental and clinical aspects. *J Hematother* 1996; **5:** 427–36.

137. Straka C, Dorken B, Kvalheim G, Polymerase chain reaction monitoring shows a high efficacy of clinical immunomagnetic purging in patients with centroblastic–centrocytic non Hodgkin's lymphoma. *Blood* 1992; **15:** 2688–90.

138. Schpall EJ, Jones RB, Bearman SI et al, Transplantation of enriched CD34-positive autologous marrow into breast cancer patients following high-dose chemotherapy: influence of CD34-positive peripheral-blood progenitors and growth factors on engraftment. *J Clin Oncol* 1994; **12:** 28–36.

139. Berenson RJ, Bensinger WI, Hill RS et al, Engraftment after infusion of CD34-positive marrow cells in patients with breast cancer or neuroblastoma. *Blood* 1991; **77:** 1717–22.

140. Kvalheim G, Pharo A, Holte H, The use of immunomagnetic beads and ISOLEX 300 gives high purity and yield of CD34$^+$ cells from peripheral blood progenitor cell products. *Bone Marrow Transplant* 1996; **17:** 57.

141. Hardy CL, Megason GC, Specificity of hematopoietic stem cell homing. *Hematol Oncol* 1996; **14:** 17–27.

142. Brugger W, Heimfeld S, Berenson RJ et al, Reconstitution of hematopoieses after high-dose chemotherapy by autologous progenitor cells generated ex vivo. *N Engl J Med* 1995; **333:** 283–7.

3

The role of cytokines in the mobilization of blood stem cells

Stefan Hohaus, Maria Teresa Voso and Rainer Haas

CONTENTS • **Introduction** • **Granulocyte and granulocyte–macrophage colony-stimulating factors** • **Other cytokines** • **Characteristics of mobilized HPC** • **Circulating tumour cells** • **Conclusions**

INTRODUCTION

The therapy for patients with solid tumours or haematological malignancies is primarily based on surgery, radiotherapy and cytotoxic chemotherapy. Depending on the type and stage of the malignant disease, the different therapeutic modalities may be used alone or in combination. The introduction of recombinant human haematopoietic growth factors (HGF) has resulted in significant improvements in the field of cytotoxic chemotherapy. Usually, these factors, which are also called 'cytokines' are given after conventional chemotherapy in order to ameliorate or circumvent treatment-related myelotoxicity.[1–3] HGF also permit an increase in dose intensity and shorter time intervals between sequential cycles of chemotherapy.[4] Moreover, HGF lead to an increase in the number of circulating progenitor and stem cells when administered during steady-state haematopoiesis or after cytotoxic chemotherapy. This finding has prompted a growing number of studies evaluating the ability of cytokines to mobilize peripheral blood progenitor cells (PBPC) for the support of high-dose therapy in the autologous as well as allogeneic setting.

The mechanisms involved in cytokine-induced PBPC mobilization are not yet clear. It could result from enhanced proliferation of early haematopoietic progenitor cells (HPC) with subsequent egress from the bone marrow. Cytokines may also decrease binding forces between HPC and components of the stromal microenvironment, which facilitates migration of HPC into the peripheral blood.[5–7] Haematopoietic progenitor and stem cells can be characterized by virtue of CD34-antigen expression.[8–10] In addition, culture assays permit the evaluation of proliferative capacity and self-renewal ability of CD34$^+$ stem cells. Dual and three-colour immunofluorescence analysis provide the basis for a CD34$^+$ subset analysis with respect to differentiation and lineage determination.

This chapter gives an overview of the methods for cytokine-based mobilization of HPC and concentrates on those cytokines that are in current clinical use. These HGF include granulocyte–macrophage colony-stimulating factor (GM-CSF), granulocyte colony-stimulating factor (G-CSF), interleukin-3 (IL-3) and stem cell factor (SCF, c-kit ligand). Particular emphasis will be put on a description of the progenitor and stem cell populations generated by the various cytokines and combinations, the yield of PBPC and patient characteristics affecting the mobilizing efficacy. The risk of mobilizing tumour cells will also be addressed, as well as methods for the detection of residual tumour cells. The chapter will conclude with an outlook on new directions for mobilization of PBPC.

GRANULOCYTE AND GRANULOCYTE–MACROPHAGE COLONY-STIMULATING FACTORS

G-CSF and GM-CSF were the first cytokines evaluated for PBPC mobilization. The respective studies were published in 1988. Socinski et al[11] found an approximately 18-fold increase of circulating colony-forming units granulocyte–macrophage (CFU-GM) over baseline levels in cancer patients who received GM-CSF during steady-state haematopoiesis, while an additional fivefold greater increase was observed when GM-CSF was given post chemotherapy. Dührsen et al[12] administered G-CSF during steady-state haematopoiesis (3–5 µg/kg/day) for 4 days, and found an up to 100-fold dose-dependent increase of CFU-GM.

First reports on the transplantation of cytokine-mobilized PBPC followed in 1989. Gianni et al[13] demonstrated that GM-CSF increased the rebound of HPC after high-dose cyclophosphamide (7 g/m^2). The cytokine-supported CD34$^+$ cell rebound post chemotherapy mostly coincided with the leukocyte recovery. The authors also showed that the addition of GM-CSF-mobilized PBPC to bone marrow accelerated haematological reconstitution after myeloablative high-dose therapy.[13]

We first mobilized PBPC using GM-CSF during steady-state haematopoiesis.[14] GM-CSF (250 µg/m^2/day, continuous i.v. infusion) led to an 8.5-fold increase of CFU-GM in the peripheral blood over baseline levels. The patients were extensively pretreated and not eligible for bone marrow harvesting. The great amount of previous cytotoxic chemotherapy might partially explain the moderate mobilizing effect. Autografting using GM-CSF-mobilized PBPC following myeloablative therapy

resulted in complete engraftment in 5 of 6 patients without additional bone marrow or cytokine support post transplantation. One patient developed relapse of disease, with bone marrow involvement interfering with haematological recovery.

Thereafter, we combined PBPC mobilization with the administration of cytotoxic chemotherapy. This approach resulted in 'disease-adapted' regimens combining effective anti-tumour therapy with the mobilization of HPC.[15–23] For instance, dexamethasone, carmustine, cytosine arabinoside, etoposide and melphalan (DexaBEAM) were given for patients with Hodgkin's disease, high-dose cytosine arabinoside with mitoxantrone (HAM) for patients with non-Hodgkin's lymphoma, and ifosfamide and epirubicin for patients with breast cancer.[15–18]

In a group of 14 patients with relapsed Hodgkin's disease who received DexaBEAM as salvage therapy, PBPC were collected during the rebound phase of leukocyte recovery.[15] The GM-CSF-supported collection resulted in a 2.2-fold greater yield of CFU-GM in comparison with harvesting without cytokine stimulation. Elias et al[23] compared the speed of haematological recovery after transplantation of PBSC harvested following GM-CSF-supported cytotoxic chemotherapy (doxorubicin, 5-fluourouracil and methotrexate) with the recovery observed after transplantation of bone marrow. The patients of both groups received the same conditioning regimen, consisting of cyclophosphamide, thiotepa and carboplatin. The time needed for haematological recovery and the time in hospital were significantly shorter in the patients autografted using PBPC.

The first reports on the transplantation of G-CSF-mobilized PBPC were published in 1992. Sheridan et al[24] collected HPC from peripheral blood between days 5 and 7 during steady-state administration of G-CSF (12 µg/kg/day) and reinfused these cells with bone marrow after high-dose therapy. The platelet recovery was significantly faster in patients who received both bone marrow and PBPC instead of bone marrow alone. Our group used cytotoxic chemotherapy and G-CSF (5 µg/kg/day) for mobilization, and transplanted the PBPC after myeloablative therapy without additional bone marrow in 10 patients with lymphoma.[16] Rapid platelet recovery was observed, given that a threshold number of 2.5×10^6 CD34$^+$ cells/kg bodyweight were reinfused. This initial observation of a relationship between the number of CD34$^+$ cells reinfused and the time needed for haematological reconstitution was confirmed in a larger group of patients and is in line with the findings of other groups (Figure 3.1).[19–22,25–40] For a review see reference 41. Haematopoietic reconstitution after transplantation of G-CSF-mobilized PBPC in general is fast, with neutrophil recovery to 0.5×10^9/litre after 9–15 days and platelet recovery to 20×10^9/litre after

9–23 days, irrespective of the addition of bone marrow after transplant.

Cytokines have also been used in normal donors for mobilization of HPC for allogeneic transplantation.[42–48] G-CSF was administered at doses between 5 and 16 µg/kg bodyweight for five to six days to mobilize HPC in human leukocyte antigen (HLA)-identical sibling donors. One to three leukaphereses were necessary for the collection of PBPC. Haematological recovery after transplantation was rapid, and, despite the approximately 10-fold greater number of reinfused T cells in comparison with bone marrow grafts, there was apparently no increase in the incidence of acute graft-versus-host disease (GVHD).[44–47] Using cytogenetic and

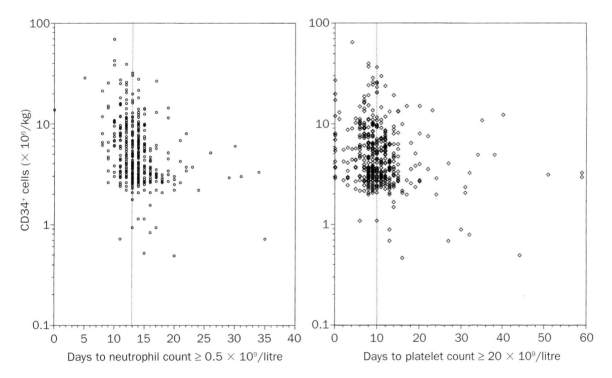

Figure 3.1 Haematological reconstitution after high-dose therapy with peripheral blood progenitor cell support. The majority of 452 cycles of high-dose therapy including total body irradiation in 152 cycles were supported with autografts containing more than 2.5×10^6 CD34$^+$ cells/kg. The median time of recovery to neutrophil counts of greater than 0.5×10^9/litre was 13 days, and 10 days to platelet counts of greater than 20×10^9/litre. The diagnoses included were Hodgkin's disease (32), non-Hodgkin's lymphoma (124), multiple myeloma (101), breast cancer (165) and other solid tumours (30).

molecular biological methods, long-term engraftment of donor cells could be demonstrated.[44,45] Acute adverse effects mostly consisted of moderate bone pain in donors that were treated with more than $10 \, \mu g/kg/day$ G-CSF.[42,48] To look for adverse effects of cytokine administration on long-term haematopoiesis of normal donors, regular follow-up examinations are required. The side-effects of GM-CSF observed in patients included low-grade fever, myalgias and flu-like symptoms.[14,49]

The kinetics of PBPC mobilization during steady-state G-CSF administration have also been examined. The peripheral blood CD34[+] cell count does not rise before 72 h after the first dose of G-CSF, while peak values are usually observed between day 4 or 6 of G-CSF administration. A decrease in the level of circulating CD34[+] cells was noted thereafter, even though G-CSF administration had been continued.[48]

Dose-finding studies were initiated to improve steady-state mobilization. Grigg et al[50] found significantly higher peak levels of circulating CD34[+] cells in normal donors when the daily dose of G-CSF (filgrastim) was $10 \, \mu g$ instead of 3 or $5 \, \mu g/kg$. Similarly, Höglund et al[51] reported that an increase in the dose of glycosylated G-CSF (lenograstim) from 3, 5, 7.5 to $10 \, \mu g/kg/day$ improved the mobilization of PBPC in healthy volunteers.[51] An increase of G-CSF (filgrastim) from 10 to 24 (2×12) $\mu g/kg/day$ significantly enhanced the harvest of PBPC in a group of patients with lymphoma and testicular cancer.[52] In the same line, a dose of $30 \, \mu g/kg/day$ G-CSF resulted in a significantly better collection efficiency compared with 5 or $10 \, \mu g/kg$.[53] Increasing the dose of G-CSF during steady state might compensate a reduction in the bioavailability of G-CSF that results from G-CSF binding to the largely expanded neutrophils. Therefore, the greater levels of PBPC observed post chemotherapy in comparison with steady-state haematopoiesis might simply reflect a better bioavailability of G-CSF because of neutropenia.

For instance, in an intra-individual comparison we observed a sevenfold greater yield of CD34[+] cells per leukapheresis after G-CSF-supported chemotherapy compared with steady-state administration of G-CSF, although the same dose of $5 \, \mu g/kg/day$ was given (Figure 3.2).[54] The high endogenous G-CSF serum levels observed during neutropenia have led some authors to propose a different scheduling of G-CSF administration.[55–57] Data of Faucher et al[58] suggest that administration of G-CSF can be delayed to day 6 after PBPC transplantation without a difference in the speed of neutrophil reconstitution, when compared with continuous G-CSF administration starting on day 1 post transplantation. However, one cannot conclude from this study whether G-CSF administration could be also delayed without affecting the rebound of HPC.

Independently of the dose administered, a wide variation in the number of circulating progenitor and stem cells has been observed in normal volunteers as well as patients.[59] In a group of 9 normal donors, an inverse correlation between age and yield of CD34[+] cells collected after G-CSF treatment has been reported by Dreger et al.[42] Factors affecting PBPC mobilization in patients are the underlying disease and the amount of previous cytotoxic treatment, including radiotherapy.[25,48,59–65] In a group of 61 patients with haematological malignancies each cycle of chemotherapy resulted in a decrease of 0.2×10^6 CD34[+] cells/kg per leukapheresis in non-irradiated patients, while large-field radiotherapy reduced the collection efficiency by $1.8 \times 10^6/kg$ CD34[+] cells, on average (Figure 3.3).[25] Dreger et al[64] found that the number of cycles of chemotherapy containing carmustine and melphalan adversely affected not only the yield of PBPC collection but also platelet engraftment. The mobilizing efficacy of a cytokine-supported cytotoxic chemotherapy is also dependent on the dose of the chemotherapeutic drug. For instance, administration of $7 \, g/m^2$ in comparison with $4 \, g/m^2$ cyclophosphamide resulted in significantly greater peak values of CD34[+] cells in the peripheral blood of patients with multiple myeloma.[66]

In a comparison between G-CSF and GM-CSF, no difference was found between these cytokines in their ability to mobilize PBPC. GM-CSF and G-CSF administered at a dose of $5 \, \mu g/kg/day$ during steady-state haemato-

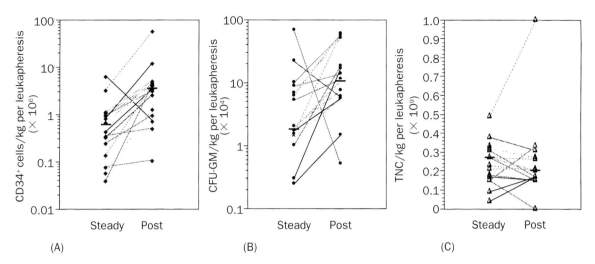

Figure 3.2 Intra-individual comparison of CD34[+] cells (A), CFU-GM (B) and total nucleated cells (TNC) (C), harvested per leukapheresis and per kg bodyweight following mobilization with G-CSF (5 µg/kg/day) during steady-state haematopoiesis or post chemotherapy. Ninety-two leukapheresis products of 17 patients (9 patients with breast cancer and 8 patients with multiple myeloma) were analysed. Mobilization chemotherapy consisted of high-dose cyclophosphamide (4 g/m² in 4 patients, 7 g/m² in 4 patients) and ifosfamide (10 g/m²) with epirubicin (100 mg/m²). The difference is statistically significant for CD34[+] cells/kg per leukapheresis ($p \leqslant 0.002$) and CFU-GM/kg per leukapheresis ($p \leqslant 0.015$, paired Wilcoxon signed rank test).

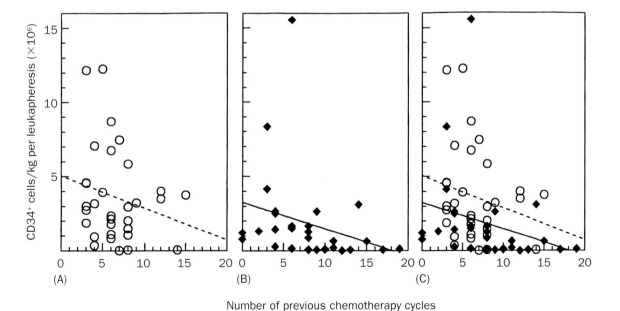

Number of previous chemotherapy cycles

Figure 3.3 Effect of chemotherapy on the collection efficiency. Separate analyses were performed for patients without (A, ○) and with previous radiotherapy (B, ◆). The number of CD34[+] cells harvested per leukapheresis decreased by 0.2 × 10⁶/kg with each cycle of chemotherapy, on average. The regression curve for the 29 irradiated patients has a similar slope (B), allowing superimposition of both graphs (C). The difference of the intercept on the ordinate is 1.8 × 10⁶/kg per leukapheresis and represents the radiotherapy-related decrease in the collection efficiency.[25]

poiesis increased the number of harvested CFU-GM 33.7- and 35.6-fold respectively over baseline values.[67] The addition of GM-CSF to G-CSF did not enhance the yield of progenitor cells. In contrast, Lane et al[49] found greater CD34$^+$ cell counts in normal volunteers on day 5 of G-CSF treatment during steady state compared with GM-CSF given at the same dose of 10 µg/kg/day. Bolwell et al[34] suggested that haematopoietic recovery after high-dose therapy was faster when G-CSF-mobilized PBPC, bone marrow and G-CSF were used post transplantation in comparison with GM-CSF-mobilized PBPC, bone marrow and GM-CSF post transplantation. In this study, the contribution of the cytokine-mobilized PBPC cannot be evaluated because of the different cytokines administered following transplantation.

OTHER CYTOKINES

In addition to G-CSF and GM-CSF, there are cytokines with a potential effect on more primitive HPC, such as IL-3, PIXY321, SCF, IL-11 and flt (fms-like tyrosine kinase)-3 ligand. The ability of these cytokines to mobilize HPC when given as single agents is apparently not better than that of G-CSF or GM-CSF, while the combination of these early acting cytokines with G- or GM-CSF is currently being evaluated in different studies.

Interleukin-3

The effects of IL-3 on HPC in vitro are similar to those of GM-CSF. Still, IL-3 promotes proliferation and differentiation of a larger number of erythroid and megakaryocytic progenitor cells than GM-CSF, which preferentially supports the growth of myeloid progenitors. Since IL-3 by itself only has a modest mobilizing efficacy,[68] we administered IL-3 and GM-CSF sequentially following salvage chemotherapy with high-dose cytosine arabinoside and mitoxantrone (HAM) in patients with high-grade non-Hodgkin's lymphoma.[69] IL-3 was given at a dose of 5 µg/kg/day subcutaneously for 6 days, followed by GM-CSF at the same dose. Compared with a historical control group who received G-CSF after HAM, no difference was observed in the number of CD34$^+$ cells mobilized. The transplantation of IL-3/GM-CSF-mobilized and G-CSF-mobilized PBPC resulted in an almost identical median time to recover a neutrophil count of 0.5×10^9/litre (14 days vs 14 days) and a platelet count of 20×10^9/litre (14 days vs 12 days).

A similar dose schedule was used by Brugger et al.[70] Sequential administration of IL-3 and GM-CSF (IL-3, days 1–5, GM-CSF, days 6–15, each at a dose of 250 µg/m^2/day) following a combination of etoposide, ifosfamide and cisplatin resulted in peak numbers of CD34$^+$ cells that were similar to the peak values observed after GM-CSF-supported chemotherapy. Still, the authors found a greater clonogenic efficiency of progenitor cells following IL-3/GM-CSF compared with GM-CSF alone.

Other authors used a combination of IL-3 with G-CSF or GM-CSF administered during steady-state haematopoiesis.[71,72] When given in combination with other cytokines, IL-3 is considered as a priming agent rendering the early stem cells more susceptible to the effect of the later-acting cytokine. Administration of IL-3 (3–5 µg/kg/day) for 4 days before G-CSF (5 µg/kg/day for 7 days) in healthy volunteers did not result in higher peak levels of circulating CD34$^+$ cells compared with a treatment with G-CSF alone, while a greater plating efficiency for CFU-GM was reported.[71] Adverse effects related to IL-3 were predominantly flu-like symptoms, including headache, fever, conjunctival and nasal congestion, facial flushing, and fatigue. Geissler et al[72] reported a potentiation of the GM-CSF-induced mobilization when IL-3 was given for a period of 7 days, while a shorter pretreatment of 5 days had no significant effect.

PIXY321

PIXY321 is a fusion protein that contains the active domains of GM-CSF and IL-3. The two parts are joined by a flexible linker sequence, resulting in better receptor affinity. PBPC harvested after cyclophosphamide and PIXY321 were similar to cyclophosphamide/GM-CSF-mobilized PBPC in their capacity to support high-dose therapy.[73] PIXY321 was moderately tolerated, and side-effects included mild-to-moderate erythema at the injection site, grade III fever, myalgias and arthralgias.

Stem cell factor

Stem cell factor is the ligand of c-kit. The endogenous serum levels of SCF and c-kit are relatively high during steady-state haematopoiesis,[74,75] while the concentration of SCF does not change during myelosuppression and leukocyte recovery.[76] In non-human primates, recombinant SCF (10–200 µg/kg/day for 7 days) resulted in a 61-fold greater number of circulating CFU-GM, which was paralleled by an increased number of $CD34^+$ cells when compared with baseline values.[77] Autografting with SCF-mobilized PBPC resulted in complete haematological reconstitution within 17–30 days.[78] The combined administration of SCF (2.5–25 µg/kg/day) and G-CSF for 7 days led to a significant increase of PBPC.[79] When baboons received low-dose rhCSF (25 µg/kg/day) with rhG-CSF (100 µg/kg/day), the harvests contained 14-fold more HPC compared with the leukapheresis products from animals treated with rhG-CSF alone.[80] Haematological reconstitution following reinfusion of rhSCF/G-CSF-mobilized PBPC was more rapid than that observed with G-CSF-mobilized PBPC.[80] Based on these animal studies, phase I/II studies in humans were performed combining G-CSF and SCF administration either during steady-state haematopoiesis or after chemotherapy.[80,81] Patients with breast cancer were treated with G-CSF alone (12 µg/kg/day) or in combination with SCF (10 µg/kg/day) either given concomitantly for 7 days or 3 days before G-CSF administration for a total of 10 days.[81] The greatest numbers of HPC were observed on days 5 and 6 of G-CSF administration, while in SCF-treated patients the increased numbers of HPC were

sustained up to day 12. Compared with patients who received G-CSF alone, the yield of CFU-GM was significantly greater in SCF-costimulated patients, with a trend towards a better mobilization in patients receiving SCF for 10 days. Weaver et al[82] administered G-CSF (5 µg/kg/day) either alone or in combination with SCF in 36 patients with ovarian cancer following 3 g/m² cyclophosphamide. The SCF dose varied between 5 and 15 µg/kg/day, and 15 µg/kg/day appeared to be most effective, resulting in a harvest of 9.9×10^6 $CD34^+$ cells/kg per leukapheresis for the combination of G-CSF and SCF, compared with 5.0×10^6 $CD34^+$ cells/kg for G-CSF alone.

Interleukin-11, flt-3 ligand

Cytokines affecting more primitive HPC include IL-11 and flt-3 ligand. These factors synergize with other cytokines in the stimulation of HPC.[83–86] IL-11 increased the number of CFU-S in murine blood, and a combination of IL-11 and SCF enhanced the mobilization of long-term repopulating cells from the marrow to the spleen in intact animals or to the blood in splenectomized mice.[87] rhIL-11 (30–240 µg/kg/day for 7 days) enhanced the number of circulating HPC in dogs.[88] Recently, the ligand for the tyrosine kinase receptor flt3/flk2 was cloned and termed the flt-3 ligand.[89,90] This cytokine is similar to SCF, since both proteins stimulate the proliferation of early progenitor cells, and a transmembrane and soluble form have been described for both. In contrast to SCF, serum levels of flt-3 ligand are low in normal individuals, whereas no data are currently available on serum concentrations during myelosuppression. The flt-3 ligand alone maintains CFU-GM and progenitors with high-proliferative potential in vitro for 3–4 weeks.[91,92] The flt-3 ligand combined with IL-1α, IL-3, IL-6 and erythropoietin synergizes in the expansion of progenitor cells.[92] Besides its potential role for ex vivo application, the mobilizing ability of the flt-3 ligand has to be examined.[92–94] Gratwohl et al[95] administered recombinant human flt-3 ligand in rabbits, and observed a

40–55-fold increase of myeloid colony-forming units. The increase was similar to that found in animals treated with human G-CSF.

Interleukin-8 and macrophage inflammatory protein-1α

Other cytokines with HPC-mobilizing ability are IL-8 and macrophage inflammatory protein-1 alpha (MIP-1α).[96,97] In contrast to the haematopoietic growth factors described so far, the peripheralization of HPC occurs rapidly within 30 minutes following administration of IL-8. In rhesus monkeys, the level of circulating HPC was 10–100-fold increased over baseline after 30 minutes following injection of 100 µg IL-8/kg bodyweight. The concentration of HPC returned to pretreatment levels within 4 hours after injection.[96] Similarly, a synthetic peptide (BB-110) derived from MIP-1α enhanced the number of circulating HPC after 30 minutes following subcutaneous injection in mice.[97] Addition of BB110 after 2 days of G-CSF administration resulted in a greater number of circulating primitive HPC in comparison with G-CSF treatment alone.

CHARACTERISTICS OF MOBILIZED HPC

There is a difference between HPC from peripheral blood and bone marrow, independent of the mobilizing agent. In most studies, the comparison between the progenitor cell populations from both haematopoietic compartments was made following the use of G-CSF.

Cytokine-based mobilization results in a greater concentration of HPC in the peripheral blood compared with bone marrow during steady-state haematopoiesis. In a group of cancer patients who underwent G-CSF-supported PBPC harvesting post chemotherapy, the peak concentration of $CD34^+$ cells in the peripheral blood during the cytokine-enhanced rebound was 3.7-fold greater than in bone marrow samples that were obtained before the start of cytotoxic chemotherapy (Figure 3.4).[98] Besides this

quantitative aspect, circulating HPC are almost exclusively in the G_0 phase of the cell cycle.[99,100] Adhesion molecules are also differentially expressed. Circulating HPC express greater levels of L-selectin, which plays a pivotal role for the first contact between HPC and endothelial cells.[101] On the other hand, bone marrow HPC express greater levels of the integrins very late antigen (VLA-4) and leukocyte function antigen (LFA-1). These molecules are presumably involved in the anchoring of HPC to stromal elements of the bone marrow.[101,102] The stage of differentiation of PBPC is different from that of bone marrow-derived HPC, since a greater proportion of G-CSF-mobilized $CD34^+$ cells express the stem cell-associated antigen Thy-1 (Figure 3.5).[98,100] Mobilized $CD34^+$ cells also differ from bone marrow $CD34^+$ cells in their lower expression of c-kit and CD45RA (Figure 3.5).[98,103] The myeloid-associated antigen CD33 is variably expressed on bone marrow and on mobilized peripheral blood $CD34^+$ cells.[16,103–105] From these immunophenotypical data, one may conclude that peripheral blood during G-CSF-enhanced recovery contains a greater number of more primitive HPC than bone marrow. These findings were confirmed by other authors using culture assays for the determination of LTCIC and pre-CFU-GM.[64,106]

Characterization of particular $CD34^+$ cell subsets might help to predict the speed of haematological reconstitution. Dercksen et al[103] found that the time to neutrophil and platelet recovery correlated better with the number of transplanted $CD34^+/CD33^-$ cells and $CD34^+/CD41^+$ (megakaryocytic HPC) respectively than with the total number of $CD34^+$ cells. They also observed that the amount of $CD34^+$ cells co-expressing the adhesion molecule L-selectin correlated better with haematological recovery than with the total $CD34^+$ cell population.[102]

Comparing the effect of sequential IL-3/GM-CSF with G-CSF administration post chemotherapy on the antigenic profile of circulating HPC, we did not find any difference in the co-expression of HLA-DR, CD38, CD33, CD71 or CD19.[69] Some characteristics of PBPC may still depend on the mobilization modality. The

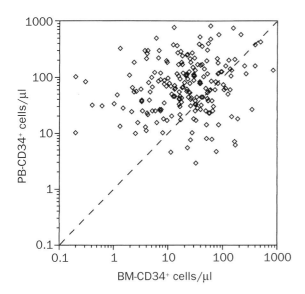

Figure 3.4 Inter-individual comparison between the concentration of CD34$^+$ cells in bone marrow (BM) samples before the start of cytotoxic chemotherapy and peripheral blood obtained during cytokine-enhanced marrow recovery in 208 patients. The comparison is based on individual peak concentrations of CD34$^+$ cells observed during cytokine-enhanced rebound. The median peak concentration of CD34$^+$ cells was 3.7-fold greater compared with BM samples (median, peripheral blood CD34$^+$ cells/μl, 70.2; median bone marrow CD34$^+$ cells/μl, 22.8).

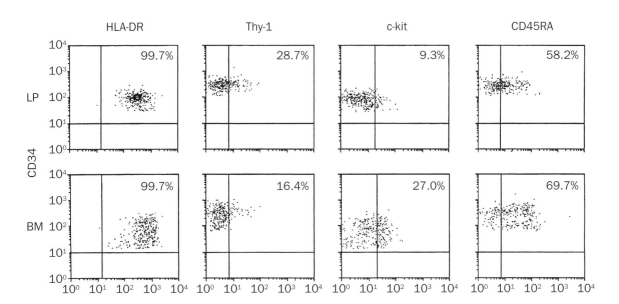

Figure 3.5 The results of a two-colour immunofluorescence analysis of CD34$^+$ cells in a representative patient are shown. During G-CSF-supported recovery, a leukapheresis product (LP) and a bone marrow sample (BM) were obtained. Immunophenotyping was performed using the following monoclonal antibodies: HPCA-2-FITC/PE (CD34), HLA-DR-PE (clone L243), c-kit-PE, Leu-18-FITC (CD45RA), and Thy-1-FITC (clone 5E10). For the analysis, 400 (BM and LP) cells were acquired into a life gate. The CD34 mean fluorescence intensity tended to be greater on blood-derived CD34$^+$ cells, whereas their level of HLA-DR expression was significantly lower compared with CD34$^+$ cells from bone marrrow. Notably, Thy-1 expression was restricted to the CD34^{bright} cell population in samples from both sources. On the basis of two-colour immunofluorescence analysis, c-kit or CD45RA expression could not be ascribed to a particular level of CD34 expression.[98]

proportion of early CD34$^+$ cells lacking HLA-DR and CD38 is greater after G-CSF mobilization during steady-state haematopoiesis than post chemotherapy. Still, the absolute amount of more primitive PBPC is greater post chemotherapy because of the greater number of CD34$^+$ cells mobilized.[54] Similar results were reported by To et al,[107] who compared CD34$^+$ cells following mobilization with chemotherapy ±GM-CSF or G-CSF, and G-CSF alone during steady state haematopoiesis with CD34$^+$ cells in the peripheral blood before mobilization. They found that CD34$^+$ cells mobilized following G-CSF administration during steady state contained a greater proportion of CD38$^-$ cells than CD34$^+$ cells induced by the other regimens.

PBPC harvesting post chemotherapy is associated with a small proportion of B-lineage progenitors as characterized by the co-expression of CD19,[16,17,54,103,108,109] while during steady-state haematopoiesis there is no difference in the proportion of CD34$^+$/CD19$^+$ between bone marrow and peripheral blood.[54,110]

The addition of a cytokine to cytotoxic chemotherapy may change the characteristics of PBPC, since Bender et al[111] reported that the administration of G-CSF during the recovery phase increased the number of CD34$^+$ cells, CFC and LTC-IC in comparison with chemotherapy alone. Data from Benbouker et al[112] indicate that GM-CSF-supported chemotherapy mobilizes fewer primitive stem cells than chemotherapy alone as assessed in long-term cultures. The authors concluded that GM-CSF predominantly exerts a mobilizing effect through differentiation and leads to an increased production of CFU-GM at the expense of more primitive stem cells.

CIRCULATING TUMOUR CELLS

The use of cytokines in patients with haematological malignancies and solid tumours is associated with a potential risk of mobilizing tumour cells, and gene-marking studies in patients with acute myeloid leukaemia (AML) and neuroblastoma have shown that reinfused tumour cells can contribute to a relapse.[113]

Molecular markers and specific genomic alterations provide the basis for detection of tumour cells. The polymerase chain reaction (PCR) can be used as a sensitive method to find translocation-bearing cells such as the t(14;18) in follicular lymphoma or the t(9;22) in chronic myeloid leukaemia (CML) and some cases of acute lymphoblastic leukaemia (ALL).[114–117] The evaluation of 29 patients with t(14;18)-positive follicular lymphoma showed that the majority of patients (22 of 29) had PCR-positive PBPC autografts that were harvested during G-CSF-supported recovery post chemotherapy.[17]

The design of clone-specific probes for immunoglobulin heavy-chain and T-cell receptor gene rearrangements permits a sensitive assessment of tumour cells in patients with multiple myeloma and other lymphoid malignancies.[118–120] Using this method, recent data suggest that circulating CD19$^+$ B cells may contain cells of the myeloma clone.[121] Gazitt et al[120] compared the content of normal HPC with those of myeloma cells in PBPC harvests of patients after high-dose cyclophosphamide and GM-CSF administration. They found the greatest proportion of CD34$^+$ cells during the first 2 days of apheresis, whereas the greatest proportion of myeloma cells was observed on days 5 and 6. In contrast, the data of Lemoli et al[122] suggest a concomitant mobilization of PBPC and myeloma cells after high-dose cyclophosphamide and G-CSF.

Most of the solid tumours lack a simple genomic alteration that could be used for monitoring of residual tumour cells. For these patients, tissue-specific gene expression could help to discriminate between normal and malignant cells. The methods include immunocytological staining and reverse-transcription (RT) PCR for the assessment of protein and mRNA expression respectively.[18,123–132] Immunocytochemical staining for epithelial antigens such as cytokeratins is widely used to look for tumour cells in peripheral blood or bone marrow in patients with breast and lung cancer.[123–126] RT-PCR assays are not always specific,[129] and immunocytochemical staining therefore represents the gold standard. Brugger et al[130] found circulating tumour cells during steady-state haematopoiesis in 29% of patients with stage IV breast cancer most of whom had bone marrow involvement by histopathological examination, and in 20% of patients with small-cell lung cancer. The incidence was greater following G-CSF-supported cytotoxic chemotherapy. Other studies suggest a relatively low risk of mobilizing malignant cells. PBPC collections after cytokine-supported chemotherapy contained fewer tumour cells than bone marrow. Before PBPC mobilization, Passos-Coelho et al[131] found tumour cells in 4% of blood samples of patients with stage III/IV breast cancer, whereas bone marrow samples were positive in 15% of the patients. After GM-CSF-supported chemotherapy, 7% of the patients had PBPC harvests containing tumour cells. Our studies suggest a reduced risk of collecting tumour cells in patients with breast cancer following repeated cycles of chemotherapy.[18] Ross et al[132] found tumour cells in only 10% of PBPC specimens of patients with locally advanced or metastatic breast cancer, whereas 62% of bone marrow harvests harboured tumour cells.

The biological potential of residual tumour cells has to be assessed in addition to molecular and immunocytochemical examination. Culture assays and animal models may help to define the proliferative capacity and relapse-inducing ability of these cells. Ross et al[132] demonstrated clonogenic tumour cell growth from most specimens of bone marrow and PBPC collections that were immunocytochemically positive. Using a semi-solid culture assay, Sharp et al[133] also found malignant clonogenic cells in the peripheral blood of patients with Hodgkin's disease and non-Hodgkin's lymphomas.

CONCLUSIONS

Haematopoietic growth factors have facilitated the mobilization and collection of HPC from peripheral blood. Moreover, CD34 immunophenotyping permitted a standardized and rapid assessment of PBPC. Using multicolour-immunofluorescence analysis, the PBPC could be characterized with respect to their stage of differentiation and their lineage-commitment, as well as expression of adhesion molecules.

This kind of assessment permits an evaluation of new mobilization protocols with SCF, IL-11 and flt-3 ligand, as well as IL-8 and MIP-1α. In clinical studies, immunophenotyping should be accompanied by culture assays to determine the proliferative capacity and lineage commitment of the PBPC generated. A new class of mobilizing agents are monoclonal antibodies that are directed against adhesion molecules expressed on CD34$^+$ HPC or endothelial cells.[134] Similarly, specific peptides may be used that represent binding motifs of adhesion molecules present on HPC, endothelial cells, stromal cells or components of the extracellular matrix. Competitive inhibition of receptor–ligand interactions that are involved in PBPC peripheralization may provide a different or synergistic way to improve cytokine-based PBPC mobilization.

The risk of mobilizing tumour cells following cytokine-supported chemotherapy is relatively low in comparison with bone marrow grafts obtained during steady state, but the likelihood of collecting tumour cells has to be addressed in the context of the underlying disease, the stage of the disease and its chemosensitivity. With the availability of ex vivo methods such as purging or positive selection of CD34$^+$ cells, a significant depletion of potentially contaminating tumour cells can be achieved. An important prerequisite for the use of these methods is a sufficient yield of CD34$^+$ cells, which can be obtained in the majority of patients when PBPC harvesting is performed early during the course of the disease. Despite the more rapid recovery in comparison with bone marrow transplantation, autografting using PBPC results in a significant reduction in the number of haematopoietic progenitor and stem cells.[135] This reduction is not associated with a functional impairment in most patients, since, with a longest observation period of eight years, there has been no evidence of graft failure following the transplantation of cytokine-mobilized PBPC.[136] Since blood-derived autograft candidates contain a significant proportion of more primitive HPC, including true stem cells, cytokine-mobilized PBPC are also suitable for ex vivo expansion as well as somatic gene therapy.

REFERENCES

1. Gianni AM, Bregni M, Siena S et al, Recombinant human granulocyte–macrophage colony-stimulating factor reduces hematologic toxicity and widens clinical applicability of high-dose cyclophosphamide treatment in breast cancer and non-Hodgkin's lymphoma. *J Clin Oncol* 1990; **8:** 768–78.

2. Crawford J, Ozer H, Stoller R et al, Reduction by granulocyte colony-stimulating factor of fever and neutropenia induced by chemotherapy in patients with small-cell lung cancer. *N Engl J Med* 1991; **325:** 164–70.

3. Pettengell R, Gurney H, Radford JA et al, Granulocyte colony-stimulating factor to prevent dose-limited neutropenia in non-Hodgkin's lymphoma: a randomized controlled trial. *Blood* 1992; **80:** 1430–6.

4. Bronchud MH, Howell A, Crowther D et al, The use of granulocyte colony-stimulating factor to increase the intensity of treatment with doxorubicin in patients with advanced breast and ovarian cancer. *Br J Cancer* 1989; **60:** 121–5.

5. Bussolino F, Ziche M, Wang JM et al, In vitro and in vivo activation of endothelial cells by colony-stimulating factors. *J Clin Invest* 1991; **87:** 986–95.

6. Levesque JP, Leavesley DI, Niutta S et al, Cytokines increase human hemopoietic cell adhesiveness by activation of very late antigen (VLA)-4 and VLA-5 integrins. *J Exp Med* 1995; **181:** 1805–15.

7. van der Loo JC, Ploemacher RE, Marrow- and spleen-seeding efficiencies of all murine hematopoietic stem cell subsets are decreased by preincubation with hematopoietic growth factors. *Blood* 1995; **85:** 2598–606.

8. Civin CI, Strauss LC, Brovall C et al, Antigenic analysis of hematopoiesis: III. A hematopoietic progenitor cell surface antigen defined by a monoclonal antibody raised against KG-1a cells. *J Immunol* 1984; **133:** 157–65.

9. Siena S, Bregni M, Brando B et al, Circulation of CD34+ hematopoietic stem cells in the peripheral blood of high-dose cyclophosphamide-treated patients: enhancement by intravenous recombinant human granulocyte–macrophage colony-stimulating factor. *Blood* 1989; **74:** 1905–14.

10. Serke S, Säuberlich S, Huhn D, Multiparameter flow-cytometrical quantitation of circulating CD34+ cells: correlation to the quantitation of circulation haematopoietic progenitor cells by in vitro colony-assay. *Br J Haematol* 1991; **77:** 453–9.

11. Socinski MA, Cannistra SA, Elias A et al, Granulocyte–macrophage colony stimulating factor expands the circulating hematopoietic progenitor cell compartment in man. *Lancet* 1988; **i:** 1194–8.

12. Dührsen U, Villeval JL, Boyd J et al, Effects of recombinant human granulocyte colony-stimulating factor on hematopoietic progenitor cells in cancer patients. *Blood* 1988; **72:** 2074–81.

13. Gianni AM, Siena S, Bregni M et al, Granulocyte–macrophage colony-stimulating factor to harvest circulating haemopoietic stem cells for autotransplantation. *Lancet* 1989; **i:** 580–4.

14. Haas R, Ho AD, Bredthauer U et al, Successful autologous transplantation of blood stem cells mobilized with recombinant human granulocyte–macrophage colony-stimulating factor. *Exp Hematol* 1990; **18:** 94–8.

15. Haas R, Hohaus S, Egerer G et al, Recombinant human granulocyte–macrophage colony-stimulating factor (rhGM-CSF) subsequent to chemotherapy improves collection of blood stem cells for autografting in patients not eligible for bone marrow harvest. *Bone Marrow Transplant* 1992; **9:** 459–65.

16. Hohaus S, Goldschmidt H, Ehrhardt R, Haas R, Successful autografting following myeloablative conditioning therapy with blood stem cells mobilized by chemotherapy plus rhG-CSF. *Exp Hematol* 1993; **21:** 508–14.

17. Haas R, Moos M, Karcher A et al, Sequential high-dose therapy with peripheral-blood progenitor-cell support in low-grade non-Hodgkin's lymphoma. *J Clin Oncol* 1994; **12:** 1685–92.

18. Haas R, Schmid H, Hahn U et al, Tandem high-dose therapy with ifosfamide, epirubicin, carboplatin and peripheral blood stem cell support is an effective adjuvant treatment for high-risk primary breast cancer *Eur J Cancer* 1997; **33:** 372–8.

19. Menichella G, Pierelli L, Scambia G et al, Low-dose cyclophosphamide in combination with cisplatin or epirubicin plus rhG-CSF allows adequate collection of PBSC for autotransplantation during adjuvant therapy for high-risk cancer. *Bone Marrow Transplant* 1994; **14:** 907–12.

20. Brugger W, Birken R, Bertz H et al, Peripheral blood progenitor cells mobilized by chemo-

therapy plus granulocyte colony-stimulating factor accelerate both neutrophil and platelet recovery after high-dose VP16, ifosamide and cisplatin. *Br J Haematol* 1993; **84**: 402–7.

21. Shimazaki C, Oku N, Ashihara E et al, Collection of peripheral blood stem cells mobilized by high-dose ara-c plus VP-16 or aclarubicin followed by recombinant human granulocyte colony-stimulating factor. *Bone Marrow Transplant* 1992; **10**: 341–6.

22. Venturini M, Del Mastro L, Melioli G et al, Release of peripheral blood progenitor cells during standard dose cyclophosphamide, epidoxorubicin, 5-fluorouracil regimen plus granulocyte colony-stimulating factor for breast cancer therapy. *Cancer* 1994; **74**: 2300–6.

23. Elias AD, Ayash L, Anderson KC et al, Mobilization of peripheral blood progenitor cells by chemotherapy and granulocyte–macrophage colony-stimulating factor for hematologic support after high-dose intensification for breast cancer. *Blood* 1992; **79**: 3036–44.

24. Sheridan WP, Begley CG, Juttner CA, Effect of peripheral-blood progenitor cells mobilised by filgrastim (G-CSF) on platelet recovery after high-dose chemotherapy. *Lancet* 1992; **339**: 640–4.

25. Haas R, Möhle R, Frühauf S et al, Patient characteristics associated with successful mobilizing and autografting of peripheral blood progenitor cells in malignant lymphoma. *Blood* 1994; **83**: 3787–94.

26. Bensinger W, Singer J, Appelbaum F et al, Autologous transplantation with peripheral blood mononuclear cells collected after administration of recombinant granulocyte colony-stimulating factor. *Blood* 1993; **81**: 3158–63.

27. Schwartzberg L, Birch R, Blanco R et al, Rapid and sustained hematopoietic reconstitution by peripheral blood stem cell infusion alone following high-dose chemotherapy. *Bone Marrow Transplant* 1993; **11**: 369–74.

28. Bensinger WI, Longin K, Appelbaum F et al, Peripheral blood stem cells (PBSCs) collected after recombinant granulocyte colony stimulating factor (rhG-CSF): An analysis of factors correlating with the tempo of engraftment after transplantation. *Br J Haematol* 1994; **87**: 825–31.

29. Weaver CH, Hazelton B, Birch R et al, An analysis of engraftment kinetics as a function of the CD34 content of peripheral blood progenitor cell collections in 692 patients after the

administration of myeloablative chemotherapy. *Blood* 1995; **86**: 3961–9.

30. Bender TG, To LB, Williams SF et al, Defining a therapeutic dose of peripheral blood stem cells. *J Hematother* 1992; **1**: 329–40.

31. Chao NJ, Schriber JR, Grimes K et al, Granulocyte colony-stimulating factor 'mobilized' peripheral blood progenitor cells accelerate granulocyte and platelet recovery after high-dose chemotherapy. *Blood* 1993; **81**: 2031–5.

32. Sheridan WP, Begley CG, To LB et al, Phase II study of autologous filgrastim (G-CSF)-mobilized peripheral blood progenitor cells to restore hemopoiesis after high-dose chemotherapy for lymphoid malignancies. *Bone Marrow Transplant* 1994; **14**: 105–11.

33. Nademanee A, Sniecinski I, Schmidt GM et al, High-dose therapy followed by autologous peripheral-blood stem-cell transplantation for patients with Hodgkin's disease and non-Hodgkin's lymphoma using unprimed and granulocyte colony-stimulating factor-mobilized peripheral-blood stem cells. *J Clin Oncol* 1994; **12**: 2176–86.

34. Bolwell BJ, Goormastic M, Yanssens T et al, Comparison of G-CSF with GM-CSF for mobilizing peripheral blood progenitor cells and for enhancing marrow recovery after autologous bone marrow transplant. *Bone Marrow Transplant* 1994; **14**: 913–18.

35. Craig JI, Anthony RS, Stewart A et al, Peripheral blood stem cell mobilization using high-dose cyclophosphamide and G-CSF in pretreated patients with lymphoma. *Br J Haematol* 1993; **85**: 210–12.

36. Bolwell BJ, Fishleder A, Andresen SW et al, G-CSF primed peripheral blood progenitor cells in autologous bone marrow transplantation: parameters affecting bone marrow engraftment. *Bone Marrow Transplant* 1993; **12**: 609–14.

37. Brice P, Divine M, Marolleau JP et al, Comparison of autografting using mobilized peripheral blood stem cells with and without granulocyte colony-stimulating factor in malignant lymphomas. *Bone Marrow Transplant* 1994; **14**: 51–5.

38. Sica S, Di Mario A, Salutari P et al, Sequential peripheral blood progenitor cell transplantation after mobilization with salvage chemotherapy and G-CSF in patients with resistant lymphoma. *Am J Hematol* 1994; **46**: 18–23.

39. Jones HM, Jones SA, Watts MJ et al,

Development of a simplified single-apheresis approach for peripheral-blood progenitor-cell transplantation in previously treated patients with lymphoma. *J Clin Oncol* 1994; **12:** 1693–1702.

40. Cortelazzo S, Viero P, Bellavita P et al, Granulocyte colony-stimulating factor following peripheral-blood progenitor-cell transplant in non-Hodgkin's lymphoma. *J Clin Oncol* 1995; **13:** 935–41.

41. Haas R, Murea S, The role of granulocyte colony-stimulating factor in mobilization and transplantation of peripheral blood progenitor and stem cells. *Cytokines Molec Ther* 1995; **1:** 249–70.

42. Dreger P, Haferlach T, Eckstein V et al, G-CSF-mobilized peripheral blood progenitor cells for allogeneic transplantation: safety, kinetics of mobilization, and composition of the graft. *Br J Haematol* 1994; **87:** 609–13.

43. Dreger P, Suttorp M, Haferlach T et al, Allogeneic granulocyte colony-stimulating factor-mobilized peripheral blood progenitor cells for treatment of engraftment failure after bone marrow transplantation. *Blood* 1993; **81:** 1404–7.

44. Bensinger WI, Weaver CH, Appelbaum FR et al, Transplantation of allogeneic peripheral blood stem cells mobilized by recombinant human granulocyte colony-stimulating factor. *Blood* 1995; **85:** 1655–8.

45. Körbling M, Przepiorka D, Huh YO et al, Allogeneic blood stem cell transplantation for refractory leukemia and lymphoma: Potential advantage of blood over marrow allografts. *Blood* 1995; **85:** 1659–65.

46. Schmitz N, Dreger P, Suttorp M et al, Primary transplantation of allogeneic peripheral blood progenitor cells mobilized by filgrastim (granulocyte colony-stimulating factor). *Blood* 1995; **85:** 1666–72.

47. Körbling M, Huh YO, Durett A et al, Allogeneic blood stem cell transplantation: peripheralization and yield of donor-derived primitive hematopoietic progenitor cells (CD34+ Thy-1dim) and lymphoid subsets, and possible predictors of engraftment and graft-versus-host disease. *Blood* 1995; **86:** 2842–8.

48. Sekhsaria S, Fleisher TA, Vowells S et al, Granulocyte colony-stimulating factor recruitment of CD34+ progenitors to peripheral blood: Impaired mobilization in chronic granulomatous disease and adenosine deaminase-deficient severe combined immunodeficiency disease

patients. *Blood* 1996; **88:** 1104–12.

49. Lane TA, Law P, Maruyama M et al, Harvesting and enrichment of hematopoietic progenitor cells mobilized into the peripheral blood of normal donors by granulocyte–macrophage colony-stimulating factor (GM-CSF) or G-CSF: potential role in allogeneic marrow transplantation. *Blood* 1995; **85:** 275–82.

50. Grigg AP, Roberts AW, Raunow H et al, Optimizing dose and scheduling of filgrastim (granulocyte colony-stimulating factor) for mobilization and collection of peripheral blood progenitor cells in normal volunteers. *Blood* 1995; **86:** 4437–45.

51. Höglund M, Smedmyr B, Simonsson B et al, Dose-dependent mobilisation of haematopoietic progenitor cells in healthy volunteers receiving glycosylated rHuG-CSF. *Bone Marrow Transplant* 1996; **18:** 19–27.

52. Zeller W, Gutensohn K, Stockschläder M et al, Increase of mobilized CD34+-peripheral blood progenitor cells in patients with Hodgkin's disease, non-Hodgkin's lymphoma, and cancer of the testis. *Bone Marrow Transplant* 1996; **17:** 709–13.

53. Weaver CH, Hazelton B, Palmer PA et al, A randomized dose finding study of filgrastim for mobilization of peripheral blood progenitor cells (PBSCs) [abstract]. *Proc Am Soc Clin Oncol* 1996; **15:** 900.

54. Möhle R, Pförsich M, Frühauf S et al, Filgrastim post-chemotherapy mobilizes more CD34+ cells with a different antigenic profile compared with use during steady-state hematopoiesis. *Bone Marrow Transplant* 1994; **14:** 827–32.

55. Haas R, Gericke G, Witt B et al, Increased serum levels of granulocyte colony-stimulating factor after autologous bone marrow or blood stem cell transplantation. *Exp Hematol* 1993; **21:** 109–13.

56. Cairo MS, Sender L, Gillan ER et al, Circulating granulocyte colony-stimulating factor (G-CSF) levels after allogeneic and autologous bone marrow transplantation: endogenous G-CSF production correlates with myeloid engraftment. *Blood* 1992; **79:** 1869–73.

57. Shimazaki C, Uchiyama H, Fujita N et al, Serum levels of endogenous and exogenous granulocyte colony-stimulating factor after autologous blood stem cell transplantation. *Exp Hematol* 1995; **23:** 1497–1502.

58. Faucher C, Le Corroller AG, Chabannon C et al, Administration of G-CSF can be delayed after

transplantation of autologous G-CSF-primed blood stem cells: a randomized study. *Bone Marrow Transplant* 1996; **17**: 533–6.

59. Roberts AW, DeLuca E, Begley CG et al, Broad inter-individual variations in circulating progenitor cell numbers induced by granulocyte colony-stimulating factor therapy. *Stem Cells* 1995; **13**: 512–16.

60. Menichella G, Pierelli L, Foddai ML et al, Autologous blood stem cell harvesting and transplantation in patients with advanced ovarian cancer. *Br J Haematol* 1991; **79**: 444–50.

61. Tarella C, Caracciolo D, Gavarotti P et al, Circulating progenitors following high-dose sequential (HDS) chemotherapy with G-CSF: short intervals between drug courses severely impair progenitor mobilization. *Bone Marrow Transplant* 1995; **16**: 223–8.

62. Bensinger W, Appelbaum F, Rowley S et al, Factors that influence collection and engraftment of autologous peripheral-blood stem cells. *J Clin Oncol* 1995; **13**: 2547–55.

63. Schneider JG, Crown JP, Wasserheit C et al, Factors affecting the mobilization of primitive and committed hematopoietic progenitors into the peripheral blood of cancer patients. *Bone Marrow Transplant* 1994; **14**: 877–84.

64. Dreger P, Kloss M, Petersen B et al, Autologous progenitor cell transplantation: prior exposure to stem cell-toxic drugs determines yield and engraftment of peripheral blood progenitor cell but not of bone marrow grafts. *Blood* 1995; **86**: 3970–8.

65. Demirer T, Buckner CD, Gooley T et al, Factors influencing collection of peripheral blood stem cells in patients with multiple myeloma. *Bone Marrow Transplant* 1996; **17**: 937–41.

66. Goldschmidt H, Hegenbart U, Haas R, Hunstein W, Mobilization of peripheral blood progenitor cells with high-dose cyclophosphamide (4 or 7 g/m^2) and granulocyte colony-stimulating factor in patients with multiple myeloma. *Bone Marrow Transplant* 1996; **17**: 691–7.

67. Winter JN, Lazarus HM, Rademaker A et al, Phase I/II study of combined granulocyte colony-stimulating factor and granulocyte–macrophage colony-stimulating factor administration for the mobilization of hematopoietic progenitor cells. *J Clin Oncol* 1996; **14**: 277–86.

68. Ottmann OG, Ganser A, Seipelt G et al, Effects of recombinant human interleukin-3 on human hematopoietic progenitors and precursor cells in vivo. *Blood* 1990; **76**: 1494–501.

69. Haas R, Ehrhardt R, Witt B et al, Autografting with peripheral blood stem cells mobilized by sequential interleukin-3/granulocyte–macrophage colony-stimulating factor following high-dose chemotherapy in non-Hodgkin's lymphoma. *Bone Marrow Transplant* 1993; **12**: 643–9.

70. Brugger W, Bross K, Frisch J et al, Mobilization of peripheral blood progenitor cells by sequential administration of interleukin-3 and granulocyte–macrophage colony-stimulating factor following polychemotherapy with etoposide, ifosfamide, and cisplatin. *Blood* 1992; **79**: 1193–200.

71. Huhn RD, Yurkow EJ, Tushinski R et al, Recombinant human interleukin-3 (rhIL-3) enhances the mobilization of peripheral blood progenitor cells by recombinant human granulocyte colony-stimulating factor (rhG-CSF) in normal volunteers. *Exp Hematol* 1996; **24**: 839–47.

72. Geissler K, Peschel C, Niederwieser D et al, Effect of interleukin-3 pretreatment on granulocyte–macrophage colony-stimulating factor induced mobilization of circulating hematopoietic progenitor cells. *Br J Haematol* 1995; **91**: 299–305.

73. Roman-Unfer S, Bitran JD, Garrison L et al, A phase II study of cyclophosphamide followed by PIXY321 as a means of mobilizing peripheral blood hematopoietic progenitor cells. *Exp Hematol* 1996; **24**: 823–8.

74. Langley KE, Bennett LG, Wypych J et al, Soluble stem cell factor in human serum. *Blood* 1993; **81**: 656–60.

75. Wypych J, Bennett LG, Schwartz MG et al, Soluble kit receptor in human serum. *Blood* 1995; **85**: 66–73.

76. Testa U, Martucci R, Rutella S et al, Autologous stem cell transplantation: release of early and late acting growth factors relates with hematopoietic ablation and recovery. *Blood* 1994; **84**: 3532–9.

77. Andrews RG, Bartelmez SH, Knitter GH et al, A c-kit ligand, recombinant human stem cell factor, mediates reversible expansion of multiple CD34$^+$ colony-forming cell types in blood and marrows of baboons. *Blood* 1992; **80**: 920–7.

78. Andrews RG, Bensinger WI, Knitter GH et al, The ligand for c-kit, stem cell factor, stimulates the circulation of cells that engraft lethally irradiated baboons. *Blood* 1992; **80**: 2715–20.

79. Andrews RG, Briddell RA, Knitter GH et al, In vivo synergy between recombinant human stem cell factor and recombinant human granulocyte colony-stimulating factor in baboons: enhanced circulation of progenitor cells. *Blood* 1994; **84:** 800–10.

80. Andrews RG, Briddell RA, Knitter GH et al, Rapid engraftment by peripheral blood progenitor cells mobilized by colony-stimulating factor in nonhuman primates. *Blood* 1995; **85:** 15–20.

81. Basser R, Begley CG, Mansfield R et al, Mobilization of PBPC by priming with stem cell factor (SCF) before filgrastim compared to concurrent administration [abstract]. *Blood* 1995; **86:** 687a.

82. Weaver A, Slowley C, Woll PJ et al, A randomized comparison of progenitor cell mobilization using chemotherapy plus stem cell factor (r-metHuSCF) and filgrastim (r-methHuG-CSF) or chemotherapy plus filgrastim [abstract]. *Proc Am Soc Clin Oncol* 1996; **15:** 269.

83. Lemoli RM, Fogli M, Fortuna A et al, Interleukin-11 stimulates the proliferation of human hematopoietic CD34$^+$ and CD33$^-$DR$^-$ cells and synergizes with stem cell factor, interleukin-3, and granulocyte–macrophage colony-stimulating factor. *Exp Hematol* 1993; **21:** 1668–72.

84. Tsuji K, Lyman SD, Sudo T et al, Enhancement of murine hematopoiesis by synergistic interactions between steel factor (ligand for c-kit), interleukin-11, and other early acting factors in culture. *Blood* 1992; **79:** 2855–60.

85. Broxmeyer HE, Lu L, Cooper S et al, Flt3 ligand stimulates/costimulates the growth of myeloid stem/progenitor cells. *Exp Hematol* 1995; **23:** 1121–9.

86. Jacobsen SE, Okkenhaug C, Myklebust J et al, The flt3 ligand potently and directly stimulates the growth and expansion of primitive murine bone marrow progenitor cells in vitro: synergistic interactions with interleukin (IL)-11, IL-12, and other hematopoietic growth factors. *J Exp Med* 1995; **181:** 1357–63.

87. Mauch P, Lamont C, Neben TY et al, Hematopoietic stem cells in the blood after stem cell factor and interleukin-11 administration: evidence for different mechanisms of mobilization. *Blood* 1995; **86:** 4674–80.

88. Nash RA, Seidel K, Storb R et al, Effects of rhIL-11 on normal dogs and after sublethal radiation. *Exp Hematol* 1995; **23:** 389–96.

89. Lyman SD, James L, Vanden Bos T et al, Molecular cloning of a ligand for the flt3/flk-2 tyrosine kinase receptor: a proliferative factor for primitive hematopoietic cells. *Cell* 1993; **75:** 1157–67.

90. Lyman SD, James L, Johnson L et al, Cloning of the human homologue of the murine flt3 ligand: a growth factor for early hematopoietic progenitor cells. *Blood* 1994; **83:** 2795–801.

91. Lyman SD, Seaberg M, Hanna R et al, Plasma/serum levels of flt3 ligand are low in normal individuals and highly elevated in patients with Fanconi anemia and acquired aplastic anemia. *Blood* 1995; **86:** 4091–6.

92. McKenna HJ, de Vries P, Brasel K et al, Effect of flt3 ligand on the ex vivo expansion of human CD34$^+$ hematopoietic progenitor cells. *Blood* 1995; **86:** 3413–20.

93. Gabianelli M, Pelosi E, Montesoro E et al, Multilevel effects of flt3 ligand on human hematopoiesis: expansion of putative stem cells and proliferation of granulomonocytic progenitors/monocytic precursors. *Blood* 1995; **86:** 1661–70.

94. Hudak S, Hunte B, Culpepper J et al, Flt3/flk2 ligand promotes the growth of murine stem cells and the expansion of colony-forming cells and spleen colony-forming units. *Blood* 1995; **85:** 2747–55.

95. Gratwohl A, Filipowicz A, Baldomero H et al, Rh-flt-3 ligand mobilizes hematopoietic progenitor cells in rabbits [abstract]. *Exp Hematol* 1996; **24:** 1039.

96. Laterveer L, Lindley IJ, Heemskerk DP et al, Rapid mobilization of hematopoietic progenitor cells in rhesus monkeys by single intravenous injection of interleukin-8. *Blood* 1996; **87:** 781–8.

97. Hunter MG, Bawden L, Brotherton D, et al, BB-10010: an active variant of human macrophage inflammatory protein-1 alpha with improved pharmaceutical properties. *Blood* 1995; **86:** 4400–8.

98. Haas R, Möhle R, Pförsich M et al, Blood-derived autografts collected during granulocyte colony-stimulating factor-enhanced recovery are enriched with early Thy-1$^+$ hematopoietic progenitor cells. *Blood* 1995; **85:** 1936–43.

99. Roberts AW, Metcalf D, Noncycling state of peripheral blood progenitor cells mobilized by granulocyte colony-stimulating factor and other cytokines. *Blood* 1995; **86:** 1600–5.

100. Donahue RE, Kirby MR, Metzger ME et al, Peripheral blood CD34$^+$ cells differ from bone marrow CD34$^+$ cells in Thy-1 expression and

cell cycle status in nonhuman primates mobilized or not mobilized with granulocyte colony-stimulating factor and/or stem cell factor. *Blood* 1996; **87**: 1644–53.

101. Möhle R, Murea S, Kirsch M, Haas R, Differential expression of L-selectin, VLA-4 and LFA1 and CD34[+] progenitor cells from bone marrow and peripheral blood during G-CSF-enhanced recovery. *Exp Hematol* 1995; **23**: 1535–42.

102. Dercksen MW, Gerritsen WR, Rodenhuis S et al, Expression of adhesion molecules on CD34[+] cells: CD34[+] L-selectin[+] cells predicts a rapid platelet recovery after peripheral blood stem cell transplantation. *Blood* 1995; **85**: 3313–19.

103. Dercksen MW, Rodenhuis S, Dirkson MKA et al, Subsets of CD34[+] cells and rapid hematopoietic recovery after peripheral-blood stem-cell transplantation. *J Clin Oncol* 1995; **13**: 1922–32.

104. Pierelli L, Teofili L, Menichella G et al, Further investigations on the expression of HLA-DR, CD33 and CD13 surface antigens in purified bone marrow and peripheral blood CD34[+] haematopoietic progenitor cells. *Br J Haematol* 1993; **84**: 24–30.

105. Teofili L, Iovino MS, Sica S et al, Characterization of peripheral blood CD34[+] progenitor cells mobilized with chemotherapy and granulocyte colony-stimulating factor. *Exp Hematol* 1994; **22**: 990–5.

106. Tarella C, Benedetti G, Caracciolo D et al, Both early and committed haemopoietic progenitors are more frequent in peripheral blood than in bone marrow during mobilization induced by high-dose chemotherapy + G-CSF. *Br J Haematol* 1995; **91**: 535–43.

107. To LB, Haylock DN, Dowse T et al, A comparative study of the phenotype and proliferative capacity of peripheral blood (PB) CD34[+] cells mobilized by four different protocols and those of steady-phase PB and bone marrow CD34[+] cells. *Blood* 1994; **84**: 2930–9.

108. Bender JG, Williams SF, Myers S et al, Characterization of chemotherapy mobilized peripheral blood progenitor cells for use in autologous stem cell transplantation. *Bone Marrow Transplant* 1992; **10**: 281–5.

109. Haas R, Möhle R, Murea S et al, Characterization of peripheral blood progenitor cells mobilized by cytotoxic chemotherapy and recombinant human granulocyte colony-stimulating factor. *J Hematother* 1994; **3**: 323–30.

110. Bender JG, Unverzagt KL, Walker DE et al,

Identification and comparison of CD34-positive cells and their subpopulations from normal peripheral blood and bone marrow using multicolor flow cytometry. *Blood* 1991; **77**: 2591–6.

111. Bender JG, Lum L, Unverzagt KL et al, Correlation of colony-forming cells, long-term culture initiating cells and CD34[+] cells in apheresis products from patients mobilized for peripheral blood progenitors with different regimens. *Bone Marrow Transplant* 1994; **13**: 479–85.

112. Benbouker L, Domenech J, Linassier C et al, Long-term cultures to evaluate engraftment potential of CD34[+] cells from peripheral blood after mobilization by chemotherapy with and without GM-CSF. *Exp Hematol* 1995; **23**: 1568–73.

113. Brenner MK, Rill DR, Moen RC et al, Gene-marking to trace origin of relapse after autologous bone marrow transplantation. *Lancet* 1994; **341**: 85–6.

114. Gribben JG, Freedman AS, Neuberg D et al, Immunologic purging of marrow assessed by PCR before autologous bone marrow transplantation for B-cell lymphoma. *N Engl J Med* 1991; **325**: 1525–33.

115. Gribben JG, Neuberg D, Freedman AS et al, Detection by polymerase chain reaction of residual cells with the bcl-2 translocation is associated with increased risk of relapse after autologous bone marrow transplantation for B-cell lymphoma. *Blood* 1993; **81**: 3449–57.

116. Lin F, Goldman JM, Cross NC. A comparison of the sensitivity of blood and bone marrow for the detection of minimal residual disease in chronic myeloid leukemia. *Br J Haematol* 1994; **86**: 683–85.

117. Maurer J, Janssen JWG, Thiel E et al, Detection of chimeric BCR-ABL genes in acute lymphoblastic leukaemia by the polymerase chain reaction. *Lancet* 1991; **337**: 1055–8.

118. Ouspenskaia MV, Johnston DA, Roberts WM et al, Accurate quantitation of residual B-precursor acute lymphobastic leukemia by limiting dilution and a PCR-based detection system: a description of the method and the principles involved. *Leukemia* 1995; **9**: 321–8.

119. Henry JM, Sykes PJ, Brisco MJ et al, Comparison of myeloma cell contamination of bone marrow and peripheral blood stem cell harvests. *Br J Haematol* 1996; **92**: 614–19.

120. Gazitt Y, Tian E, Barlogie B et al, Differential mobilization of myeloma cells and normal hematopoietic stem cells in multiple myeloma

after treatment with cyclophosphamide and granulocyte–macrophage colony-stimulating factor. *Blood* 1996; **87:** 805–11.

121. Bergsagel PL, Smith AM, Szczepek A et al, In multiple myeloma, clonotypic B lymphocytes are detectable among CD19[+] peripheral blood cells expressing CD38, CD56, and monotypic Ig light chain. *Blood* 1995; **85:** 436–47.

122. Lemoli RM, Fortuna A, Motta MR et al, Concomitant mobilization of plasma cells and hematopoietic progenitors in peripheral blood of multiple myeloma patients: positive selection and transplantation of enriched CD34[+] cells to remove circulating tumor cells. *Blood* 1996; **87:** 1625–34.

123. Schlimok G, Funke I, Holzmann BB et al, Micrometastatic cancer cells in bone marrow, in vitro detection with anticytokeratin and in vivo labeling with anti-17-1A monoclonal antibodies. *Proc Natl Acad Sci* 1987; **84:** 8672–6.

124. Diel IJ, Kaufmann M, Goerner R et al, Detection of tumor cells in bone marrow of patients with primary breast cancer: a prognostic factor for distant metastasis. *J Clin Oncol* 1992; **10:** 1534–9.

125. Cote RJ, Rosen PP, Lesser ML et al, Prediction of early relapse in patients with operable breast cancer by detection of occult bone marrow micrometastases. *J Clin Oncol* 1991; **9:** 1749–56.

126. Pantel K, Izbicki J, Passlick B et al, Frequency and prognostic significance of isolated tumor cells in bone marrow of patients with non-small-cell lung cancer without overt metastases. *Lancet* 1996; **347:** 649–53.

127. Datta YH, Adams PT, Drobyski WR et al, Sensitive detection of occult breast cancer by the reverse-transcriptase polymerase chain reaction. *J Clin Oncol* 1994; **12:** 475–82.

128. Fields KK, Elfenbein GJ, Trudeau WL et al, Clinical significance of bone marrow metastases as detected using the polymerase chain reaction in patients with breast cancer undergoing high-dose chemotherapy and autologous bone marrow transplantation. *J Clin Oncol* 1996; **14:** 1868–76.

129. Krismann M, Todt B, Schröder J et al, Low specificity of cytokeratin 19 reverse transcriptase-polymerase chain reaction analyses for detection of hematogenous lung cancer dissemination. *J Clin Oncol* 1995; **13:** 2769–75.

130. Brugger W, Bross KJ, Glatt M et al, Mobilization of tumor cells and hematopoietic progenitor cells into peripheral blood of patients with solid tumors. *Blood* 1994; **83:** 636–40.

131. Passos-Coelho JL, Ross AA, Moss TJ et al, Absence of breast cancer cells in a single-day peripheral blood progenitor cell collection after priming with cyclophosphamide and granulocyte–macrophage colony-stimulating factor. *Blood* 1995; **85:** 1138–43.

132. Ross AA, Cooper BW, Lazarus HM et al, Detection and viability of tumor cells in peripheral blood stem cell collections from breast cancer patients using immunocytochemical and clonogenic assay techniques. *Blood* 1993; **82:** 2605–10.

133. Sharp JG, Kessinger A, Vaughan WP et al, Detection and clinical significance of minimal tumor cell contamination of peripheral stem cell harvests. *Int J Cell Cloning* 1992; **10:** 92–7.

134. Papayannopoulou T, Nakamoto B, Peripheralization of hemopoietic progenitors in primates treated with anti-VLA-4 integrin. *Proc Natl Acad Sci USA* 1993; **90:** 9374–8.

135. Voso MT, Murea S, Goldschmidt H et al, High-dose chemotherapy with PBSC support results in a significant reduction of the hematopoietic progenitor cell compartment. *Br J Haematol* 1996; **94:** 757–63.

136. Haas R, Witt B, Möhle R et al, Sustained long-term hematopoiesis after myeloablative therapy with peripheral blood progenitor cell support. *Blood* 1995; **85:** 3754–61.

4

Collection and processing of peripheral blood hematopoietic progenitor cells

Adrian P Gee

CONTENTS • **Introduction** • **Collection of blood-derived grafts** • **Collection targets** • **Collection complications** • **Processing** • **Cryopreservation and storage** • **Thawing and reinfusion** • **Conclusions**

INTRODUCTION

Sources of stem cell grafts

Hematopoietic progenitor cell (HPC) transplantation has found widespread application in the treatment of marrow failure and myelodysplastic syndromes, and in the hematological rescue of patients who receive high-dose therapy for a variety of malignant diseases.[1] Historically this approach was pioneered, after early failures, using bone marrow cells obtained from HLA-matched sibling donors as the source of the graft. These grafts are available to only one-quarter to one-third of suitable patients, and considerable effort has been exerted to find alternative donors for patients lacking a matched sibling donor. Approaches have included the use of hematopoietic cells obtained from matched unrelated donors (obtained through national and international marrow registries),[2] partially mismatched related marrow donors,[3] placental and umbilical cord blood[4] and autologous bone marrow.[5]

Transplantation of allogeneic marrow cells from alternative donors has usually resulted in an increased incidence of graft failure and/or graft-versus-host disease (GVHD), depending on the source of the graft and the use of ex vivo manipulation to deplete T cells as prophylaxis against GVHD.[6] In addition, in cases where T-cell depletion has achieved a decrease in the incidence and severity of GVHD, this has usually been obtained at the expense of an increase in the incidence of relapse of disease post transplant, due to the parallel abrogation of a potentially beneficial graft-versus-leukemia effect.[7] Placental and umbilical cord blood is a rich source of hematopoietic cells that is readily available and can be easily HLA-typed, tested and banked for possible autologous use, or for allogeneic transplantation.[8] In spite of difficulties with respect to the restricted size of the graft and ethical questions regarding informed consent and donor/recipient linkage, it is clear that this material is an important new source of stem cells for transplantation. There is some early evidence that there is a reduced risk of GVHD with these grafts, due presumably to the relative naiveté of the T cells; however, there is still limited clinical experience in cord blood transplantation, and such conclusions may prove to be premature.

Use of blood-derived grafts

As a result, the majority of alternative donor transplants have used autologous HPC. Recently published European data[9] show that over the course of 11 years the percentage of transplants using autologous grafts has increased from 35% in 1983 to 65% in 1994. Hidden within these numbers is another important trend – the change in the source of HPC from the marrow to the peripheral circulation. In 1991, 85% of European autologous transplants were performed using marrow grafts, whereas in 1994, 65% used blood-derived HPC and another 6% used a combination of HPC from blood and marrow.[9] A similar revolution appears to be underway in allogeneic transplantation, where the percentage of allogeneic transplants performed using blood-derived grafts has increased from zero in 1991 in Europe, to nearly 6% three years later.[9]

This increase has been paralleled by the number of publications appearing in the literature on blood stem cells. The reader is directed to articles by Fliedner[10] and Körbling and Fliedner[11] for detailed overviews and reference material on the historical development of the field; however, the major milestones can be briefly summarized. The first preclinical study was published in 1973 by Fliedner et al on a therapy model for the use of blood stem cells in the treatment of a radiation-induced marrow failure; however, the existence of these cells had been proposed as early as 1909 by Maximow. The prevailing belief among hematologists was, nonetheless, that pluripotent stem cells did not enter the peripheral circulation under normal physiological conditions – a notion that was disproved by experiments in which labeled DNA-synthesizing cells were shown to traffic between marrow sites. Subsequently, in 1962, peripheral blood cells were shown to be capable of restoring hematopoiesis in irradiated mice,[12] and studies by Thomas' group[13] in dogs confirmed these observations and ruled out the possibility that these cells were not derived from extramedullary sites of hematopoiesis. Colony-forming cells were identified in human peripheral blood in the early 1970s.[14]

Collections of stem cells were performed by continuous flow centrifugation in human volunteers in the late 1970s by Körbling et al[15] in Heidelberg, and in 1986 six independent studies appeared in the literature in which blood stem cells were used for clinical transplantation.

Early collections were performed during steady-state hematopoiesis, with the result that many aphereses had to be performed. This made the procedure costly and tedious for both the patient and the collection staff, required freezing and storage of each apheresis product, and necessitated the infusion of large volumes of cells and cryoprotectant at the time of the transplant. The approach would, therefore, have probably have remained restricted to use in patients with overt metastatic involvement of the marrow, or with marrow fibrosis, because of its impracticality. This situation was changed irreversibly, however, by the use of chemotherapy[16] and/or hematopoietic growth factors[17] to mobilize HPC into the peripheral circulation (see Chapters 3 and 4), thereby dramatically reducing the required number of collections, and the final graft volume. This has resulted in a dramatic growth in this type of autologous transplantation, and the way in which transplantation is performed.[9] The graft is procured by one to three apheresis procedures, usually in an outpatient setting,[18] without the necessity for general anaesthesia. The rapid engraftment characteristics of peripheral blood HPC have also prompted the trend towards performing the infusion in the outpatient environment, in which the patient is only admitted to hospital at the first sign of a potential clinical complication. The apparent relative simplicity of this approach to autologous transplantation has also fueled the spread of transplant therapy from traditional tertiary care health centers into community hospitals, health centers and clinics.

This approach is now being extended to the use of peripheral blood HPC for allogeneic transplantation.[19] This has been prompted by the possibility of using recombinant human growth factors alone to mobilize normal donors and by the finding that the higher burden of mature T lymphocytes in blood-derived grafts[20] does not result in a concomitant increase in the incidence and severity of acute GVHD.[21] Preliminary results have indicated, however, that chronic GVHD may be higher in the recipients of these grafts[22] (see also Chapter 10). Ongoing clinical studies should resolve this question.

COLLECTION OF BLOOD-DERIVED GRAFTS

Introduction and overview

In the vast majority of transplants, peripheral blood HPC are collected within an erythrocyte-depleted leukocyte population, in much the same way that marrow HPC may be collected within a buffy coat or 'mononuclear' cell fraction of the bone marrow. In contrast to marrow HPC, however, the collection and enrichment of this population is automated by connecting the donor to an apheresis machine and performing a modified leukapheresis procedure (Figure 4.1)[23] Although a variety of machines are available for this purpose, they all function using the same principle. Blood is drawn from the donor (who has been mobilized using chemotherapy and/or recombinant human growth factors), anticoagulated, and pumped into a spinning chamber. Here the blood separates into its component elements on the basis of cell size and density, forming distinct bands or layers within the vessel. The leukocyte-rich layer is harvested into a collection vessel and the remaining elements returned to the patient. This procedure takes place either continuously or in a batch mode (discontinuous flow), and is maintained until the required volume of blood has been processed. There is evidence that the collection procedure itself recruits HPC into the peripheral circulation, although this finding has been disputed and attributed to inadequate mobilization.

Leukapheresis is repeated on subsequent days until the target number of cells has been collected. The parameters according to which the adequacy of the collection is evaluated vary between centers (see later).[24] For determining whether additional collections need to be performed, only assays that provide results within a few hours can be used. This effectively limits the assays to nucleated cell counts and/or total numbers of CD34+ cells (Figure 4.2) (and/or

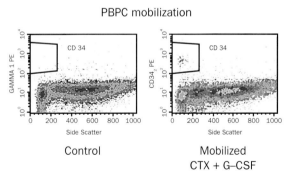

PBPC mobilization

Control / Mobilized CTX + G–CSF

Figure 4.2 Mobilization of CD34+ cells into the peripheral circulation following administration of cyclophosphamide and recombinant human granulocyte colony-stimulating factor. Flow cytometry 'dot-plot' of orthogonal light scatter (abscissa) and staining with anti-CD34 monoclonal antibody conjugated to phycoerythrin (ordinate). 'Stem cells' characterized by low orthogonal light scatter and positive staining are mobilized into the peripheral blood, and appear as the discrete population in the upper left quadrant of the right-hand panel.

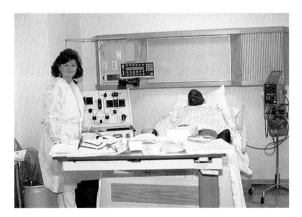

Figure 4.1 Donor undergoing stem cell collection using the COBE BCT Spectra.

PBPC evaluation – available assays

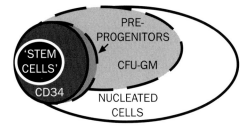

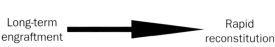

Long-term engraftment → Rapid reconstitution

Figure 4.3 Assays used for characterization of peripheral blood stem cell collections. The interrelationship between the assays is indicated as well as their relationship to the engraftment potential of the product. Preprogenitor cell assays include long-term culture-initiating cells and cobblestone area forming cells.

CD34$^+$ subpopulations). In most cases, within a center, the number of CD34$^+$ cells correlates with the colony-forming unit granulocyte–macrophage (CFU-GM) and long-term culture-initiating cell (LTC-IC) content of the cell suspension (Figure 4.3), and relates, up to a threshold value, with the time to engraftment.[24,25]

Each apheresis product is cryopreserved while the remainder of the graft is collected, and the patient goes on to receive high-dose therapy. In most centers, the product is frozen without any additional manipulation. If there is a concern that an autologous graft contains tumor cells, it may be subjected to purging or to antibody-based enrichment of CD34$^+$ cells.[26] In the case of allogeneic collections, T-cell depletion may be considered.[27]

For storage prior to infusion, the cells are usually frozen following one of two protocols. In the first, 10% v/v of dimethyl sulfoxide (DMSO) is added as a cryoprotectant, freezing is achieved using a controlled-rate programmable freezer, and the cells are stored in the liquid or vapour phase of liquid nitrogen.[28] In the second method,[29] 5% DMSO, 6% hydroxyethyl starch and albumin are added, and the cells are frozen and stored at −80°C. For infusion, cells

are usually thawed rapidly at the bedside and infused quickly, without washing, but frequently after addition of acid–citrate–dextrose, through a blood administration set.

Donor preparation

Procedures for mobilization of donors are described in Chapters 3 and 4. For autologous collections this is often achieved using a combination of chemotherapy and growth factors. Collection is usually initiated during the rebound that follows the nadir in the leukocyte count. Traditionally, apheresis was started when a count of ~10^9/liter was achieved, but is increasingly being delayed until the count reaches more than 2×10^9/liter. Alternatively, some centers monitor the concentration of CD34$^+$ cells in the circulation,[30] and initiate apheresis once the count starts to increase (e.g. to more than 15 CD34$^+$ cells/µl). At least one center has reported a correlation between the steady-state CD34 count and the yield following mobilization,[31] although this finding has not been universal.[32]

A number of organizations have developed guidelines and standards for the evaluation of prospective donors of PBHPC. These include the BCSH Blood Transfusion Task Force in the United Kingdom,[33] and the American Association of Blood Banks[34] and the Foundation for the Accreditation of Hematopoietic Cell Therapy[35] (FAHCT) in the United States and Canada. These relate primarily to the timing and performance of infectious disease screening, HLA typing and general health evaluation, and differ for autologous and allogeneic collections. The following is a summary of the standards developed by the FAHCT:

- There must be a documented evaluation by medical history, physical examination and laboratory testing for the risks of apheresis donation, including the possible need for central venous access and/or mobilization therapy.
- An interim health assessment must be performed immediately before each collection procedure.

- A complete blood count, including platelet count, must be performed within 72 hours prior to the first collection, and within 24 hours before each subsequent apheresis.
- For allogeneic donors, the medical history (including a vaccination and blood transfusion history, pregnancy assessment and identification of persons at high risk for HIV infections and for HIV transmission) must be obtained, and a physical examination and laboratory tests (to include HLA-A, -B and -DR type, ABO group and Rh type, tests for anti-HIV-1, anti-HIV-2, HIV-1-Ag, anti-HTLV, HBsAg, anti-HBc, anti-HCV and anti-CMV, and a serological test for syphilis) must be performed. In the case of multiple collections, these tests must be performed within 30 days prior to each collection. The tests must be performed and suitability documented before the recipient's high-dose therapy has begun.
- For autologous donors, the HLA typing is not required, and tests must be performed no more than 30 days prior to collection or on the day of the first collection.
- Abnormal findings must be reported to the prospective donor; however, a donor not meeting criteria may be used, but the rationale for the selection of such a donor must be documented and requires the informed consent of the donor and the recipient.
- Informed consent is required prior to commencing high-dose therapy, and the procedure must be explained in terms that the donor can understand.
- Growth factor administration must be under the supervision of a physician experienced in the management of persons receiving these agents.
- Central venous catheters must be placed by a licensed physician qualified to perform the procedure, and adequacy of line placement must be documented radiographically.
- There must be a written request from the recipient's physician before collection is begun. This includes timing and procedural details of collection.
- The cells must be packaged in transfer packs approved for human cells.

Fewer than half of the patients from whom peripheral blood HPC are to be collected will have adequate peripheral venous access.[36] The remainder require placement of catheters of a design that permits repeated use and high flow rates, for example the double-lumen polyurethane Quinton-Mahurkar (Quinton Instrument Company, Seattle, WA), the silicone rubber double-lumen PermCath (also from Quinton), and the silicone rubber, apheresis/hemodialysis, single- or double-lumen Hickman (Bard Access Systems, Salt Lake City, UT). Subclavian Quinton-Mahurkar catheters can be used for up to 3 weeks and are then removed, whereas silicone rubber catheters can be left in place for longer periods, but are associated with venous thrombosis in 10–40% of donors. The use of short-term large-bore (2.7–3.5 mm) polyurethane catheters (Pellethane, Fresenius St Wendel, St Wendel, Germany) inserted via the internal jugular vein has also been described, and resulted in a 5% incidence of thrombosis.[37]

Access for withdrawal and return can be achieved using a variety of types of catheters, although autologous collections usually employ a catheter that can also be used for supportive care over a longer period (e.g. a silicone rubber catheter) unless there is to be a substantial delay between collection and transplant. The placement of catheters and the use of antithrombotic therapy during collection has recently been expertly reviewed by Haire and Sniecinski,[38] and the following recommendations are summarized from that review:

- For continuous-flow apheresis a double-lumen silicone rubber apheresis/hemodialysis catheter is recommended. This is placed with the tip in the lower third of the superior vena cava via the subclavian vein.
- For discontinuous-flow apheresis, or when a peripheral vein is used for return, a single-lumen apheresis/hemodialysis catheter is recommended. This is placed in the subclavian vein with the tip positioned in the lower third of the superior vena cava, where inferior vena cava placement is not possible.

• If catheter-related thrombosis is a potential problem, aspirin should be administered at a dose of 325 mg/day, when GM-CSF is not used for mobilization, and should be discontinued when collection has been completed. If subclavian catheters and cytokine mobilization are used, warfarin, at a dose of 1 mg/day, should be administered starting 48 hours prior to catheter placement. This can be continued until initiation of the preparative regimen for transplantation. There is no published safe and effective method for thromboprophylaxis for inferior vena cava catheters used with cytokines.

Anticoagulation during collection is routinely achieved using anticoagulant–citrate–dextrose Formula A (ACD-A).[36] Heparin is usually restricted to donors with allergies to citrate, although combinations of heparin and ACD-A have been used. The major side-effect associated with the use of ACD-A is hypocalcemia, which is manifested as tingling of the extremities and around the mouth. This can be prevented by oral administration of milk or calcium citrate or carbonate (e.g. calcium-rich indigestion remedies) before apheresis.[39] If symptoms appear during collection, calcium gluconate (45 mg calcium in 5 ml 2.25 mEq) can be slowly administered over 5–10 minutes.[38] Adverse reactions to this infusion appear as a burning sensation or a metallic taste.

Anticoagulation is achieved by mixing blood to ACD-A solution at a ratio of about 11–13:1, which results in an adult patient receiving up to a liter of ACD-A when 10–12 liters of blood are processed. This results in marked decreases in calcium levels;[38,39] however, these usually return to normal levels within 1–2 hours after the procedure. A higher ratio of blood to anticoagulant (e.g. 15:1) may be used in donors with low precollection hematocrits and low platelet counts (e.g. below 150 000/µl), and allows a faster inlet flow rate. Lower ratios of 9–12:1 are appropriate for donors with hematocrits above 36% and platelet counts above 150 000/µl. Vital signs should be monitored every 30 minutes during collection and patients should be advised of the signs of hypocalcemia. The platelet count and hematocrit should also be closely followed.

Collection

As described previously, peripheral blood HPC are obtained within a leukapheresis product obtained on an automated blood cell separator. Collection may be either discontinuous/intermittent, in which collection proceeds in a series of batches, or continuous, in which blood is processed in a closed continuous-flow mode. The most commonly used machines are the Haemonetics V50 Plus,[40] which operates using the discontinuous-flow mode, and the Baxter Fenwal CS-3000 (Figure 4.4),[41] the COBE BCT Spectra (Figure 4.5),[42] the DIDECO Vivacell[43] and the Fresenius AS104 (Figure 4.6),[44] which use continuous/intermittent flow mode. All of the machines use a similar principle in which cell layers are established in a spinning vessel, under the influence of centrifugal force (with or

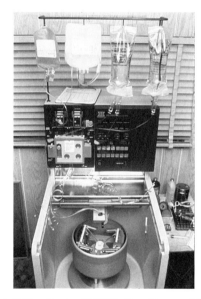

Figure 4.4 The Baxter CS300 Plus. The centrifuge bowl containing the two opposing separation and collection chambers can be seen. Note that in the United States, peripheral blood stem cell collection using apheresis machines may require regulatory approval under an Investigational Device Exemption (IDE). Investigators are advised to consult the Center for Biologics Evaluation and Research of the Food and Drug Administration. (Photograph courtesy of Baxter Biotech.)

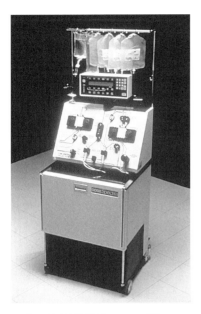

Figure 4.5 The COBE BCT Spectra. (Photograph courtesy of COBE BCT.)

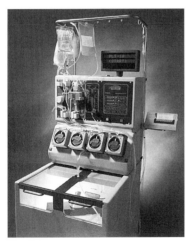

Figure 4.6 The Fresenius AS104. (Photograph courtesy of Fresenius.)

without counterflow) and harvested continuously or intermittently. The following provides an overview of the basics of the most commonly used machines; however, detailed instructions, performance parameters and the latest operating procedures should be obtained directly from the manufacturers.

In the V50, blood enters a spinning bell-shaped rigid (Latham) bowl and separates into plasma, buffy coat and red cell layers. The leukocytes are harvested by progressively pumping more blood into the bowl, forcing the layer to the apex and out of the chamber under the control of optic fiber detectors mounted at the bowl shoulder. The remaining contents of the bowl are then returned to the patient and the entire procedure repeated[40] – normally for 8–10 cycles in an adult donor. The collected leukocytes may be reprocessed to reduce the red cell content using the lymphosurge protocol, in which the entire collection is returned to the bowl, the mononuclear cell-rich fraction is collected and the red cell fraction returned to the patient. The discontinuous technique is slower, and patients may react to the bolus of ACD-A received with the red cells after each pass.

The Fenwal CS-3000[45] and CS3000 Plus (Figure 4.4) (a later version with more features and a modified control panel) separators pump blood into a flexible pack contained within a rigid mold of defined configuration. The layers are established, and, under the control of a system of detectors, the mononuclear white cell layer and plasma are pumped into a second spinning collection container in the opposing centrifuge bucket. Here the cells are separated from the plasma, which is returned, together with the red cells, to the donor. Platelet contamination of the product can be reduced by the use of a small volume collection chamber.[45] More blood enters the separation chamber and the process continues. The entire collection procedure is automated and shepherded by a system of sensors; however, the separation process cannot be viewed by the operator, which is a source of concern to some. Unlike some separators, the CS3000 does not use a rotating seal, which can fail, resulting in leakage of blood into the centrifuge bowl.

The COBE BCT Spectra (Figure 4.5) performs the separation in a spinning, flexible, belt-shaped disposable. The height of the leukocyte layer within the belt can be adjusted manually by controlling the flow of plasma. The cells are harvested by bringing the interface into contact with the collection outlet channel through which the cells exit the chamber. The layer is continuously established and harvested. The system (Version 4, MNC Program) allows operator control of the depth of collection within the mononuclear cell layer. A fully automated procedure for the Spectra has recently been described.[46] In the Fresenius AS104 (Figure 4.6) the separation is carried out in a two-chambered rigid disposable in four phases.[46] In the *separation phase*, the layers are established in the first chamber, platelets and plasma are continuously pumped into the second chamber and on to the air detector, where they are joined by red cells exiting the first chamber; the blood flow is then reduced to concentrate the leukocytes. In the *spillover phase*, the leukocytes are drawn into the second chamber, where they are concentrated during the *resting phase*. Finally, in the *collection phase*, the leukocytes are transferred to the collection bag.

In most cases, two to three blood volumes (10–12 liters) are processed during a 3–4 hour collection. Due to the relatively large 'dead volume' of most cell separator disposables, the separation chamber may require priming with red cells when small children (15–20 kg) are apheresed.[47] Large-volume leukaphereses, in which 20–25 liters of inlet volume (blood plus anticoagulant) are processed, have been described in both adults[48] and children.[49]

Overall, the products obtained by the newer machines, using recent protocols, are similar in cellular composition.[50,51] The volume of the final product ranges from 50 ml (using the CS3000 small-volume collection chamber),[45] through 150–400 ml for the Spectra, ~250 ml for the AS104, and up to 300–800 ml (30–50 ml per pass) for the V50. The products are, however, different in cellular composition from marrow-derived grafts. In an analysis of 16 products harvested at the Netherlands Red Cross in Amsterdam, following mobilization by chemotherapy and cytokines, the products consisted of 40% (±22%) lymphocytes, 31% (±15%) monocytes, 26% (±19%) myeloid (band cells, myelocytes, metamyelocytes and promyelocytes)

cells and 2.7% (±1.5%) CD34[+] cells. There were 15 ± 12 erythrocytes and 21 ± 15 platelets per leukocyte (I Slaper-Cortenbach, personal communication). Platelets and myeloid elements can cause problems if the product is to be manipulated, and following cryopreservation and thawing. Platelets may be removed by slow-speed centrifugation after product collection,[51] or as part of the automated collection procedure.[45]

COLLECTION TARGETS

Experience with marrow harvesting and transplantation has indicated that a target cell dose of $(1–2) \times 10^8$ nucleated cells should be harvested per kilogram of recipient body weight. If ex vivo manipulation of the graft is to be performed, two to three times that number of cells may be required, to compensate for anticipated losses during harvesting. In the case of peripheral blood HPC collections, the identity and number of cells to be collected have yet to be definitively established. Presently available assays are surrogate measurements of engraftment potential,[24,31] which is multifactorial, depending upon both the composition of the graft and the clinical status of the patient. Three parameters have been widely used to evaluate collection adequacy: total nucleated cells, colony-forming assays (CFU-GM, long-term culture-initiating cells and cobblestone area-forming cells) and CD34[+] cells and cell subsets (Figures 4.2 and 4.3).[24,31,32] Recently, CFU content has also been shown to correlate with numbers of mononuclear cells in DNA synthesis.[53] The 12-day to >14-day incubation period required for colony-forming assays means that they cannot be used in real time to determine when to discontinue apheresis. In spite of the variability in colony-forming assays between centers, most can correlate CFU content with numbers of CD34[+] cells in the product and the engraftment time.[24,25,31,32] As a result, the most widely used target parameter is the total number of CD34[+] cells collected.[24,54] With time, the target dose has declined from 1×10^7/kg to $1.5–2.0 \times 10^6$/kg recipient body weight. These numbers must, however, be interpreted with great caution. There is tremendous variability between laboratories assaying CD34$^+$ cells, due primarily to technical variables, such as the choice of anti-CD34 monoclonal antibody, the choice of conjugate, the gating strategy used during flow cytometric analysis, and the denominator used (e.g. total events acquired, CD45$^+$ events). These problems have been revealed in a variety of national and international multicenter studies[55–57] in which stained and unstained cell samples, and data were exchanged. Tremendous variability has been reported, to the extent that some centers would have terminated collections while others would have required multiple additional aphereses. Careful standardization of methodology and analysis can produce substantial improvements in reproducibility both within and between centers;[58] however, a single approach has yet to be adopted universally. The following is a brief summary of the guidelines developed by the Stem Cell Enumeration Subcommittee of the International Society for Hematotherapy and Graft Engineering:[58]

- Samples should be anticoagulated with ACD-A and transported at ambient temperature. Adjust the leukocyte count to <10^{10}/liter.
- Set up four tubes for staining:
  (i) and (ii) CD45-FITC/CD34-PE;
  (iii) CD45-FITC/Isotype control-PE;
  (iv) optional: Isotype-FITC/Isotype-PE.
  Specificities and suggested sources of the antibodies are given in the guidelines.
- Add 100 µl blood to each tube, and the appropriate antibodies. Incubate for 20–30 min at 4°C. Lyse red cells or lyse/fix samples and resuspend for analysis.
- CD34$^+$ cells are identified as cells (i) staining with anti-CD34; (ii) staining with anti-CD45 with an intensity characteristic of blast cells, i.e. lower than lymphocytes and monocytes; and (iii) with low side and low-to-intermediate forward light scatter.
- A sequential gating strategy is employed to identify the CD34$^+$ population. This is described in detail in the guidelines.[58]

Standardization should also be facilitated by the development of automated analysis and enumeration systems, such as the ProCOUNT Progenitor Cell Enumeration Kit from Becton Dickinson Immunocytometry Systems (San Jose, CA).

It is also clear that the CD34$^+$ cell population is heterogenous, containing both early committed and pluripotent stem cells (PSC)[59] and that the phenotype may be affected by the mobilization used and prior therapy received by the patient.[60] Recent studies have even suggested that PSC may be CD34 low or negative.[61] The rapid engraftment seen following peripheral blood HPC transplantation is undoubtedly a reflection of this heterogeneity. Measurement of a single common parameter cannot be expected to reflect this diversity, and attempts have been made, with some success, to correlate engraftment time to the numbers of CD34$^+$ cell subsets (e.g. CD34$^+$, CD38$^-$) infused.[62] Ongoing studies have indicated that enumeration of total CD34$^+$ cells is mainly of value as a crude measure of the likely minimum number of cells required to achieve engraftment,[24] in a manner analogous to the historical use of total nucleated cell numbers as the collection parameter in bone marrow harvests. This is supported by the widespread finding that patients will often engraft satisfactorily when large numbers of nucleated cells, containing 'inadequate' numbers of CD34$^+$ cells, are infused. As a result, many programs have adopted duel criteria for collection adequacy, in which target doses of nucleated (usually $(2–6) \times 10^8$/kg) and CD34$^+$ (usually $(1–3) \times 10^6$/kg)[54] cells are established, and apheresis is discontinued when either target is achieved. If the CD34 target is not reached, a decision may be made to go ahead with the transplant, to attempt remobilization or to harvest a back-up bone marrow.

COLLECTION COMPLICATIONS

The number of complications associated with collection of peripheral blood HPC has declined as the procedure has become more efficient and the number of aphereses per patient has declined. As described previously, citrate toxicity can be a problem, but it is usually easily prevented or resolved. Hypovolemia may be avoided by interrupting the procedure and subsequently reducing the flow rate. Thrombocytopenia is sometimes the result of platelets adhering to the surfaces of the disposable set, and can be reversed by returning platelet-rich plasma to the patient, or by a platelet transfusion. In a review of 554 mobilized and non-mobilized collections performed on 75 consecutive candidates between 1990 and 1994 on a V50 Plus, Goldberg et al[63] described catheter complications in 15.9% of collections. This required cessation of collection or thrombolytic therapy, which was successful in 85% of cases. Anemia or transient thrombocytopenia requiring transfusion therapy were observed in 30.7% and 14.7% of patients respectively. Sixteen percent of patients experienced infectious complications during harvesting; however, this was increased in patients mobilized using chemotherapy, whereas cytokine mobilization was protective. In this study, a median of nine collections were performed on each patient, and a lower incidence of complications would be expected using newer protocols for mobilization and collection.

PROCESSING

Routine processing

Routine processing of apheresis products usually occurs on the day of collection, although there is increasing evidence that products may be held overnight or as long as 72 hours.[64,65] The conditions for optimal storage have not been rigorously established; however, CFU appear to be maintained adequately at 4°C when the cell concentration is kept below $5 \times 10^7/ml$ and the pH is kept above 7.0.

Quality control mandates that each product should be assayed for sterility, qualitative and quantitative cellular composition, and progenitor cell content (using the assay in place to assess collection adequacy). CFU assays may also be employed to evaluate viability and functional activity of the cells by measuring their ability to proliferate. Viability assays that employ dye exclusion provide limited information related to membrane integrity, rather than proliferate potential. Information from these laboratory tests can be used to assess the efficiency of cell collection, aseptic technique and adequacy of mobilization, as well as providing indicators for ongoing quality improvement.

The high content of mononuclear cells in apheresis products obviates the necessity to perform density-gradient centrifugation. Erythrocytes do not survive cryopreservation, and hemoglobinuria is frequently seen post infusion of thawed grafts. This is not serious, and usually does not warrant further reduction of the erythrocyte content of the apheresis product before freezing. Platelets may cause cellular aggregation during downstream processing, but can be removed by slow-speed centrifugation.

EXTENSIVE PROCESSING

Peripheral blood HPC may be further manipulated in a number of ways. Tumor can be depleted from autologous grafts either actively, by the use of CD34$^+$ progenitor cell enrichment,[66] or by varying the type and timing of mobilization.[67] These stem cells may be infused directly, expanded and differentiated ex vivo, or used as the targets for gene therapy. In the allogeneic setting, T-cell depletion may be used as prophylaxis against GVHD, and may be similarly achieved by active depletion or HPC enrichment.[27]

Most types of extensive processing have been pioneered on marrow grafts, which contain fewer total cell numbers and have a different cellular composition. When these techniques are adapted for use with apheresis collections, the product may be (i) variable in composition, containing higher numbers of 'problem' cells, such as platelets and granulocyte precursors, and (ii) collected over several days requiring decisions on whether separate collections should be stored, pooled and then manipulated.

Autologous collections

The clinical relevance of tumor cells within autologous HPC grafts as a source of relapse of disease remains largely unresolved.[66] Evidence from gene-marking and purging studies, and from retrospective outcome analyses in patients receiving purged versus non-purged marrow grafts, support the hypothesis that removal of tumor from the graft may improve disease-free survival.[66,68] Others have failed to show any benefit to purging, as judged by patterns and incidence of disease relapse in patients receiving tumor-free or overtly contaminated grafts.[66,68] At present, the consensus appears to be in favor of purging or using grafts with an innately lower level of tumor involvement. The level of tumor infiltration in the bone marrow has been found to be consistently higher than in the peripheral blood in a variety of cancers,[66,68,69] making blood-derived grafts an attractive alternative. Studies using paired samples of marrow and peripheral blood HPC have confirmed this observation,[70] although there is no simple relationship between the stage of disease and the incidence of contamination,[70] and there are reports of tumor contamination of apheresis collections from patients who had undetectable marrow involvement.[67] These findings must be interpreted with caution, since they are critically dependent on the sensitivity and reproducibility of the assay that was used, and a negative finding may simply indicate that the tumor is present at levels below the sensitivity of detection. In most cases, immunocytochemical or molecular methods have been used for detection,[70–72] and these provide no information on the proliferative potential of the cells. Clonogenic assays[70,72] can provide this information; however, similar caution must be used in interpretation, since a negative result may indicate that the ex vivo culture conditions could not support tumor cell growth. An additional factor that must be taken into consideration is that the level of tumor contamination must be converted to total tumor burden within the graft. Historically, patients have tended to receive larger total cell numbers of cells when the graft is derived from the blood rather than the marrow. When this is factored into the calculations, the overall tumor burden may approach that in a marrow transplant.[66] This problem can be circumvented, however, by the use of more efficient mobilization regimens, thereby reducing the size of the peripheral blood HPC graft.[66]

An emerging concern is that tumor cells may be recruited into the peripheral circulation by protocols used for HPC mobilization.[66] This has been reported in both epithelial cancers[73] and multiple myeloma,[74] but has not been a universal finding.[75] However, there is increasing use of ex vivo techniques to reduce tumor burden within apheresis products. This has been achieved either by actively depleting the tumor (negative selection)[68] or by specifically enriching the CD34$^+$ cell population (positive selection).[74,76] Numerous techniques are available for each approach,[76] and these have recently been extensively reviewed elsewhere.[66,68] Negative selection is capable of high levels of tumor depletion;[68] however, the procedure is relatively expensive, there can be significant losses of nucleated cells, and most procedures are long and would have to be repeated on each apheresis product. Although storage of products is possible,[64,65] allowing pooling for manipulation, stored cells are frequently more difficult to manipulate.

Enrichment of CD34$^+$ cells provides an attractive alternative, in that there are a number of systems available commercially,[76,77] and these are usually automated and relatively rapid, making daily use more realistic. In general, the results obtained in terms of CD34$^+$ cell yield and purity have been more variable with blood than with marrow,[26] leading to an increased risk of tumor contamination of the product. In addition, there have been reports that certain tumor cells may bear the CD34 antigen,[78] and would co-purify with the stem cell population. Ultimately, combinations of positive and negative selection may achieve optimal levels of tumor depletion,[66] however, the ratio of cost/risk to clinical benefit must be considered when designing these types of extensive manipulations.

Allogeneic collections

Experience in the use of allogeneic peripheral blood HPC is accruing,[19,21,22] and it appears that, despite the approximately 10-fold higher burden of T cells in these grafts,[20] the incidence of acute GVHD is unexpectedly low. This may be achieved at the expense of an increased incidence of chronic GVHD,[22] which is prompting consideration of the use of T-cell depletion. Numerous methods (including positive and negative selection) have been developed for this purpose,[27] although they have been used almost exclusively on bone marrow.[79] There are reports that they can be adapted successfully for the depletion of blood-derived grafts;[27,80] however, careful optimization will be required due to the higher T-cell numbers and different cellular compositions of leukapheresis products.

The use of procedures that achieve tumor cell or T-lymphocyte depletion by extensive purification of HPC raises the concern that potentially beneficial cell subpopulations are also depleted. These may facilitate engraftment and immune reconstitution and/or provide graft-versus-disease activity. This may be of particular concern in peripheral blood HPC, where immunological activity within the graft may explain an increase in failure-free survival in lymphoma patients who received blood-versus-marrow grafts.[81]

CRYOPRESERVATION AND STORAGE

Although there are a few reports that apheresis products may be stored successfully for several days in liquid form,[64,65] the normal practice is to cryopreserve each collection. This requires the addition of a cryoprotectant, to maintain cell integrity, and controlled transition to the storage temperature.[28] Two methods are in widespread use;[28,29] they have been reviewed elsewhere,[28] but are summarized below. In both cases, careful attention should be paid to labeling of the product. It has been difficult to find labels that withstand low-temperature storage and thawing; however, freezing bags are now available that have a top pocket into which the label may be sealed.

DMSO and programmed freezing

In the first method,[28] DMSO alone is used as the cryoprotectant and the cells are frozen using a controlled-rate programmable freezer. The cells are suspended in autologous plasma or in physiological salt solutions containing plasma proteins (e.g. human serum albumin (HSA), 2–4 g%) or plasma protein fraction (0.5% v/v) at *final* concentrations ranging from $3 \times 10^7/ml$ to $8 \times 10^8/ml$. The cells are split into aliquots in freezing bags (e.g. Baxter Cryocyte containers) at volumes that should not exceed half the recommended capacity of the container. To this suspension is slowly added, with mixing, a chilled physiological salt solution containing 20% v/v clinical grade DMSO (Figure 4.7). The bags are heat-sealed and rapidly placed into canisters that maintain the thin-layer configuration of the cell suspension and protect the bags during freezing and storage. The canisters are placed in a controlled-rate freezer (e.g. from Cryomed-Forma, Gordinier or Planer) (Figure 4.8) and are frozen at −1 to −2°C/min to about −50°C, with eutectic-point compensation, and then at −5°C/min to about −90°C, at which

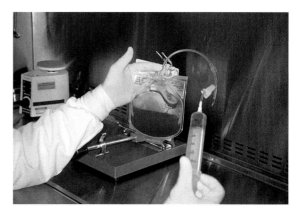

Figure 4.7 Addition of cryopreservation medium to a stem cell product. Freezing medium is added slowly with mixing to the stem cell product (shown here as whole blood to assist visualization). The plasma expressor in the background is used to expel air from the freezing bag prior to sealing, placing into a canister and freezing.

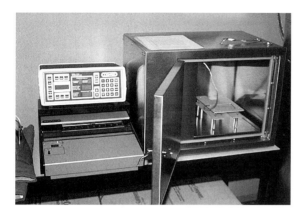

Figure 4.8 Programmable freezer. The canisters containing the product are stacked horizontally in the freezing chamber, shown to the right. Liquid nitrogen is pumped into the chamber to achieve the preprogrammed temperature stored in the control device (upper left). The temperature of the chamber and a 'dummy' product during cryopreservation are printed out by the chart recorder (lower left).

point they are transferred to the liquid or vapor phase of liquid nitrogen for long-term storage. In our laboratory, we have used a simplified protocol in which the chilled product is routinely split into four 60 ml aliquots in Cryocyte bags to each of which is added, with mixing, 6 ml of chilled, undiluted DMSO. This method is faster and results in uniformly high cell viabilities on thawing. Recently, variations have been described in which cells were frozen in 10% DMSO alone and stored at −80°C,[82] or frozen using a methanol bath.[83]

DMSO, starch and 'dump' freezing

In the second technique, the final concentration of DMSO is reduced to 5% v/v and 6% hydroxyethyl starch (HES) is added to the cell suspension, which also contains HSA.[29] The starch solution is prepared by adding 42 g of intermediate-weight HES (obtained in the United States under an FDA investigational new drug exemption from Dupont Chemical Corporation, Wilmington, DE; molecular

weight ~250 000) to 140 ml Normosol (Abbott Laboratories, North Chicago, IL). The solution is autoclaved for 20 minutes, cooled, and aseptically supplemented with 100 ml 25% HSA and 70 ml 50% DMSO; 300 ml of the solution are then added to an equal volume of cells (the final cell concentration should not exceed 1×10^8/ml, to avoid clumping). The suspension is then divided between freezing bags which are placed horizontally in a −80°C freezer for cryopreservation and storage. Although this method is frequently referred to as non-controlled-rate freezing, the cell suspension does in fact cool at a predictable and reproducible rate.

Storage

There is still some controversy regarding the optimal conditions for long-term storage. Successful engraftment has been obtained using HPC stored in liquid nitrogen banks for at least 5 years,[28] and in mechanical freezers at −80°C (in DMSO/HES) for at least $2\frac{1}{2}$ years[29] (P Stiff, personal communication). Storage by immersion in liquid nitrogen provides a greater degree of temperature stability[28] and security in the event of a failure of the nitrogen supply; however, it also provides a means for the transmission of infectious agents between products,[84] and poses increased thermal stress on the freezing bags during banking and removal. The risk of transmission of infections between bags can be reduced by the use of double-bagging or by storage in the vapor phase, or in mechanical freezers equipped with a back-up supply of liquid nitrogen. In all cases, the banks should be fitted with a 24-hour alarm system and the temperature recorded continuously (for mechanical and vapor-phase freezers) or at regular intervals (for liquid-phase freezers).

Frozen products are increasingly being transported between centers, and this activity is likely to increase with the use of allogeneic peripheral blood HPC. This can be achieved using 'dry shippers' in which the temperature can be maintained for several days by liquid nitrogen that has been absorbed into material lining the shipping container. Wherever possible, the shipment should be accompanied by a courier, although most express delivery services will accept these shipments. There have, however, been incidences where such shipments have gone temporarily astray, and the product temperature has not been maintained. For this reason, temperature monitoring indicators should accompany all shipments and form part of the permanent processing record.[35]

THAWING AND REINFUSION

Prior to infusion of the thawed product, the patient should be well hydrated and premedicated with antihistamine to reduce the risk of vascular collapse and hypotension.[85] This may result from DMSO-induced histamine release. Although serious reactions to DMSO are infrequent, they have been reported, and range from cardiovascular effects (bradycardia and hypertension) and encephalopathy,[86] to sudden death.[85] Headache, nausea, vomiting and hematuria are frequently seen. In some centers, the amount of DMSO infused is restricted to 1 g/kg recipient weight on any one occasion.[28,85] In the case of large-volume grafts, it may be necessary to spread infusion over several days or to wash the cells before infusion to remove cryoprotectant and cell debris. This requires slow dilution of the cells to avoid osmotic shock,[28] and the addition of ACD-A to prevent clumping. Washing may result in substantial cell losses.

Thawing is usually achieved rapidly by immersion of the frozen product in a 37–40°C bath. The bath should always be scrupulously clean, and may be filled with sterile water to avoid the risk of product contamination due to water entering the sampling ports of the container. Preparations should be made to deal with bags that rupture during thawing. This may be avoided by allowing canisters stored in the liquid phase to remain in the vapor phase for several hours before removal from the bank, and by not attempting to remove a frozen bag from a canister before immersion in the waterbath. Precautions against loss of the product include the use of double-bagging during thawing, and thawing in a container of prewarmed

sterile saline placed in the water bath. The delay between thawing and infusion should be minimized, and, for that reason, most products are transported frozen to the bedside, thawed rapidly and infused.

Once the product is thawed, it is infused rapidly through a blood administration set. Aggregates resulting from cells that do not survive freezing may be removed by filtration through a 170 µm blood filter.[85] If cells are frozen at high concentrations, ACD-A is frequently added to the thawed product to reduce the risk of cell clumping.[28,85] Deoxyribonuclease may be added to digest aggregates; however, this should be used as a final resort due to the potential for reactions when infused. A pharmaceutical-grade recombinant formulation of this enzyme is now available.[87]

Samples for quality control should be taken directly from the thawed bags, rather than from small vials frozen and stored alongside the product. Tests on these samples should be performed as soon as possible to avoid changes in cell viability.

CONCLUSIONS

The use of blood-derived HPC for transplantation has already revolutionized the way in which these grafts are collected and processed. Sufficient cells can be collected in a single apheresis, and can be relatively easily manipulated, frozen and stored for many years. Future developments will continue to exploit this source of HPC, and promise to simplify further both collection and processing.

ACKNOWLEDGEMENTS

The author thanks Karin Mauldin of the Stem Cell Apheresis Unit, and Carlos Lee and Mary Brouillette of the Stem Processing Laboratory of the Division of Transplantation Medicine at the University of South Carolina for their valuable assistance in the preparation of this chapter.

REFERENCES

1. Armitage JO, Antman KH, *High-Dose Cancer Therapy: Pharmacology, Hematopoietins, Stem Cells.* Baltimore: Williams & Wilkins, 1992.
2. Anasetti C, Hansen J, Bone marrow transplantation from HLA-partially matched related and unrelated volunteer donors. In: *Bone Marrow Transplantation* (Forman SJ, Blume KG, Thomas ED, eds). Boston: Blackwell, 1994: 665–79.
3. Fleming DR, Henslee-Downey PJ, Romond EH et al, Allogeneic bone marrow transplantation with T cell-depleted partially matched related donors for advanced acute lymphoblastic leukemia in children and adults: a comparative matched cohort study. *Bone Marrow Transplant* 1996; **17:** 917–22.
4. Kurtzberg J, Umbilical cord blood: a novel source of hematopoietic stem cells for bone marrow transplantation [Editorial]. *J Hematother* 1996; **5:** 95–6.
5. Keating A, Autologous bone marrow transplantation. In: *High-Dose Cancer Therapy: Pharmacology, Hematopoietins, Stem Cells* (Armitage JO, Antman KH, eds). Baltimore: Williams & Wilkins, 1992: 162–81.
6. Kernan N, T-Cell depletion for the prevention of graft-versus-host disease. In: *Bone Marrow Transplantation* (Forman SJ, Blume KG, Thomas ED, eds). Boston: Blackwell, 1994: 124–35.
7. Horowitz MM, Gale RP, Sondel PM et al, Graft-versus-leukemia reactions following bone marrow transplantation in humans. *Blood* 1990; **75:** 555–62.
8. Rubinstein P, Rosenfield RE, Adamson JV et al, Stored placental blood for unrelated bone marrow reconstitution. *Blood* 1993; **81:** 1679–90.
9. Gratwohl A, Schmitz N, First International Symposium on Allogeneic Peripheral Blood Precursor Cell Transplants. *Bone Marrow Transplant* 1996; **17:** S1–S3.
10. Fliedner TM, Blood stem cell transplantation: from preclinical to clinical models. *Stem Cells* 1995; **13**(Suppl 3): 1–12.
11. Körbling M, Fliedner TM, Historical perspective: the evolution of clinical peripheral blood stem cell transplantation. *Bone Marrow Transplant* 1996; **17:** 675–8.
12. Goodman JW, Hodgson GS, Evidence for stem cells in the peripheral blood of mice. *Blood* 1962; **19:** 702–14.
13. Cavins JS, Scheer SC, Thomas ED, Ferrebee JW, The recovery of lethally irradiated dogs given infusions of autologous leukocytes preserved at −80°C. *Blood* 1964; **23:** 38–43.
14. McCredie K, Hersh EM, Freireich EJ, Cells capable of colony formation in the peripheral blood of man. *Science* 1971; **171:** 293–4.
15. Körbling M, Ross WM, Pliegler H et al, Procurement of human blood stem cells by continuous-flow centrifugation – further comment. *Blood* 1977; **50:** 753–4.
16. Richman CM, Weiner RS, Yankee RA, Increase in circulating stem cells following chemotherapy in man. *Blood* 1976; **47:** 1031–4.
17. Socinski MA, Cannistra SA, Elias A et al, Granulocyte–macrophage colony-stimulating factor expands the circulating progenitor cell compartment in man. *Lancet* 1988; **28:** 1194–8.
18. Schwartzberg LS, Peripheral blood stem cell mobilization in the outpatient setting. In: *Peripheral Blood Stem Cell Autografts* (Wunder EW, Hénon PR, eds). Berlin: Springer-Verlag, 1993: 177–84.
19. Körbling M, Przepiorka D, Hug YO et al, Allogeneic blood stem cell transplantation for refractory leukemia and lymphoma: potential advantage of blood over marrow cells. *Blood* 1995; **85:** 1659–65.
20. Dreger P, Oberböster K, Schmitz N, PBPC grafts from healthy donors: analysis of CD34$^+$ and CD3$^+$ subpopulations. *Bone Marrow Transplant* 1996; **17**(Suppl 2): S22–S27.
21. Bensinger WI, Buckner CD, Demirer T et al, Transplantation of allogeneic peripheral blood stem cells [abstract]. *Bone Marrow Transplant* 1996; **17**(Suppl 2): S56–S57.
22. Champlin RE, Anderlini P, Przepiorka D et al, Allogeneic transplantation of peripheral blood progenitor cells [abstract]. In: *Proceedings of the Fourth International Symposium on Blood Cell Transplantation*, 1996: 18.4.
23. Kessinger A, McMannis JD (eds), *Practical Considerations of Apheresis in Peripheral Blood Stem Cell Transplantation.* Lakewood: COBE BCT, 1994.
24. Bender JG, To LB, Williams SF, Schwartzberg L, Defining a therapeutic dose of peripheral blood stem cells. *J Hematother* 1992; **1:** 329–41.
25. Bender JG, Lum L, Unverzagt KL et al, Correlation of colony-forming cells, long-term culture initiating cells and CD34$^+$ cells in apheresis products from patients mobilized for peripheral blood progenitors with different regimens. *Bone Marrow Transplant* 1994; **13:** 479–85.

26. Heimfeld S, Berenson RJ, Clinical transplantation of CD34+ hematopoietic progenitor cells: Positive selection using a closed, automated avidin–biotin immunoadsorption system. In: *Hematopoietic Stem Cells: The Mulhouse Manual* (Wunder E, Sovalat H, Hénon PR, Serke S, eds). Dayton: AlphaMed Press, 1994: 231–9.

27. Dreger P, Viehman K, Steinmann J et al, G-CSF-mobilized peripheral blood progenitor cells for allogeneic transplantation: Comparison of T cell depletion strategies using different CD34+ selection systems or CAMPATH-1. *Exp Hematol* 1995; **23**: 147–54.

28. Rowley SD, Hematopoietic stem cell cryopreservation: a review of current techniques. *J Hematother* 1992; **1**: 233–50.

29. Stiff PJ, Simplified bone marrow cryopreservation using dimethylsulfoxide and hydroxyethyl starch as cryoprotectants. In: *Bone Marrow Processing and Purging: A Practical Guide* (Gee AP, ed.). Boca Raton: CRC Press, 1991: 341–50.

30. Nowicki B, Sniecinski I, Val H et al, Peripheral blood CD34 % as an indicator for CD34+ cell content in leukapheresis products [abstract]. *J Hematother* 1995; **4**: 239.

31. Fruehauf S, Haas R, Conradt C et al, Peripheral blood progenitor cell (PBPC) counts during steady state hematopoiesis allow to estimate the yield of mobilized PBPC after filgrastim (R-metHuG-CSF)-supported cytotoxic chemotherapy. *Blood* 1995; **85**: 2619–26.

32. Husson B, Ravoet C, Dehon M et al, Predictive value of the steady-state peripheral blood progenitor cell (PBPC) counts for the yield of PBPC collected by leukapheresis after mobilization by granulocyte colony-stimulating factor (G-CSF) alone or chemotherapy and G-CSF [Letter]. *Blood* 1996; **87**: 3526–8.

33. BCSH Blood Transfusion Task Force, Guidelines for the Collection. Processing and Storage of Human Bone Marrow and Peripheral Blood Stem Cells. *Transfus Med* 1994; **4**: 165–72.

34. American Association of Blood Banks, *Standards for Blood Banks and Transfusion Services: Section Q Bone Marrow and Peripheral Blood Progenitor Cells*, 17th edn. Bethesda: American Association of Blood Banks 1996.

35. Foundation for the Accreditation of Hematopoietic Cell Therapy (FAHCT), *Standards for the Collection, Processing and Transplantation of Hematopoietic Progenitor Cells*, 1st edn. Omaha: FAHCT, 1996.

36. Haire WD, Lieberman RP, Lund GB et al, Translumbar inferior vena cava catheters, safety and efficacy in peripheral blood stem cell transplantation. *Transfusion* 1990; **30**: 511–15.

37. Hahn U, Goldschmidt H, Salwender H et al, Large-bore central venous catheters for the collection of peripheral blood stem cells. *J Clin Apheresis* 1995; **10**: 12–16.

38. Haire W, Sniecinski I, Venous access, anticoagulation, and patient care during apheresis. In: *Practical Considerations of Apheresis in Peripheral Blood Stem Cell Transplantation* (Kessinger A, McMannis JD, eds). Lakewood: COBE BCT, 1994.

39. Cassidy MJD, Wood L, Jacobs P, Hypocalcemia during plateletpheresis. *Transfus Sci* 1990; **11**: 217–21.

40. Schouten HC, Kessinger A, Smith DM et al, Counterflow centrifugation apheresis for the collection of autologous peripheral blood stem cells from patients with malignancies: a comparison with a standard centrifugation apheresis procedure. *J Clin Apheresis* 1990; **5**: 140–4.

41. To LB, Stemmelin GR, Haylock DN et al, Collection efficiency on the Fenwal CS3000 when using filgrastim (recombinant methionyl human granulocyte colony-stimulating factor) as a peripheral blood stem cell mobilization agent. *J Clin Apheresis* 1994; **9**: 1991–5.

42. James P, Collection of peripheral blood stem cells on Spectra. *J Clin Apheresis* 1994; **9**: 33–4.

43. Del Monte C, Basso P, Consoli P et al, Collection of peripheral blood stem cells by apheresis with continuous flow blood cell separator DIDECO Vivacell. *Hematologica* 1990; **75**(Suppl 1): 18–21.

44. Pierelli L, Menichella G, Paolini A et al, Evaluation of a novel automated protocol for the collection of peripheral blood stem cells mobilized with chemotherapy plus G-CSF using the Fresenius AS104 cell separator. *J Hematother* 1993; **2**: 145–53.

45. Bender JG, Harvesting of peripheral blood stem cells with the Fenwal CS-3000 Plus® cell separator and a small volume collection chamber. *Int J Cell Cloning* 1992; **10**(Suppl 1): 79–81.

46. Shpall EJ, Sanford C, Hami L et al, A randomized study of the standard versus a new automated leukapheresis procedure using the COBE Spectra™ [abstract]. *Blood* 1996; **88**: 642a.

47. Takaue Y, Kawano Y, Abe T et al, Collection and transplantation of peripheral blood stem cells in very small children weighing 20 kg or less. *Blood* 1995; **86**: 372–80.

48. Hillyer CD, Large-volume leukapheresis to max-

imize peripheral blood stem cell collection. *J Hematother* 1993; **2**: 529–32.

49. Alegre A, Díaz MA, Madero L et al, Large-volume leukapheresis for peripheral blood stem cell collection in children: a simplified single-apheresis approach. *Bone Marrow Transplant* 1996; **17**: 923–7.

50. Menichella G, Pierelli L, Vittori M et al, Five year experience in PBSC collection: results of the Catholic University of Rome. *Int J Artif Organs* 1993; **16**(Suppl 5): 39–44.

51. Hénon PR, Wunder E, Zingsem J, Lepers M, Siegert W, Eckstein R, Collection of peripheral blood stem cells apheresis monitoring and procedure. In: *Peripheral Blood Stem Cell Autografts* (Wunder EW, Hénon PR, eds). Berlin: Springer-Verlag, 1993: 185–93.

52. Breems D, van Hennik PB, Kusadasi N et al, Individual stem cell quality in leukapheresis products is related to the number of mobilized stem cells. *Blood* 1996; **87**: 5370–8.

53. Legros M, Fleury J, Cure H et al, New method for stem cell quantitation: application to the management of peripheral blood stem cell transplantation. *Bone Marrow Transplant* 1995; **15**: 1–8.

54. van der Wall E, Richel DJ, Holtkamp MJ et al, Bone marrow reconstitution after high-dose chemotherapy and autologous peripheral blood cell transplantation: Effect of graft size. *Ann Oncol* 1994; **5**: 795–802.

55. Siena S, Di Nicola M, Danova M et al, Intergroup standardization of absolute CD34$^+$ cell count assay for blood cell transplants for cancer therapy [abstract]. In: *Proceedings of the Fourth International Symposium on Blood Cell Transplantation*, 1996: 6.4.

56. Wunder E, Sovalat H, Fritsch G et al, Report on the European workshop on peripheral blood stem cell determination and standardization. *J Hematother* 1992; **1**: 131–42.

57. Lowdell MW, Bainbridge DR, External quality assurance for CD34 cell enumeration – results of a preliminary national trial. *Bone Marrow Transplant* 1996; **17**: 849–53.

58. Sutherland DR, Anderson L, Keeney M et al, The ISHAGE guidelines for CD34$^+$ cell determination by flow cytometry. *J Hematother* 1996; **5**: 213–26.

59. Olweus J, Lund-Johansen F, Terstappen LWMM, Expression of cell surface markers during differentiation of CD34$^+$, CD38$^{-/lo}$ fetal and adult bone marrow cells. *Immunomethods* 1995; **5**: 179–88.

60. Tricot G, Jagganath S, Vesole D et al, Peripheral blood stem cell transplants for multiple myeloma: identification of favorable variables for rapid engraftment in 22 patients. *Blood* 1995; **85**: 588–96.

61. Osawa M, Hanada K, Hamada H, Nakauchi H, Long-term lymphohematopoietic reconstitution by a single CD34-low/negative hematopoietic stem cell. *Science* 1996; **273**: 242–5.

62. Hénon P, Sovalat H, Becker M et al, Determination of the number of infused CD34$^+$/CD38$^-$ cells for accurate prediction of both early and sustained multilineage hematopoietic engraftment [abstract]. In: *Proceedings of the Fourth International Symposium on Blood Cell Transplantation*, 1996: 10.7.

63. Goldberg SL, Mangan KF, Klumpp TR et al, Complications of peripheral blood stem cell harvesting: review of 554 PBSC leukaphereses. *J Hematother* 1995; **4**: 85–90.

64. Jestice HK, Scott MA, Ager S et al, Liquid storage of peripheral blood progenitor cells for transplantation. *Bone Marrow Transplant* 1994; **14**: 991–4.

65. Ruiz Arguelles GJ, Ruiz Arguelles A, Perez Romano B et al, Filgrastim mobilized peripheral blood stem cells can be stored at 4°C and used in autografts to rescue high-dose chemotherapy. *Am J Hematol* 1995; **48**: 100–3.

66. Gee A, Purging of peripheral blood stem cell grafts. *Stem Cells* 1995; **13**(Suppl 3): 52–62.

67. Carella AM, Frassoni F, Podestá M et al, Idarubicin, intermediate-dose cytarabine, etoposide and granulocyte-colony-stimulating factor are able to recruit CD34$^+$/HLA-DR$^-$ cells during early hematopoietic recovery in accelerated and chronic phases of chronic myeloid leukemia. *J Hematother* 1994; **3**: 199–202.

68. Gee AP, Purging tumor from autologous stem cell grafts. In: *The Clinical Practice of Stem Cell Transplantation* (Barrett J, Treleaven J, eds). Oxford: Isis Medical Media, 1997.

69. Dwenger A, Lindeman A, Mertelsmann R, Minimal residual disease: detection, clinical relevance and novel treatment – a goal within the reach of gene- and immunotherapy. *J Hematother* 1996; **537–48.**

70. Ross AA, Cooper BW, Lazarus HM et al, Detection and viability of tumor cells in peripheral blood stem cell collections from breast cancer patients using immunocytochemical and clonogenic assay techniques. *Blood* 1993; **82**: 2605–10.

71. Moss TJ, To LB, Pantel K, Evaluation of grafts for occult tumor cells [Editorial]. *J Hematother* 1994; **3:** 163–4.

72. Chan WC, Wu GQ, Greiner TC et al, Detection of tumor contamination of peripheral stem cells in patients with lymphoma using cell culture and polymerase chain reaction technology. *J Hematother* 1994; **3:** 175–84.

73. Brugger W, Bross KJ, Glatt M et al, Mobilization of tumor cells and hematopoietic progenitor cells into peripheral blood of patients with solid tumors. *Blood* 1994; **83:** 636–40.

74. Lemoli RM, Fortuna A, Motta MR et al, Concomitant mobilization of plasma cells and hematopoietic progenitors into peripheral blood of multiple myeloma patients: positive selection and transplantation of enriched CD34$^+$ cells to remove circulating tumor cells. *Blood* 1996; **87:** 1625–34.

75. Passos-Coelho JL, Ross AA, Moss TJ et al, Absence of breast cancer cells in a single day peripheral blood progenitor cell collection after priming with cyclophosphamide and granulocyte–macrophage colony-stimulating factor. *Blood* 1995; **85:** 1138–43.

76. de Wynter EA, Coutinho LH, Pei X et al, Comparison of purity and enrichment of CD34$^+$ cells from bone marrow, umbilical cord and peripheral blood (primed for apheresis) using five separation systems. *Stem Cells* 1995; **13:** 524–32.

77. Shpall EJ, Gehling U, Cagnoni P et al, Isolation of CD34-positive hematopoietic progenitor cells. *Immunomethods* 1994; **5:** 197–203.

78. Reading CL, Gazitt Y, Estrov Z, Juttner C, Does CD34$^+$ cell selection enrich malignant cells in B cell (and other) malignancies [Letter]? *J Hematother* 1996; **5:** 97–8.

79. Collins NH, Gee AP, Henslee-Downey PJ, T cell depletion of allogeneic bone marrow transplants by immunologic and physical techniques. In: *Marrow and Stem Cell Processing for Transplantation* (Lasy L, Warkentin P, eds). Bethesda: American Association of Blood Banks, 1995: 149–68.

80. Suzue T, Kawano Y, Takaue Y, Kuroda Y, Cell processing protocol for allogeneic peripheral blood stem cells mobilized by granulocyte colony-stimulating factor. *Exp Hematol* 1994; **22:** 888–92.

81. Verbik DJ, Jackson JD, Pirruccello J et al, Functional and phenotypic characterization of human peripheral blood stem cell harvests: a comparative analysis of cells from consecutive harvests. *Blood* 1995; **85:** 1964–70.

82. Galmes A, Besalduch J, Bargay J et al, A simplified method for cryopreservation of hematopoietic stem cells with −80°C mechanical freezer with dimethylsulfoxide as the sole cryoprotectant. *Leuk Lymphoma* 1995; **17:** 181–4.

83. Hernandez Navarro F, Ojeda E, Arrieta R et al, Single-centre experience of peripheral blood stem cell transplantation using cryopreservation by immersion in a methanol bath. *Bone Marrow Transplant* 1995; **16:** 71–7.

84. Tedder RS, Zuckerman MA, Goldstone AH et al, Hepatitis B transmission from contaminated cryopreservation tank. *Lancet* 1995; **346:** 137–40.

85. Rowley SD, Secondary processing, cryopreservation, and reinfusion of the collected product. In: *Practical Considerations of Apheresis in Peripheral Blood Stem Cell Transplantation* (Kessinger A, McMannis JD, eds). Lakewood: COBE BCT, 1994: 53–62.

86. Dhodapkar M, Goldberg SL, Tefferi A, Gertz MA, Reversible encephalopathy after cryopreserved peripheral stem cell infusion. *Am J Hematol* 1994; **45:** 187–8.

87. Rowley SD, Recombinant human deoxyribonuclease for hematopoietic stem cell processing. *J Hematother* 1995; **4:** 99–104.

5 Clinical results in peripheral blood stem cell autografting

5.1

Chronic myeloid leukaemia

Stephen G O'Brien and John M Goldman

CONTENTS • Introduction • Residual normal cells in CML • Rationale for autografting • Blood versus marrow as source of stem cells • Peripheral blood stem cell mobilization and autografting • Autografting using 'in vivo' purged bone marrow • Current multicentre prospective randomized trials • Prospects for the future

INTRODUCTION

Since the beginning of the decade, there has been renewed interest in the possibility that chronic myeloid leukaemia (CML) patients can be treated effectively with autografting. Allogeneic stem cell transplantation (allo-SCT) remains the only treatment that offers a reasonable chance of long-term disease-free survival – tantamount to 'cure' – but allo-SCT is available to a small proportion of all patients with CML. At present, we can reasonably expect to cure only 15–20% of all CML patients (Figure 5.1.1). A series of prospective studies including large numbers of patients performed in different countries suggest that treatment with interferon-α (IFN-α) in the chronic phase of CML can significantly prolong survival.[1–6] However, although there are occasional case reports of prolonged remissions induced by this agent, molecular evidence of disease persists even in complete cytogenetic responders,[7] and it seems unlikely that IFN-α can routinely cure any patient.

The use of high-dose cytoreduction with autografting may therefore prove superior to IFN-α, but again it is unlikely to cure patients. Whilst many of the autografting data described below are encouraging, no large clinical trials have yet been carried out to address the question whether autografting in CML extends the duration of chronic phase or prolongs survival. Such studies have, however, been implemented, and we should be in a position to answer this important question in due course.

Here we will briefly consider the possible rationale for autografting in CML and then review some of the clinical and laboratory data and explore various autografting methods

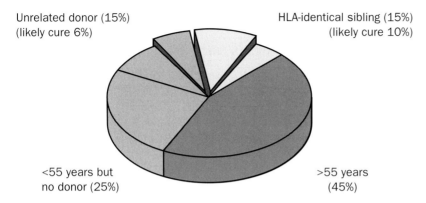

Figure 5.1.1 Eligibility of CML patients for allogeneic bone marrow transplantation. The figure shows an estimate of donor availability and probability of cure as a percentage of all patients with CML, assuming that median age of presentation is 50 years and the average number of siblings in a family is two.[66] About 70% of all CML patients are ineligible for a potentially curative allograft procedure.

Table 5.1.1 Sources of cells for autografting in CML

- Unmanipulated cells:
  PBSC (leukapheresis at diagnosis)
  bone marrow

- In vitro manipulated cells:
  bone marrow
  PBSC

- Mobilized PBSC following chemotherapy
  and/or growth factor

- Bone marrow collected from patients
  rendered Ph-negative

PBSC = peripheral blood stem cells.

(Table 5.1.1). We will identify the more contentious issues and finally suggest a synthesis for how autografting might fit into a general management plan for a patient with CML.

RESIDUAL NORMAL STEM CELLS IN CML

Until recently, autografting has not been widely employed in CML, partly because prolonged cytogenetic remission is rarely obtained and partly because the use of autologous haemopoietic stem cells that are obviously leukaemic might not be expected to benefit the patient. However, the exploration of autografting techniques has been vindicated by recent insights into the biology of CML and the new understanding of some of the features of the haemopoietic stem cell.

A number of different lines of clinical evidence suggest that Philadelphia (Ph)-negative stem cells are present in patients with CML at diagnosis.[8] First, it has been known for some years that some Ph-positive CML patients 'overtreated' with busulphan and a proportion of those treated with combination chemotherapy recover with entirely or predominantly Ph-negative haemopoiesis, which may continue for long periods.[9–14] Results from 'straight' autografting (in which no attempt was made to separate Ph-positive and Ph-negative progenitor cells) have yielded a similar pattern of results in terms of response rates and degree and duration of Ph-negativity.[15,16] Secondly, IFN-α can induce partial or complete cytogenetic responses in CML[1,17] and prolongation of survival has recently been demonstrated in some[2,4] but not all[3] clinical trials. This induction of Ph-negativity must mean that at least a proportion of CML patients have residual Ph-negative haemopoietic cells. Thirdly, it is possible in some cases to mobilize Ph-negative peripheral blood progenitor cells (PBPC) in CML patients using high-dose chemotherapy.[15,18–20] Thus, in summary, these different clinical approaches can all restore some degree of Ph-negativity in about 20–40% of patients with Ph-positive CML.

In vitro data also support the notion that Ph-negative cells survive in CML marrow. Chervenick et al[21] first reported the then surprising finding that some colony-forming unit granulocyte–macrophage (CFU-GM) colonies from CML patients contained Ph-negative metaphases. The Vancouver group have developed this theme further.[22–24] They observed that in some cases marrow cells from CML patients placed into Dexter-type long-term bone-marrow culture produce increasing numbers of Ph-negative haemopoietic cells with time.[25] They then developed a clinical autografting program to exploit these findings (see below). The presence of non-clonal haemopoietic progenitors among cells in such long-term cultures was also supported by analysis of a glucose-6-phosphate dehydrogenase (G6PD) heterozygote.[26] Since it is now generally accepted that the presence of the *BCR–ABL* fusion gene and its transcript is the definitive marker of CML,[27,28] it may be concluded from these in vitro studies that loss of the Ph chromosome and the *BCR–ABL* gene implies a return to non-malignant haemopoiesis. Whilst most data appear to support this statement, there are some confounding observations. For example, about 5% of patients with the clinical syndrome of CML have Ph-negative disease and only about half of these patients have the *BCR–ABL* chimaeric gene.[29] Furthermore, some patients have been described with a clinical CML syndrome who were initially Ph-negative but later had

detectable Ph-positive cells.[30] Some small studies, analysing G6PD heterozygotes, have suggested the presence of clonal Ph-negative cells in Ph-positive CML patients,[31–33] but 'pseudo-clonality' or artefactual skewing towards one or other isoenzyme is a possible explanation. One may therefore conclude that Ph-negative haemopoietic cells are present in a significant proportion of patients with CML and, notwithstanding some of the observations above, they are almost certainly not part of the leukaemic population.

RATIONALE FOR AUTOGRAFTING

Given that some 'normal' haemopoietic stem cells persist in CML patients, there are at least three possible interrelated reasons why autografting might prolong life:

1. If progression from chronic phase to transformation depends in part on 'random' genetic events occurring in primitive *BCR–ABL*-positive stem cells, any manoeuvre that reduced their number might delay transformation.
2. There is some evidence that steps that reduce both normal and leukaemic stem cells to low levels favour regeneration of normal stem cells – at least in the short term; occasionally this proliferative advantage for normal cells is prolonged.[9,10]
3. It may be possible to develop reliable techniques for collection of and subsequent autografting with Ph-negative-enriched or Ph-positive-depleted stem cells from patients with Ph-positive CML.[8,34]

A theoretical objection to the use of autografting in CML is the lack of any 'graft versus leukaemia' (GVL) effect that seems to be an essential component of the curative potential allo-SCT.[35] Some would therefore argue that the best result that could be expected with autografting would be similar to results with syngeneic transplants, where, although there are moderate numbers of long-term disease-free survivors, relapse rates are considerably higher than non-twin allo-SCT. It may well be true that an ongoing immune-mediated antileukaemia effect is a major factor in achieving long-term disease-free survival after allo-SCT, but this syngeneic/auto-BMT comparison is not entirely relevant and ignores the possibilities that a second autograft may be curative or that autografting may modulate the response to IFN-α. Furthermore, if relapse of leukaemia after autografting for CML originated mainly from the grafted cells and not from residual leukaemic haemopoiesis, it is conceivable that improvements in ex vivo purging together with more effective cytoreduction could produce results approaching those presently achieved with allo-SCT but with less procedure-related morbidity and mortality.

BLOOD VERSUS MARROW AS SOURCE OF STEM CELLS

It has been known for many years that, occasionally, patients whose marrow became hypoplastic after treatment with apparently conventional doses of busulphan could, when they recovered, display long periods of completely or partially Ph-negative haemopoiesis.[9,10] These observations and other speculations led workers in the 1970s to explore the proposition that treating patients in chronic phase with high doses of cytotoxic drugs – such as those then in vogue for the treatment of acute myeloid leukaemia – could restore Ph-negativity and prolong life.[12–14] The largest series was reported from the Memorial Sloan Kettering Cancer Center in New York; about one-third of the patients achieved some degree of Ph-negative haemopoiesis: and these patients survived longer than non-responders.[14] It was not clear that this association was causal, and the use of high-dose chemotherapy alone for CML in chronic phase in CML has not been widely adopted.

In parallel with these chemotherapy-only approaches, Buckner and colleagues in Seattle in the early 1970s treated some patients with CML in blastic transformation by high-dose chemoradiotherapy and autografting with marrow cells.[36] These endeavours antedated the widespread use of allogeneic bone-marrow transplantation (BMT) in CML; the approach evolved from experience of autografting in acute myeloid leukaemia. The Hammersmith group in London showed that similar results could be obtained with blood-derived stem cells, and others confirmed these results during the late 1970s and 1980s.[37–39] Some patients were then treated electively by autografting in chronic phase.[16,40] Since then, CML patients in many centres throughout the word have undergone autograft procedures, with various attempted refinements.

Results of autografting using unmanipulated haemopoietic stem cells

A number of recent studies have also addressed the value of 'straight' autografting (i.e. using unmanipulated stem cells) to treat patients with CML in chronic phase. Meloni et al[41] reported a study of 34 patients autografted in chronic phase. All patients engrafted, and there was only one procedure-related death from interstitial pneumonitis. Although the duration of follow-up was short, 31 of the 34 patients were alive at the time of analysis, and 18 of 32 patients evaluated had a reduction in the proportion of Ph-positive marrow metaphases of greater than 50%.[41] At the Hammersmith Hospital, the five-year survival after autografting with unmanipulated blood-derived stem cells for a group of 21 patients was 56%. Eleven of 17 patients studied during the first year posttransplant had some degree of cytogenetic conversion, and there was a suggestion of prolonged survival in this subgroup.[16] The Bordeaux group reported a series of 23 patients with 'poor prognosis' CML (i.e. a Sokal score at diagnosis of greater than 1.2 or no response to IFN-α) who were transplanted with peripheral blood stem cells (PBSC) collected at diagnosis.[42] The three-year probability of transformation-free survival was 67%, a value similar to the Rome and London series. Khouri et al[43] from Houston have recently published details of a larger series of patients ($n = 73$ in total), 22 of whom were transplanted in chronic phase.

These patients were resistant to, or intolerant of, IFN-α. Eighteen achieved a complete haematological response and 5 a partial or complete cytogenetic response. The median survival from transplantation for these 22 patients was 34 months.[43]

McGlave et al[44] conducted an overview analysis of 142 patients autografted for CML in eight major transplant centres. The four-year probability of survival for the selected group of patients transplanted in chronic phase was about 60%, but a more recent analysis of the same patient population showed inferior results. Although patient age affected transplant outcome, neither the source of stem cells (blood or marrow) nor the use of ex vivo purging techniques influenced survival.

In a retrospective analysis from the registry of the European Group for Blood and Bone Marrow Transplantation (EBMT), 174 patients who underwent blood (66%) or marrow (34%) stem cell transplantation during chronic phase have been evaluated[45] (J Reiffers, personal communication). The patients received a variety of cytoreduction regimens and most were treated with IFN-α after transplantation. The actuarial probability of survival at five years was 68.4 ± 11%; it was significantly higher for younger patients and for those who achieved cytogenetic and/or haematological responses following autograft. As with the McGlave overview, the source of stem cells and the use of techniques for purging cells in vitro did not affect the clinical outcome. Interestingly, some patients became responsive to IFN-α following autografting when they had not been so prior to the procedure.

It is important to emphasize that these individual studies and overview analyses can only give the broadest indication of efficacy, and none of the studies cited provides statistically rigorous evidence that autografting can prolong survival. Furthermore, the patients in these studies in whom autografting was carried out were almost universally highly selected and often had had their disease for some time. It is possible that, simply by virtue of having survived a certain length of time with CML, individuals in these studies may be a self-selected group of 'good prognosis' patients. Thus the need for large prospective randomized trials is self-evident.

In vitro techniques for removing Ph-positive stem cells

A number of in vitro methods are currently being used to separate Ph-positive from Ph-negative haemopoietic stem cells in blood or marrow collected from patients with CML (Table 5.1.2). One of the best-studied approaches is that pioneered by the group in Vancouver. They have attempted to exploit the differences in behaviour in 10-day culture between normal and CML cells in order to select normal cells. CML cells appear to be more 'delicate' in such conditions, with the result that normal cells predominate after 10 days in liquid culture. The group have developed an autografting protocol using such cultured cells. Patients were selected by virtue of their ability to generate adequate numbers of long-term culture-initiating cells prior to entry.[46] Over a five-year period, the Vancouver group evaluated 87 patients and selected 36 for the 10-day marrow culture, of whom 22 were autografted. Although 5 patients failed to engraft, 16 were alive up to 68 months post autograft and 5 were in complete or partial cytogenetic remission at the time of their most recent report.[46] The laboratory methods necessary for the 10-day incubation require considerable care and experience, and would not be suitable for general use.

In a study conducted jointly by the Hammersmith Hospital in London and the University of Pennsylvania in Philadelphia, bone-marrow cells have been collected from patients with CML and subjected to an in vitro purging procedure using a 24mer phosphorothioate antisense oligomer directed against codons 2–7 of the human *MYB* proto-oncogene. So far, 12 patients have been recruited to this study, and 4 were entirely or predominantly Ph-negative at the 3-month post-autograft assessment. This Ph-negativity has been transient in all cases, but 1 patient has been followed up for over a year without requiring any further therapy and the study is ongoing.[47,48]

Table 5.1.2 Current and potential approaches to in vitro purging in CML

In vitro purging method	Present status	Reference
Antibodies to BCR–ABL encoded fusion peptides	Basic research	67
Antisense oligonucleotides	Clinical trials recently started in Philadelphia, London and Rome	47, 68–71
Aptameric inhibition of p210[BCR–ABL] tyrosine kinase	Basic research	72
Benzoporphyrin derivative (BPD) photosensitization	Not yet used in clinical practice	73
Chemoprotectants, e.g. MIP-1α	Clinical trial in progress	52
Differential stromal adherence	Small recent pilot study	74, 75
Exploitation of differences in cytokine receptors, e.g. Epo-R	Basic research	76
Hyperthermia $\pm$ drugs	Basic research	77
IFN (alone or in combination) purging	Considerable laboratory evaluation; small clinical pilot study	78, 79
Mafosfamide/4HC	Small clinical trial	80, 81
Oncogene repression by DNA binding protein	Basic research	51
Positive selection on basis of CD34^{+}, HLA DR^{-} phenotype	Good laboratory results in chronic but not advanced-phase disease	82
Ribozyme cleavage of BCR–ABL mRNA	Basic research	83–85
Selective cytotoxicity using alkyl-lysophospholipid	Early studies with patient-derived material	86
Short-term culture	Clinical study running for some time	46
Stimulation of tumoricidal activity with IL-2 and other cytokines	Early in vitro data	87, 88
Various classes of p210[BCR–ABL] tyrosine kinase inhibitors	Basic research; possible clinical trial in the near future	89–91

Few methods have reached clinical trial, and probably the most extensive clinical experience is that of the Vancouver group with short-term marrow culture. Most other approaches are still some way from clinical application. MIP-1α = macrophage inflammatory protein-1α; EpoR = erythropoietin receptor; 4HC = 4-hydroperoxycyclophosphamide.

In Rome, 8 patients with advance-phase CML (7 accelerated phase, 1 second chronic phase) have been treated with a 26mer phosphorothioate oligomer directed symmetrically at the *BCR–ABL* junction. In this study, as in the *MYB* study, the stem cells were purged in vitro before being returned to the patient as an autograft.[49] The purging procedure did not appear to have an adverse effect on engraftment.[50] Between 30 and 100% of marrow metaphases were Ph-negative following the purging procedure, and in 2 patients complete Ph-negativity was achieved post-autograft, albeit transiently. Two further patients achieved a major cytogenetic response, which again was transient. Six patients received IFN-α post-autograft, and it is not possible at present to make any meaningful comment about the impact of this procedure upon survival.

The use of ribozymes, differential stromal adherence, purging with IFN-α or IFN-γ, phenylaminopyrimidine tyrosine kinase inhibitors and purging with mafosfamide is also at the early stage of clinical evaluation (Table 5.1.2). Those methods that target the *BCR–ABL* transcript or its p210 tyrosine kinase product in CML cells are potentially the most specific, but progress has been relatively slow. However, exciting new genetic targeting methods are being investigated.[51]

Another concept for in vitro purging, as well as in vivo usage, is to employ an agent that would preferentially protect normal progenitors from the effects of chemotherapy. Macrophage inflammatory protein-1α (MIP-1α) is a candidate molecule that has an inhibitory effect on normal but not CML progenitors, and may have clinical potential as a protective agent during chemotherapy or for chemotherapeutic purging of CML autograft material.[52] This approach is being evaluated in a clinical trial.

PERIPHERAL BLOOD STEM CELL MOBILIZATION AND AUTOGRAFTING

It has been known for some time that in patients with CML, progenitors released from the marrow into the circulation during the earliest stages of haemopoietic reconstitution following chemotherapy appear to be predominantly Ph-negative (Figure 5.1.2). This may therefore be considered as a form of in vivo stem/progenitor cell purging. These progenitors seem to have the capacity to reconstitute haemopoiesis in an autograft setting – an observation that has been validated in a murine system.[53] Korbling et al, in 1981, were probably the first to clinically explore this concept in CML.[54.] Reiffers et al, in 1985, again evaluated this novel autografting technique.[55] They collected bone marrow from CML patients recovering from chemotherapy-induced marrow aplasia and autografted one patient whose marrow was 25% Ph-positive at the time of collection. A prolonged cytogenetic remission was obtained.[55]

Subsequently, the group in Genoa have further developed this approach. They have the widest experience to date using chemotherapy/growth-factor-mobilized progenitor cell autografts. They have mobilized PBSC from 145 CML patients in total, 79 of whom were in chronic phase[56] (Prof AM Carella, personal communication). They stratified their chronic phase patients as follows: (a) mobilized within 1 year of diagnosis and not pretreated with IFN-α ($n = 31$); (b) pretreated with IFN-α for less than 12 months ($n = 26$); and (c) pretreated with IFN-α for more than 12 months ($n = 22$). Perhaps the most interesting aspect of their data is the results achieved in chronic-phase patients mobilized soon after diagnosis (Table 5.1.3). Seventeen patients received idarubicin, cytarabine and etoposide (ICE) chemotherapy and 14 received reduced-dose 'mini-ICE' (total 31 patients) together with G-CSF starting on day +8 from the end of chemotherapy. There was no serious toxicity and there were no deaths attributable to the mobilization procedure. Eighteen of 31 patients (58%) yielded Ph-negative leukapheresis collections and 7 (23%) yielded predominantly Ph-negative collections (major cytogenetic response). These proportions were much higher than in patients with longer disease duration.[56] Eighteen of these cytogenetic remitters successfully underwent autografting, again with no procedural mortality. Patients

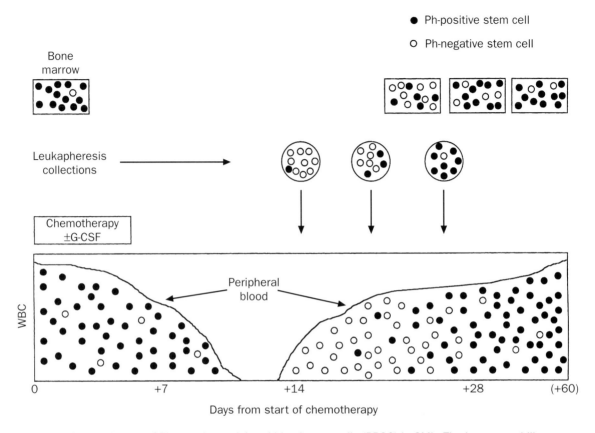

Figure 5.1.2 Mobilization of Ph-negative peripheral blood stem cells (PBSC) in CML. The lower panel illustrates the pattern of peripheral white blood cell (WBC) regeneration following a course of mobilization chemotherapy with or without G-CSF. In many patients, at the earliest stages of regeneration, the peripheral blood contains predominantly or entirely Ph-negative cells. Such Ph-negative cells can be collected either from the bone marrow or from the peripheral blood by leukapheresis. Why predominantly Ph-negative progenitors should be released into the circulation at the beginning of regeneration is currently poorly understood. (Reproduced with permission from F. Frassoni, Genoa.)

were subsequently treated with IFN-α and interleukin-2 (IL-2), and the median survival from autograft was 18 months (range 2–55 months). One patient was lost to follow-up, but 17 maintained a complete haematological remission with 5 in complete cytogenetic remission and 9 in partial cytogenetic remission 3–28 months post-autograft. The benefit of mobilizing early in the course of the disease seems to be borne out in other studies.[57]

A number of other groups are attempting to refine these methods using different chemotherapy and growth factor combinations, PBPC collection technologies and autografting cyto-

reduction regimens[15] (Table 5.1.2). No single protocol has emerged as clearly superior, and the mobilization procedure itself is not without risk. There is much heterogeneity in the ability of patients to mobilize Ph-negative progenitors even in early chronic phase, and even from an individual patient the degree of Ph-negativity can vary between individual collections separated by only a matter of days. Furthermore, as yet there seems to be no way of predicting which patients will respond best. However, the general principle of autografting with mobilized PBPC has been quite widely adopted, and this approach may translate into improved

Table 5.1.3 Overview of some peripheral blood stem cell mobilization/autografting studies in CML: published experience known to the authors at the time of writing

Centre	No. of patients in study	Mobilization regimen	Autografted	Reference
Adelaide	23	Cy, G-CSF	—	92
Birmingham	8 CP, 1 CP3, 2 AP	DAT (10), ICE (1)	6	93
		G-CSF (1)		
Bordeaux	23	G-CSF alone (in IFN responders)	NA	58
Genoa	145 in total 38 BC, 28 AP, 79 CP (31 early CP)	ICE, G-CSF 'Mini-ICE'	(18 in early CP)	56, 94
Glasgow (multicentre)	40 CP	IC(E), G-CSF	20	57, 95
Houston	6 CP, 5 AP	FAM (8) dauno-HDAC (3)	—	20
Leeds	19 CP	HD-HU	7	96
London (London Hospital)	19	IC, G-CSF	8	97
London, Hammersmith	18 CP	IC(E), G-CSF	13	63
London, Marsden	6 CP, 4 AP	ICE, G-CSF	4	98
Mainz	1 BC, 13 CP	IC + G-CSF ± IL-3	0	99
Minneapolis	15	Cy, GM-CSF	15	100
Mulhouse	5 CP, 3 AP	ARP	3	101
Newcastle	16 CP, 1 AP	DOAP	—	102
Palermo	4 CP, 2 AP	Cy	6	103
Woodville, Australia	5	HD-HU	NA	104

AP = accelerated phase; ARP = ara-C, rubidazone, prednisolone; BC = blast crisis; CP = chronic phase; Cy = cyclophosphamide; DAT = daunorubicin, cytarabine and thioguanine; dauno-HDAC = daunorubicin, high-dose ara-C; DOAP = daunorubicin, vincristine, ara-C, prednisolone; FAM = fludarabine, high-dose ara-C, mitoxantrone; HD-HU = high-dose hydroxyurea; IC = idarubicin, ara-C; ICE = idarubicin, cytarabine, etoposide (VP16). Not all ICE regimens use identical doses; 'Mini-ICE' = reduced-dose ICE; NA = data not available.

survival for certain patients with chronic-phase CML.

Ph-negative blood progenitors can be mobilized with haemopoietic growth factors alone without necessarily using additional chemotherapy. Reiffers et al[58] have recently treated 23 patients (either major or complete responders with IFN-α therapy) with G-CSF

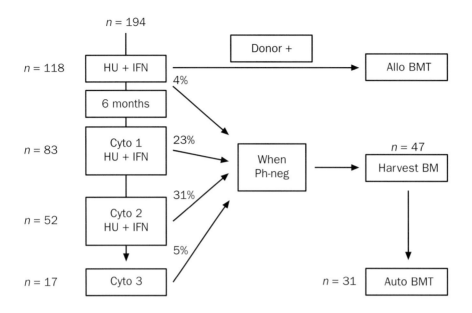

Figure 5.1.3 Design of the Swedish CML Study Group trial. Patients are subjected to treatment regimens of increasing intensity with the aim of inducing Ph-negative haemopoiesis in the bone marrow.[60] Cyto 1, 2 and 3 indicate AML-type regimens of increasing intensity. *n* values indicate the number of patients that have completed each stage of treatment and percentages indicate those in whom bone-marrow Ph-negativity was achieved (see text for details).

(lenograstim 150 µg/m²/day). Leukaphereses performed after 5–12 days of G-CSF contained no Ph-positive metaphases in 57% of cases. Interestingly, Ph-negative collections were obtained in some patients who had not achieved a complete cytogenetic response following IFN-α.[58] Carreras et al[59] have reported similar results suggesting that, at least in some patients, G-CSF may be able to preferentially mobilize Ph-negative cells. As yet, the follow-up on the small number of patients transplanted using such cells is too short to allow meaningful evaluation, but the concept is attractive.

AUTOGRAFTING USING 'IN VIVO' PURGED BONE MARROW

The Swedish CML study group have adopted an interesting alternative approach to so-called in vivo purging (Figure 5.1.3). In a study that opened in 1989, CML patients were subjected to

chemotherapy of increasing intensity with the aim of achieving Ph-negativity in the bone marrow.[60] Once Ph-negativity was achieved, patients proceeded to bone-marrow harvest, which despite a period on IFN-α did not present any technical difficulties; 194 patients have been recruited to this study (Figure 5.1.3). Four percent of the 118 patients who have received IFN-α and hydroxyurea for 6 months became completely Ph-negative. Larger proportions became Ph-negative following subsequent cycles of chemotherapy. Overall, 47 patients achieved Ph-negativity, and 31 of these have undergone autografting with Ph-negative bone marrow. Of these 31, 15 remain completely Ph-negative 35–65 months post transplant, 4 are minimally Ph-positive (<35%), 6 predominantly Ph-positive (>65%) and 6 died (5 in blast crisis) (B Simonsson, personal communication). Although this is clearly a selected group of patients, the outcome of this method of autografting is impressive, and indeed the overall probability of survival at 6 years of all patients entered into the study is equally impressive at 68%. A proportion of all patients entered into the study have undergone allografting, which may significantly modify the survival data. This approach to autografting remains attractive, and a somewhat modified version of this method has been adopted in a prospective randomized trial (see below).

SOME CONTENTIOUS ISSUES

When should patients be autografted?

There are occasional reports of patients who have been autografted soon after diagnosis being rendered Ph-negative for considerable periods of time.[61] Such early application of autografting is somewhat at odds with the traditional much gentler approach to the initial management of CML. However, there may be some merit in this concept, and it seems from some of the recent mobilization studies that outcome is better for those patients treated within the first year.[56] Some haematologists will quite reasonably wish to explore the possibilities of allografting for those of suitable age, but if this option is unavailable, autografting may then be reasonably considered for those under 60–65 years, within one year of diagnosis.

Which patients should be autografted?

There is a small minority of patients who achieve a particularly good response to IFN-α, and in various studies patients achieving a complete cytogenetic remission had a probability of survival at five years in excess of 90%. It would be reasonable to offer newly diagnosed patients a trial period of IFN-α therapy and to suggest that non-responding or poorly responding patients should proceed to an autograft. In addition, there is a suggestion that autografting may be useful in restoring IFN-α sensitivity in patients who had previously been insensitive to IFN-α.[43,45] Given the poor outcome from conventional autografting in blast crisis, it would seem optimal to perform the procedure in chronic phase. There

may be a temporary palliative role in advanced disease (see below).

The relative merits of autografting versus unrelated (or mismatched family donor) allografting can be debated. For patients over the age of 35–40 years, a reasonable case could be made for reserving such high-risk allograft procedures for those who did not respond to IFN-α or autografting.

Which cytoreduction regimen should be used before the autograft?

There is no general agreement as to the optimal approach to cytoreduction. Various combinations and doses of cyclophosphamide, total body irradiation, melphalan and busulphan have been used. Given that the need for profound immunosuppression is less than with allografting, that cure is not the current aim of autografting and that early studies indicate that the autograft material itself is the usual source of relapse,[62] minimal toxicity would seem to be the most pressing concern. At the Hammersmith Hospital, 37 patients have been autografted using busulphan alone (BU-only) for cytoreduction.[63] Although moderately severe mucositis is common, the duration of neutropenia appeared to be shorter than with other regimens, and the outcome was no worse than with more intensive regimens. BU-only is being increasingly adopted by other centres and is being used in multicentre trials.

Is there a role for autografting in accelerated phase/blast crisis?

Autografting in patients with transformed disease is generally unsuccessful, but one new approach to palliation in such patients involves 'mini-autografting' whereby patients are treated with intermediate doses of busulphan (8 mg/kg over 4 days) before autografting.[64] This approach may avoid the toxicity usually associated with higher-dose acute-leukaemia-type treatment and reduces the time the patient spends in hospital. The procedure can be repeated if successful.

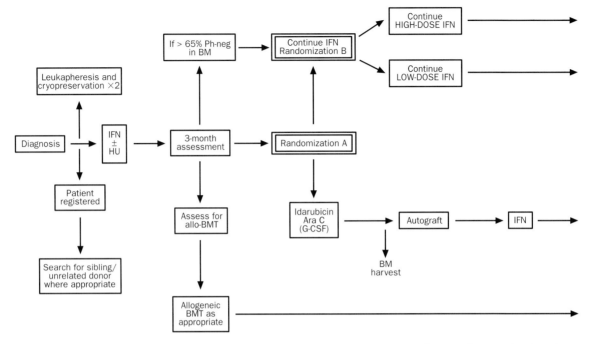

Figure 5.1.4 United Kingdom Medical Research Council (MRC) and United States Eastern Cooperative Oncology Group (ECOG)-designed prospective study to compare a modified autograft procedure followed by IFN-α with standard or low-dose IFN-α.[65] The 'best responders' to IFN-α are excluded from randomization by an initial trial of IFN-α. BM = bone marrow; BMT = bone-marrow transplantation; Ara C = cytosine arabinoside; IFN = interferon.

CURRENT MULTICENTRE PROSPECTIVE RANDOMIZED TRIALS

There are at least two multicentre prospective randomized trials underway to evaluate autografting in CML. The European Group for Blood and Marrow Transplantation (EBMT) has implemented a study comparing autografting with IFN-α. The IFN-α may be given with or without cytarabine. The autograft is performed either with unmanipulated blood stem cells or with cells collected by leukapheresis in the recovery phase after high-dose chemotherapy. The United Kingdom Medical Research Council (MRC) and the United States Eastern Cooperative Oncology Group (ECOG) have designed a prospective study to compare a modified autograft procedure followed by IFN-α with standard or low-dose IFN-α (Figure 5.1.4).[65] The 'best responders' to IFN-α are excluded from randomization by an initial trial of IFN-α. Both these studies should come to

fruition by the year 2003 and should provide long-overdue answers to a number of important questions in CML.

PROSPECTS FOR THE FUTURE

There may well be very exciting developments in the area of autologous stem cell purging, particularly as genetically targeted approaches evolve. These may offer the possibility of considerably reducing or eliminating leukaemia from the autograft material. Harvesting stem cells from patients rendered Ph-negative on IFN-α is increasingly being explored, and sequential double autografting (collecting mobilized PBSC following the first autograft to be used for the second) may have some merit. Only time, and large prospective randomized trials, will tell if autografting can prolong survival in CML.

REFERENCES

1. Ozer H, George SL, Schiffer CA et al, Prolonged subcutaneous administration of recombinant alpha 2b interferon in patients with previously untreated Philadelphia chromosome-positive chronic-phase chronic myelogenous leukemia: effect on remission duration and survival: Cancer and Leukemia Group B study 8583. *Blood* 1993; **82:** 2975–84.

2. The Italian Cooperative Study Group on Chronic Myeloid Leukemia, Interferon alfa-2a as compared with conventional chemotherapy for the treatment of chronic myeloid leukemia. *N Engl J Med* 1994; **330:** 820–5.

3. Hehlmann R, Heimpel H, Hasford J et al, Randomized comparison of interferon-alpha with busulfan and hydroxyurea in chronic myelogenous leukemia (CML). *Blood* 1994; **84:** 4064–77.

4. Allan NC, Richards SM, Shepherd PCA, UK Medical Research Council randomised, multi-centre trial of interferon-alpha n1 for chronic myeloid leukaemia: improved survival irrespective of cytogenetic response. *Lancet* 1995; **345:** 1392–7.

5. Guilhot F, Chastang C, Michallet M et al, Interferon alfa-2b combined with cytarabine versus interferon alone in chronic myelogenous leukemia. *N Engl J Med* 1997; **337:** 223–9.

6. CML Trials Collaborative Group, Interferon alpha versus chemotherapy for chronic myeloid leukemia: a meta analysis of 7 randomized trials. *J Natl Cancer Inst* 1997 (in press).

7. Hochhaus A, Lin F, Reiter A et al, Quantification of residual disease in chronic myelogenous leukemia patients on interferon-alpha therapy by competitive polymerase chain reaction. *Blood* 1996; **87:** 1549–55.

8. Dunbar CE, Stewart FM, Separating the wheat from the chaff: selection of benign hematopoietic cells in chronic myeloid leukemia [Editorial]. *Blood* 1992; **79:** 1107–10.

9. Finney R, McDonald GA, Baikie AG, Douglas AS, Chronic granulocytic leukaemia with Ph 1 negative cells in bone marrow and a ten year remission after busulphan hypoplasia. *Br J Haematol* 1972; **23:** 283–8.

10. Weinberger A, Benjamin D, Douer D, Barabash G, Djaldetti M, Pinkhas J, A 13-years remission in chronic myelocytic leukemia after a single course of busulphan. *Acta Haematol* 1978; **59:** 354–9.

11. Smalley RV, Vogel J, Huguley CM, Jr, Miller D, Chronic granulocytic leukemia: cytogenetic conversion of the bone marrow with cycle-specific chemotherapy. *Blood* 1977; **50:** 107–13.

12. Sharp JC, Joyner MV, Wayne AW et al, Karyotypic conversion in Ph1-positive chronic myeloid leukaemia with combination chemotherapy. *Lancet* 1979; **i:** 1370–2.

13. Cunningham I, Gee T, Dowling M et al, Results of treatment of Ph-positive chronic myelogenous leukemia with an intensive regimen (L-5 protocol). *Blood* 1979; **53:** 375–95.

14. Goto T, Nishikori M, Arlin Z et al, Growth characteristics of leukemic and normal hematopoietic cells in Ph-positive chronic myelogenous leukemia and effects of intensive treatment. *Blood* 1982; **59:** 793–808.

15. O'Brien SG, Goldman JM, Autografting in chronic myeloid leukaemia. *Blood Rev* 1994; **8:** 63–9.

16. Hoyle CF, Gray R, Goldman JM, Autografting for patients with CML in chronic phase: an update. *Br J Haematol* 1994; **86:** 76–81.

17. Talpaz M, Kantarjian HM, Kurzrock R, Interferon-alpha produces sustained cytogenetic responses in chronic myelogenous leukemia. *Ann Intern Med* 1991; **114:** 532–8.

18. Carella AM, Gaozza E, Raffo MR et al, Therapy of acute phase chronic myelogenous leukemia with intensive chemotherapy, blood cell autotransplant and cyclosporine A. *Leukemia* 1991; **5:** 517–21.

19. Carella AM, Podesta M, Frassoni F et al, Collection of 'normal' blood repopulating cells during early hemopoietic recovery after intensive conventional chemotherapy in chronic myelogenous leukemia. *Bone Marrow Transplant* 1993; **12:** 267–71.

20. Kantarjian HM, Talpaz M, Hester J et al, Collection of peripheral blood diploid cells from chronic myelogenous leukemia patients early in the recovery phase from myelosuppression induced by intensive chemotherapy. *J Clin Oncol* 1995; **13:** 553–9.

21. Chervenick PA, Ellis LD, Pan SF, Lawson AL, Human leukemic cells: in vitro growth of colonies containing the Philadelphia (Ph) chromosome. *Science* 1971; **174:** 1134–6.

22. Coulombel L, Kalousek DK, Eaves CJ, Gupta CM, Eaves AC, Long-term marrow culture reveals chromosomally normal hematopoietic

progenitor cells in patients with Philadelphia chromosome-positive chronic myelogenous leukemia. *N Engl J Med* 1983; **306**: 1493–8.

23. Dube ID, Kalousek DK, Coulombel L et al, Cytogenetic studies of early myeloid progenitor compartments in Ph1-positive chronic myeloid leukemia. II. Long-term culture reveals the persistence of Ph1-negative progenitors in treated as well as newly diagnosed patients. *Blood* 1984; **63**: 1172–7.

24. Petzer AL, Eaves CJ, Lansdorp PM et al, Characterization of primitive subpopulations of normal and leukemic cells present in the blood of patients with newly diagnosed as well as established chronic myeloid leukemia. *Blood* 1996; **88**: 2162–71.

25. Turhan AG, Humphries RK, Eaves CJ et al, Detection of breakpoint cluster region-negative and nonclonal hematopoiesis in vitro and in vivo after transplantation of cells selected in cultures of chronic myeloid leukemia marrow. *Blood* 1990; **76**: 2404–10.

26. Hogge DE, Coulombel L, Kalousek DK et al, Nonclonal hemopoietic progenitors in a G6PD heterozygote with chronic myelogenous leukemia revealed after long-term marrow culture. *Am J Hematol* 1987; **24**: 389–94.

27. Daley GQ, Van Etten RA, Baltimore D, Blast crisis in a murine model of chronic myelogenous leukemia. *Proc Natl Acad Sci USA* 1991; **88**: 11 335–8.

28. Gishizky ML, Johnson-White J, Witte ON, Efficient transplantation of *BCR–ABL*-induced chronic myelogenous leukemia-like syndrome in mice. *Proc Natl Acad Sci USA* 1993; **90**: 3755–9.

29. Martiat P, Michaux JL, Rodhain J, Philadelphia-negative (Ph⁻) chronic myeloid leukemia (CML): comparison with Ph⁺ CML and chronic myelomonocytic leukemia. *Blood* 1991; **78**: 205–11.

30. Lisker R, Casas L, Mutchinick O, Perez Chavez F, Labardini J, Late-appearing Philadelphia chromosome in two patients with chronic myelogenous leukemia. *Blood* 1980;**56**: 812–14.

31. Fialkow PJ, Martin PJ, Najfeld V et al, Evidence for a multistep pathogenesis of chronic myelogenous leukemia. *Blood* 1981; **58**: 158–63.

32. Ferraris AM, Canepa L, Melani C et al, Clonal B lymphocytes lack bcr rearrangement in Ph-positive chronic myelogenous leukaemia. *Br J Haematol* 1989; **73**: 48–50.

33. Raskind WH, Ferraris AM, Najfeld V et al, Further evidence for the existence of a clonal Ph-negative stage in some cases of Ph-positive chronic myelocytic leukemia. *Leukemia* 1993; **7**: 1163–7.

34. O'Brien SG, Goldman JM, Current approaches to hemopoietic stem cell purging in chronic myeloid leukemia. *J Clin Oncol* 1995; **13**: 541–6.

35. Gale RP, Butturini A, How do transplants cure chronic myelogenous leukemia? [Editorial]. *Bone Marrow Transplant* 1992; **9**: 83–5.

36. Buckner CD, Stewart P, Clift RA et al, Treatment of blastic transformation of chronic granulocytic leukemia by chemotherapy, total body irradiation and infusion of cryopreserved autologous marrow. *Exp Hematol* 1978; **6**: 96–109.

37. Goldman JM, Catovsky D, Hows JM et al, Cryopreserved peripheral blood cells functioning as autografts in patients with chronic granulocytic leukaemia in transformation. *Br Med J* 1979; **i**: 1310–13.

38. Haines ME, Goldman JM, Worsley AM et al, Chemotherapy and autografting for chronic granulocytic leukaemia in transformation: probable prolongation of survival for some patients. *Br J Haematol* 1984; **58**: 711–21.

39. Goldman JM, Catovsky D, Goolden AWG et al, Buffy coat autografts for patients with chronic granulocytic leukaemia in transformation. *Blut* 1981; **42**: 149–55.

40. Brito-Babapulle F, Bowcock SJ, Marcus RE et al, Autografting for patients with chronic myeloid leukaemia in chronic phase: peripheral blood stem cells may have a finite capacity for maintaining haemopoiesis. *Br J Haematol* 1989; **73**: 76–81.

41. Meloni G, de Fabritiis P, Alimena F et al, Autologous bone marrow transplantation or peripheral blood stem cell transplantation for patients with chronic myelogenous leukemia in chronic phase. *Bone Marrow Transplant* 1990; **4**(Suppl 4): 92–4.

42. Reiffers J, Cahn JY, Montrastruc M et al, Peripheral blood stem cell transplantation followed by recombinant alpha interferon for chronic myelogenous leukemia in chronic phase: preliminary results. *Stem Cells Dayt* 1993; **11**: 23–4.

43. Khouri IF, Kantarjian HM, Talpaz M et al, Results with high-dose chemotherapy and unpurged autologous stem cell transplantation in 73 patients with chronic myelogenous leukemia: the MD Anderson experience. *Bone Marrow Transplant* 1996; **17**: 775–9.

44. McGlave PB, de Fabritiis P, Deisseroth A et al, Autologous transplants for chronic myelogenous leukaemia: results from eight transplant groups. *Lancel* 1994; **343:** 1486–8.

45. Reiffers J, Goldman JM, Meloni JM et al, Autologous stem cell transplantation in chronic myelogenous leukemia: a retrospective analysis of the European Group for Bone Marrow Transplantation. *Bone Marrow Transplant* 1994; **14:** 407–10.

46. Barnett MJ, Eaves CJ, Phillips GL et al, Autografting with cultured marrow in chronic myeloid leukemia: results of a pilot study. *Blood* 1994; **84:** 724–32.

47. Luger SM, Ratajczak MZ, Stadtmauer EA et al, Autografting for chronic myeloid leukemia (CML) with C-MYB antisense oligodeoxynucleotide purged bone marrow: a preliminary report [Abstract]. *Blood* 1994; **84**(Suppl 1): 151a.

48. O'Brien SG, Gewirtz AM, Rule SA et al, Autografting for CML using bone marrow purged with MYB antisense oligonucleotide [Abstract]. *Exp Hematol* 1995; **23:** 804.

49. de Fabritiis P, Montefusco M, Avvisati G et al, Bone marrow purging with BCR–ABL antisense oligonucleotides and autograft for patients with chronic myelogenous leukaemia. *Bone Marrow Transplant* 1995; **15**(Suppl 2): S107.

50. de Fabritiis P, Amadori S, Petti MC et al, In vitro purging with BCR–ABL antisense oligodeoxynucleotides does not prevent haematologic reconstitution after autologous bone marrow transplantation. *Leukemia* 1995; **9:** 662–4.

51. Choo Y, Sanchez-Garcia I, Klug A, In vivo repression by a site-specific DNA-binding protein designed against an oncogenic sequence. *Nature* 1994; **372:** 642–5.

52. Dunlop DJ, Wright EG, Lorimore S et al, Demonstration of stem cell inhibition and myeloprotective effects of SCI/rhMIP1 alpha in vivo. *Blood* 1992; **79:** 2221–5.

53. Craddock CF, Apperley JF, Wright EG et al, Circulating stem cells in mice treated with cyclophosphamide. *Blood* 1992; **80:** 264–9.

54. Korbling M, Burke P, Braine H et al, Successful engraftment of blood derived normal hemopoietic stem cells in chronic myelogenous leukemia. *Exp Hematol* 1981; **9:** 684–90.

55. Reiffers J, Maraninchi D, Marit G et al, Autologous transplantation of Ph-positive cell depleted marrow in chronic granulocytic leukemia. In: *Autologous Bone Marrow Transplantation* (Dicke K, Spitzer G, Jagannath S, eds). Houston: The University of Texas MD Anderson Hospital and Tumor Institute, 1987: 199–203.

56. Carella AM, Chimirri F, Podesta M et al, High-dose chemo-radiotherapy followed by autologous Philadelphia chromosome-negative blood progenitor cell transplantation in patients with chronic myelogenous leukemia. *Bone Marrow Transplant* 1996; **17:** 201–5.

57. Chalmers EA, Franklin IM, Kelsey SM et al, Duration of chronic phase correlates with the ability to mobilize peripheral blood stem cells in chronic myeloid leukemia. *Exp Hematol* 1995; **23:** 791–9.

58. Reiffers J, Taylor K, Gluckman E et al, Ph-negative blood progenitor cells can be successfully collected with lenograstim in patients with chronic myeloid leukemia good responders to alpha-interferon [Abstract]. *Bone Marrow Transplant* 1996; **17**(Suppl 1).

59. Carreras E, Sierra J, Rovira M et al, Successful autografting in chronic myeloid leukaemia using Philadelphia-negative blood progenitor cells mobilized with rHu G-CSF alone in a patient responding to alpha-interferon. *Br J Haematol* 1997; **96:** 421–3.

60. Simonsson B, Oberg G, Killander A et al, Intensive treatment in order to minimize the Ph-positive clone in chronic myelogenic leukemia (CML). *Bone Marrow Transplant* 1994; **14**(Suppl 3): S55–S56.

61. Brito-Babapulle F, Apperley JF, Rassool F et al, Complete remission after autografting for chronic myeloid leukaemia. *Leuk Res* 1987; **11:** 1115–7.

62. Deisseroth AB, Zu Z, Claxton D et al, Genetic marking shows that Ph[+] cells present in autologous transplants of chronic myelogenous leukemia (CML) contribute to relapse after autologous bone marrow in CML. *Blood* 1994; **83:** 3068–76.

63. O'Brien SG, Apperley JF, Szydlo R et al, High dose busulfan alone as cytoreduction before autografting in chronic myeloid leukemia – a feasibility study [Abstract]. *Blood* 1996; **88:** 200b.

64. Rule SA, Savage D, O'Brien SG et al, Intermediate dose busulphan before autografting for advanced phase chronic myeloid leukaemia. *Br J Haematol* 1996; **94:** 694–8.

65. Spencer A, O'Brien SG, Goldman JM, Options for therapy in chronic myeloid leukaemia. *Br J Haematol* 1995; **91:** 2–7.

66. Goldman JM, Management of chronic myeloid leukaemia. *Blood Rev* 1994; **8:** 21–9.

67. van Denderen J, ten Hacken P, Berendes P et al, Antibody recognition of the tumor-specific b3–a2 junction of bcr–abl chimeric proteins in Philadelphia-chromosome-positive leukemias. *Leukemia* 1992; **6:** 1107–12.

68. Ratajczak MZ, Hijiya N, Catani L et al, Acute- and chronic-phase chronic myelogenous leukemia colony-forming units are highly sensitive to the growth inhibitory effects of c-myb antisense oligodeoxynucleotides. *Blood* 1992; **79:** 1956–61.

69. Kirkland MA, O'Brien SG, McDonald C, Davidson RJ, BCR–ABL antisense purging in chronic myeloid leukaemia [Letter]. *Lancet* 1993; **342:** 614.

70. de Fabritiis P, Lisci E, Montefusco M et al, Autograft after in vitro purging with BCR–ABL antisense oligonucleotides for patients with CML in advanced phase. *Bone Marrow Transplant* 1994; **14**(Suppl 3): S80.

71. O'Brien SG, Rule SA, Ratajczak MZ et al, Autografting for CML using bone marrow purged with MYB antisense oligonucleotide [Abstract]. *Br J Haematol* 1995; **89**(Suppl 1): 12.

72. Bergan RC, Kyle E, Connell Y, Neckers L, Inhibition of protein-tyrosine kinase activity in intact cells by the aptameric action of oligodeoxynucleotides. *Antisense Res Dev* 1995; **5:** 33–8.

73. Keating A, Jamieson C, Hornby A et al, Photodynamic elimination of clonogenic Ph$^+$ chronic myeloid leukemia cells. *Leuk Lymphoma* 1993; **11**(Suppl 1): 265–9.

74. Carlo Stella C, Mangoni L, Piovani G et al, Identification of Philadelphia-negative granulocyte–macrophage colony-forming units generated by stroma-adherent cells from chronic myelogenous leukemia patients. *Blood* 1994; **83:** 1373–80.

75. Rizzoli V, Mangoni L, Piovani G et al, Fractionation of chronic myelogenous leukemia marrow cells by stroma adherence: implications for marrow purging. *Leuk Lymphoma* 1993; **11**(Suppl 1): 109–12.

76. Wognum AW, Krystal G, Eaves CJ et al, Increased erythropoietin-receptor expression on CD34-positive bone marrow cells from patients with chronic myeloid leukemia. *Blood* 1992; **79:** 642–9.

77. Osman Y, Moriyama Y, Shibata A, Enhanced elimination of Ph$^+$ chromosome cells in vitro by combined hyperthermia and other drugs (AZT, IFN-alpha and quercetin): its application to autologous bone marrow transplantation for CML. *Exp Hematol* 1995; **23:** 444–52.

78. McGlave PB, Arthur D, Miller WJ et al, Autologous transplantation for CML using marrow treated ex vivo with recombinant human interferon gamma. *Bone Marrow Transplant* 1990; **6:** 115–20.

79. Carlo Stella C, Cazzola M, Ganser A et al, Synergistic antiproliferative effect of recombinant interferon-gamma with recombinant interferon-alpha on chronic myelogenous leukemia hematopoietic progenitor cells (CFU-GEMM, CFU-Mk, BFU-E, and CFU-GM). *Blood* 1988; **72:** 1293–9.

80. Carlo Stella C, Mangoni L, Piovani G et al, In vitro marrow purging in chronic myelogenous leukemia: effect of mafosfamide and recombinant granulocyte–macrophage colony-stimulating factor. *Bone Marrow Transplant* 1991; **8:** 265–73.

81. Rizzoli V, Mangoni L, Douay L et al, Pharmacological-mediated purging with mafosfamide in acute and chronic myeloid leukemias. The Italian Study Group. *Prog Clin Biol Res Exp Hematol* 1989; **17:** 429–32.

82. Verfaillie CM, Miller WJ, Boylan K, McGlave PB, Selection of benign primitive hematopoietic progenitors in chronic myelogenous leukemia on the basis of HLA-DR antigen expression. *Blood* 1992; **79:** 1003–10.

83. Snyder DS, Wu Y, Wang JL et al, Ribozyme-mediated inhibition of *bcr–abl* gene expression in a Philadelphia chromosome-positive cell line. *Blood* 1993; **82:** 600–5.

84. Leopold LH, Shore SK, Newkirk TA et al, Multi-unit ribozyme-mediated cleavage of *bcr–abl* mRNA in myeloid leukemias. *Blood* 1995; **85:** 2162–70.

85. James H, Mills K, Gibson I, investigating and improving the specificity of ribozymes directed against the *BCR–ABL* translocation. *Leukemia* 1996; **10:** 1054–64.

86. Verdonck LF, Witteveen EO, van Heugten HG et al, Selective killing of malignant cells from leukemic patients by alkyl-lysophospholipid. *Cancer Res* 1990; **50:** 4020–5.

87. Verma UN, Bagg A, Brown E, Mazumder A, Interleukin-2 activation of human bone marrow in long-term cultures: an effective strategy for purging and generation of anti-tumor cytotoxic effectors. *Bone Marrow Transplant* 1994; **13:** 115–23.

88. Charak BS, Agah R, Gray D, Mazumder A, Interaction of various cytokines with interleukin 2 in the generation of killer cells from human bone marrow: application in purging of leukemia. *Leuk Res* 1991; **15:** 801–10.

89. Anafi M, Gazit A, Zehavi A et al, Tyrphostin-induced inhibition of p210bcr–abl tyrosine kinase activity induces K562 to differentiate. *Blood* 1993; **82:** 3524–9.

90. Geissler JF, Roesel JL, Meyer T et al, Benzopyranones and benzothiopyranones: a class of tyrosine protein kinase inhibitors with selectivity for the v-abl kinase. *Cancer Res* 1992; **52:** 4492–8.

91. Druker BJ, Tamura S, Buchdunger E et al, Effects of a selective inhibitor of the Abl tyrosine kinase on the growth of Bcr–Abl positive cells. *Nature Medicine* 1996; **2:** 561–6.

92. Hughes TP, Grigg A, Szer J et al, Mobilization of predominantly Philadelphia chromosome-negative blood progenitors using cyclophosphamide and rHUG-CSF in early chronic-phase chronic myeloid leukaemia: correlation with Sokal prognostic index and haematological control. *Br J Haematol* 1997; **96:** 635–40.

93. Butler M, Larkins S, Kyei Mensah P et al, Peripheral blood stem cells (PBSC) harvested post-chemotherapy for autologous bone marrow transplantation (ABMT) in chronic granulocytic leukaemia. *Stem Cells Dayt* 1993; **11**(Suppl 1): 135.

94. Carella AM, Cunningham I, Lerma E et al, Mobilization and transplantation of Philadelphia-negative peripheral-blood progenitor cells early in chronic myelogenous leukemia. *J Clin Oncol* 1997; **15:** 1575–82.

95. Chalmers EA, Franklin IM, Kelsey S et al, Treatment of chronic myeloid leukaemia in chronic phase with idarubicin and cytarabine: mobilisation of Ph-negative peripheral blood stem cells [Abstract]. *Br J Haematol* 1997; **96:** 627–34.

96. Johnson RJ, Owen RG, Child JA et al, Mobilization of Philadelphia-negative peripheral blood mononuclear cells in chronic myeloid leukaemia using hydroxyurea and G-CSF (figrastim). *Br J Haematol* 1996; **93:** 863–8.

97. Hazel DL, Kelsey SM, Baksh N et al, Peripheral blood stem cell transplantation (PBSCT) for chronic granulocytic leukaemia [Abstract]. *Br J Haematol* 1996; **93**(Suppl 1): 17.

98. Mehta J, Mijovic A, Powles R et al, Myelosuppressive chemotherapy to mobilize normal stem cells in chronic myeloid leukemia. *Bone Marrow Transplant* 1996; **17:** 25–9.

99. Aulitzky WE, Neubauer A, Kolbe K et al, Preliminary results of stem cell mobilization in chronic myeloid leukemia with a moderate intensity chemotherapy regimen and G-CSF or G-CSF plus IL-3. *Bone Marrow Transplant* 1996; **17**(Suppl 3): S67–S69.

100. McGlave PB, Bhatia R, Verfaillie C, Cyclophosphamide/GM-CSF priming in auto-transplant therapy for CML. *Bone Marrow Transplant* 1996; **17**(Suppl 3): S65–S66.

101. Henon PR, Eisenmann JC, Becker M et al, Difficulties in collecting peripheral blood stem cells in chronic myeloid leukemia related to persistence of the leukemic cell clone. *Stem Cells Dayt* 1993; **11**(Suppl 3): 43–7.

102. Storey N, Lennard AL, Dickinson AM et al, Is there a future for peripheral blood progenitor cell mobilisation and transplantation in CML? [Abstract]. *Br J Haematol* 1996; **93**(Suppl 1): 15.

103. Tringali S, Santoro A, Scime R et al, High-dose cyclophosphamide for mobilization of circulating stem cells in chronic myeloid leukemia. *Eur J Haematol* 1994; **53:** 1–5.

104. Kuss BJ, Sage RE, Shepherd KM et al, High dose hydroxyurea in collection of Philadelphia chromosome-negative stem cells in chronic myeloid leukaemia. *Leuk Lymphoma* 1993; **10:** 73–8.

5.2

Acute myeloid leukaemia

Gérald Marit, Jean-Michel Boiron and Josy Reiffers

CONTENTS • **Introduction** • **Mobilization–collection** • **Haematological reconstitution** • **Survival of patients** • **Conclusion**

INTRODUCTION

Blood cell transplantation (BCT) has become the standard form of autologous transplantation. For example, 8243 autologous transplants were performed in Europe in 1995, 6504 of them with blood stem cells alone (79%) and only 1384 using bone marrow (17%); 355 other patients having been transplanted with both bone marrow and blood cells.[1] However, for patients with acute leukaemias, the number of patients undergoing BCT was lower ($n = 485$) than that of patients undergoing bone-marrow transplantation (BMT) ($n = 563$). Therefore, BCT is not yet the standard for leukaemic patients who need an autologous transplantation. Many factors could explain these differences between leukaemic patients and those with other haematological malignancies. They include the difficulty in mobilizing sufficient numbers of blood stem cells in some patients with acute myeloid leukaemia (AML), and consequently the existence of delayed engraftment in these poor mobilizers, the possible adverse effects of granulocyte colony-stimulating factor (G-CSF) or of granulocyte–macrophage colony-stimulating factor (GM-CSF) when used to improve chemotherapy-induced mobilization, and finally the possibility of an increase in the risk of leukaemic relapse following BCT as compared with BMT. Other factors could contribute to the lack of enthusiasm for BCT in patients with acute lymphoblastic leukaemia (ALL), since most ALL patients are children, for whom blood cell collection has some technical drawbacks requiring more expertise than blood cell collection in adults.

In this chapter, we summarize the main data concerning blood cell mobilization and collection, haematological reconstitution following BCT, and clinical results for patients with AML. We conclude that BCT has more advantages over BMT than disadvantages. Acute lymphoblastic leukaemia is not discussed, since very few publications to date have concerned BCT in this disease.

MOBILIZATION–COLLECTION

In leukaemic patients with AML, as in patients with other malignant diseases, blood cells can be mobilized by using chemotherapy alone, chemotherapy followed by haematopoietic growth factors (HGF) and more recently HGF alone. During the late 1980s, the Adelaide

Group in Australia and our own group reported that intensive chemotherapy such as that used as induction chemotherapy in AML was able to dramatically increase the concentration of granulocyte–macrophage precursors (CFU-GM) during haematopoietic recovery following chemotherapy-induced marrow aplasia. For example in 1984, To et al[2] reported that a mean 25-fold increase in levels of CFU-GM was observed after induction chemotherapy (as the patients achieved complete remission).[2] Leukaphereses performed during this recirculation period made it possible to collect $(15–60) \times 10^4$ CFU-GM/kg.[2] In the first two patients that we treated during the same period with a very intensive consolidation during first remission, we were able to collect 128.5 and 9.3×10^4 CFU-GM/kg respectively.[3] A few years later, and as found in other reports,[4] we noted that blood cell mobilization was significantly influenced by the number of chemotherapy courses administered to AML patients before collection,[5] and subsequently that the yield of blood cells to be collected was significantly higher after induction chemotherapy than after intensification/consolidation or during relapse treatment.[6] For example, after induction chemotherapy for de novo AML, we found that the highest recorded peak level of CFU-GM was 2274/ml (median; 1133–3796), and was higher than that observed after similar chemotherapy regimens given for relapse treatment or consolidation (median 1286/ml; 240–2279).[7] Some results have also suggested that for AML patients, the combination of an anthracycline with standard doses of cytosine arabinoside (Ara-C) is a better mobilizing treatment than other chemotherapy regimens such as those including high-dose Ara-C.[8]

A large interpatient variability in the number of CFU-GM collected was found in most studies.[9] This could be due, at least in some cases, to interlaboratory variations in methods used to assay CFU-GM and to assess post-thaw viability. However, interpatient variability could also be seen within the same institution for patients mobilized under homogeneous conditions. We observed in our institution that the total number of CFU-GM collected with six leukaphere-

ses could vary from 9.4×10^4 to 190.5×10^4/kg although the patients were mobilized with the same induction chemotherapy.[6] However, although the number of cells collected could be variable, it could be predicted by several factors such as the duration of thrombocytopenia following chemotherapy,[5] a synchronous recovery of monocytes and platelets,[8] and the absolute number of circulating monocytes at the time of blood collection.[10]

When HGF became available, they were successfully combined with chemotherapy to increase the yield of cells harvested in patients with non-myeloid diseases.[11,12] However, as HGF such as G-CSF or GM-CSF could be responsible for leukaemic growth, they were not used in patients with AML for many years. In fact, G-CSF or GM-CSF were used for blood cell collection in AML after it was reported that their administration following induction or consolidation chemotherapy was not followed by an increase in the risk of leukaemia relapse.[13] However, up to now, very few studies have reported the results of blood cell collection after chemotherapy and G-CSF. In the studies by the Bordeaux–Grenoble–Marseille–Toulouse (BGMT) Cooperative Group, 13 patients received during first remission high-dose Ara-C (3 g/m²/12 h; 4 days) and daunorubicin (45 mg/m²/day; 3 days) followed by G-CSF (lenograstim, 263 μg/day). The median numbers of CFU-GM and CD34$^+$ cells collected were 36.5×10^4/kg (range 2–129) and 12.7×10^6/kg (range 5.8–79.8) respectively, and were significantly higher than those observed in a similar group of patients mobilized with the same chemotherapy without G-CSF[7] (Table 5.2.1). More recently, Lévy et al[14] and Reichle et al[15] reported similar numbers of cells collected after mobilization with Ara-C and anthracyclines plus G-CSF. As for CFU-GM collected after chemotherapy alone, a very large interpatient variability was seen in these studies (Table 5.2.1).

The administration of G-CSF (or GM-CSF) during steady state to mobilize and collect blood stem cells is not routinely used in AML, unlike in patients with other types of cancer. In the report by Demirer et al,[16] 15 patients with AML in first or second complete remission (CR)

Table 5.2.1 Number of CFU-GM and CD34$^+$ cells collected in AML patients after different types of mobilization

Type of mobilization[a]	CFU-GM ($\times 10^4$/kg)	CD34$^+$ cells ($\times 10^6$/kg)	Ref
Induction chemotherapy	76.7 (9.4–190.5)	Not done	6
High-dose Ara-C + DNR	14.6 (0.3–29.4)	5.9 (1.3–16.3)	7
High-dose Ara-C + DNR + G-CSF	36.5 (2–129)	12.7 (5.8–79.8)	7
Intermediate-dose Ara-C + ANT + G-CSF	88.1 (0.5–520)	2.3 (0.1–27.3)	14
TAD + G-CSF	13.8 (0.1–28.5)	1.3 (1–2.9)	15
G-CSF (16–32 µg/kg)	Not given	4.8 (0.04–34.8)	16

[a]ANT = anthracycline; DNR = daunorubicin; Ara-C = aracytine; TAD = thioguanine + aracytine + DNR.

were given G-CSF at a dose of 16 ($n = 13$) or 32 ($n = 2$) µg/kg/day × 4–7 subcutaneously. Two to five (median of four) leukaphereses performed after the third dose of G-CSF made it possible to collect 4.81×10^6 CD34-positive cells/kg (range 0.04–34.8). This number is similar to that obtained after mobilization with chemotherapy and lower doses of G-CSF (see above).

Blood cell collection in children with AML needs more technical expertise than in adults, especially in very small children weighing less than 20 kg,[17] but the techniques used for mobilization are similar to those used for adults.[18] Takaue et al[18] reported patients who were treated with high-dose Ara-C alone or followed by lenograstim, and concluded that an increase in the progenitor yields was observed in heavily pretreated children when lenograstim was combined with chemotherapy. They also observed that the use of growth factors could decrease the volume of blood to be processed.[18]

HAEMATOLOGICAL RECONSTITUTION (Table 5.2.2)

Most initial reports on successful haematological reconstitution following BCT have con-

cerned patients with AML.[19–21] In these patients who were given myeloablative conditioning regimens including total body irradiation (TBI), it was demonstrated that chemotherapy-mobilized blood stem cells were able to restore a complete and sustained haematopoiesis, and that this haematological reconstitution was probably quicker than that observed after autologous BMT. In the retrospective analysis of the EBMT registry, the median time to recovery to 0.5×10^9 neutrophils/l was 15.5 days after BCT (range 9–60) and was significantly shorter than that observed after unpurged BMT (median 27 days; range 9–389).[22] In the report by Körbling et al[23] comparing BCT and purged BMT in standard risk AML, the median time to reach 0.5×10^9 neutrophils/l was 14 versus 42 days respectively. However, following BCT, some patients were reported to have a very delayed platelet engraftment, so the median time for platelet reconstitution was not statistically different between BMT and chemotherapy-mobilized BCT.[22,23] In some other cases, haematological reconstitution appeared to be unstable, since after a platelet transfusion independence was achieved within 15–20 days, there was a subsequent drop in the platelet count lasting several weeks or months.[24] Such delayed or

Table 5.2.2 Patients with AML undergoing autologous transplantation: haematopoietic recovery (according to the source of stem cells)

	ANC 500[a]	P1 20 000[a]	Reference
Purged BMT	42 (not given)	46 (not given)	23
Unpurged BMT	27 (9–389)	50 (10–700)	22
Chemotherapy-mobilized BCT	15.5 (9–60)	58.5 (11–713)	22
	14 (not given)	30 (not given)	23
	13 (11–51)	92 (12–293)[b]	41
HGF + chemotherapy-mobilized BCT	15 (11–35)	16 (8–153)	31
	14 (10–27)	11 (5–210)	14
	14 (11–55)	57 (10–635)[b]	30
HGF-mobilized BCT	12 (8–27)	15 (8–103)	17

[a] ANC 500 and P1 20 000 signify the median number of days to achieve an absolute neutrophil count and platelet count of 500 and 20 000/mm^3 respectively.
[b] Time to recover 50 000 platelets/mm^3.

unstable platelet reconstitution was preferentially seen in patients transplanted with fewer than 25×10^4/kg CFU-GM, and, was rarely observed in patients transplanted for other haematological malignancies.[24,25] The unstable engraftment seen in some AML patients has been considered by some investigators as an indirect demonstration that blood stem cells might not contain very primitive progenitors with a self-renewal capacity. These authors have suggested that the early phase of haematopoietic reconstitution following BCT is due to mature blood precursors, but that long-term haematopoiesis is due to endogenous primitive progenitors that have been spared by the conditioning regimen.[25] However, it has been shown that this hypothesis is invalid, since after transplantation of CD34$^+$ blood cells transduced with a retroviral marking gene, the marker gene persisted for over 18 months post transplantation, suggesting that progeny of mobilized blood cells contribute in the long term to engraftment.[26]

The factors capable of influencing significantly haematological reconstitution after BCT have been analysed in some reports. They include those found to influence blood cell mobilization and collection as well as other disease-related (remission or relapse), patient-related (age or sex) or transplant-related variables (conditioning regimen).[27,28] In a series of 118 patients transplanted in our institution, we found that the use of busulfan prior to BCT had a negative influence on the rate of neutrophil and platelet reconstitution. However, the most important factor was the dose of progenitor cell infused.[28] This was confirmed in other studies, and so a minimum threshold of about $(15–25) \times 10^4$/kg CFU-GM to ensure a safe stable and complete engraftment was proposed.[25,29]

The kinetics of haematological reconstitution

has changed with the use of HGF as part of the mobilizing treatment. In our institution, we have performed BCT in 11 patients with AML in first CR who were included in the BGMT 91 prospective study. These patients were given busulfan (4 mg/kg/day × 4) and melphalan (140 mg/m^2) before the reinfusion of blood cells mobilized with both chemotherapy (high-dose Ara-C + daunorubicin) and G-CSF (lenogras-tim 263 µg/day).[7] The median number of days to reach $0.5 \times 10^9/l$ polymorphonuclears (PMN) and $50 \times 10^9/l$ platelets was 14 (range 11–55) and 57 days (range 10–635), and was not significantly shorter than that observed after chemotherapy-mobilized BCT.[30] In the study by Schiller et al,[31] in 48 patients mobilized with high-dose Ara-C (2 g/m^2 × 8), mitoxantrone (10 mg/m^3/day × 3) and G-CSF (5 µg/kg/day) and transplanted after a preparatory regimen consisting of TBI and cyclophosphamide (60 mg/kg/day × 2), haematopoietic recovery was observed after a median number of 15 (range 11–35) and 16 days (range 8–153) for achieving more than 500 neutrophils/mm^3 and 20 000 platelets/mm^3 respectively. In the series by Demirer et al,[16] haematopoietic recovery was achieved within 12 (median, 8–27) and 15 days (median, 8–103) for PMN and platelets respec-tively. In most of the latter studies, HGF were not administered after transplant; however, it is probable that G-CSF is able to significantly shorten the duration of neutropenia (by 2–3 days) as well as that shown in patients under-going BCT for non-AML diseases.[32] As for chemotherapy-mobilized BCT, the dose of CFU-GM and CD34$^+$ cells infused was the most significant factor that significantly affected haematopoietic recovery.

SURVIVAL OF PATIENTS

When blood stem cells were initially proposed for use instead of bone marrow to perform autologous transplants, the hypothesis was that their use could lead to a decrease in the risk of relapse, since they could be less contaminated by residual leukaemic cells than their marrow counterparts. Many years later, neither this hypothesis nor its contrary has been verified: first it is still uncertain whether relapse is due to failure to eradicate all leukaemic cells from the patient or to the re-infusion of malignant cells present in the graft (as suggested by gene-marking studies); second, it is not known if tumour contamination in AML is greater or lesser in the blood than in bone marrow. Although many biological studies have com-pared tumour contamination in bone marrow versus peripheral blood in patients with multi-ple myeloma, non-Hodgkin's lymphoma or breast cancer, few studies have been performed in AML. Using culture or cytogenetic studies, conflicting results have been reported on the presence of residual leukaemic cells within leukapheresis products.[33,34] With more recent and sensitive molecular techniques, residual leukaemic cells have been found in blood sam-ples from patients with AML or ALL during remission,[35,36] but it is not known whether or not this contamination is greater or lesser than in bone marrow.

Therefore the question whether the source of stem cells to be used for transplantation can affect the survival of patients can only be exam-ined from the results of clinical studies. In 15 patients transplanted in our institution for AML in second CR, the three-year relapse incidence (RI) and disease-free survival (DFS) were 60 ± 28% and 37 ± 26% (95% confidence inter-val, CI) respectively.[7] These results look similar to those usually reported with purged or unpurged BMT.

In patients with AML in first CR, the results are very difficult to analyse. Some preliminary reports involving a low number of patients have suggested that the RI could be higher after BCT than BMT. Laporte et al[37] reported four patients transplanted with blood cells, of whom three had relapsed within four months from transplant. Mehta et al[38] also reported four patients who presented early relapse after BCT and suggested that the higher cell dose used for BCT (with more residual leukaemic cells) could explain an increase in the RI. Körbling et al[23] reported 20 patients transplanted with unpurged blood cells for whom the two-year DFS was 35% (14–56%; 95% CI) and was lower (although not significantly) than that observed in a group of 23 patients with similar characteristics transplanted during the same period with mafosfamide-purged marrow.

Two larger series of patients have more recently been published. Sanz et al[39] have transplanted 24 AML patients with blood cells reinfused after a preparatory regimen of busulfan (4 mg/kg/day $\times$ 4) and cyclophosphamide (200 mg/kg). Actuarial DFS and RI at 30 months were 35 (25–45%; 95% CI) and 60% (50–72%; 95% CI) respectively.[39] In the study by Schiller et al,[31] 48 patients were transplanted with blood cells after TBI and cyclophosphamide; after a median follow-up of 24 months, 29 of them were still in continuous CR. Interestingly, in this latter study, although blood cells were collected after mobilization with chemotherapy and G-CSF (whereas G-CSF was not used in other studies), the incidence of relapse was not higher than that observed in the studies where G-CSF was not used for mobilization.[23,37–39] From these studies, there are no apparent differences in the long-term results of BCT versus BMT for AML patients in first CR. To address this point in a larger number of patients, we retrospectively reviewed the data of 1393 patients reported in the European Blood and Marrow Transplantation (EBMT) registry.[40] They underwent either BCT (n = 100) or BMT (n = 1293). The two-year RI and DFS were more favourable after BMT (51 $\pm$ 2% and 43 $\pm$ 1% respectively) than after BCT (44 $\pm$ 6% and 50 $\pm$ 6%) but the differences were not statistically significant (p = 0.12 and 0.045). Using multivariate analysis, the source of stem cells did not significantly influence the RI or DFS, showing that the poorer results observed after BCT were due to the presence of unfavourable prognostic factors in the population of BCT patients (greater age and shorter interval between CR and transplant);[40] when we compared the BCT patients with a double number of patients undergoing BMT and matched for the main prognostic factors (age, FAB morphology, intervals between diagnosis and CR or CR

and transplant), there was no statistically significant difference between BCT and BMT for RI, DFS or overall survival. Moreover, this study did not show any prognostic factor significantly influencing the survival of BCT patients. The use of G-CSF for mobilization or the number of chemotherapy courses given before stem cell collection did not significantly affect RI or DFS. However, prospective studies are needed to better compare BCT and BMT. In the prospective multicentric BGMT 87 study, the patients who were randomized to receive autologous stem cell transplantation were transplanted with blood stem cells in Bordeaux (n = 16) and bone marrow (n = 17) in the other centres. As reported elsewhere,[41] there was no statistical difference in the RI or DFS of the patients according to the origin (blood or marrow) of stem cells. A recent update of these results drew similar conclusions in that the three-year DFS and RI were similar after BCT (52.3 $\pm$ 12.1% and 43.7 $\pm$ 12.4%, respectively) and after BMT (56.3 $\pm$ 12.4% and 46.4 $\pm$ 9.8% respectively).[42] In the prospective BGMT 91 study, similar results were observed for patients undergoing BCT or BMT, since the actuarial percentage of patients surviving at three years without disease was 53.6 $\pm$ 18% and 47.2 $\pm$ 10.4% respectively. A summary of results observed in the BGMT 87 and 91 studies is shown in Figure 5.2.1.

CONCLUSION

Although there is a large interpatient variability, blood stem cells can be easily collected in AML patients in first remission after a mobilization with intensive chemotherapy and HGF (or even HGF alone). The use of blood cells has the advantage of a quicker neutrophil and platelet engraftment, which could lead to a decrease in morbidity but not mortality. The long-term survival of patients after either BMT or BCT is similar.

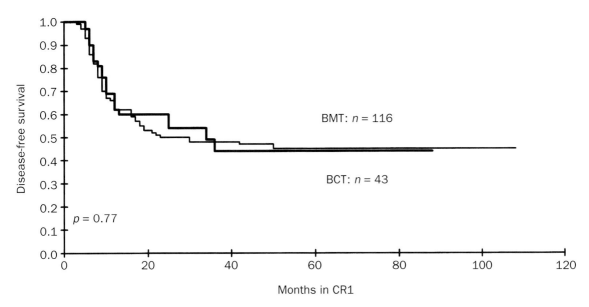

Figure 5.2.1 Disease-free survival of patients undergoing BCT (43 patients) or BMT (116 patients) in the prospective BGMT 87 and BGMT 91 studies. Patients aged ≤55 years.

REFERENCES

1. Gratwohl A, Hermans J, Baldomero H, for the EBMT, Blood and marrow transplantation activity in Europe 1995. *Bone Marrow Transplant* 1997; **19**: 407–19.

2. To LB, Haylock DN, Kimber RJ, Juttner CA, High levels of circulating hemopoietic stem cells in very early remission from acute non-lymphoblastic leukemia and their collection and cryopreservation. *Br J Haematol* 1984; **58**: 399–410.

3. Bernard Ph, Reiffers J, Vezon G et al, Collection of circulating haemopoietic cells after chemotherapy in acute non-lymphocytic leukaemia. *Br J Haematol* 1985; **61**: 577–8.

4. Reid CDL, Kirk A, Muir J, Chanarin I, The recovery of circulating progenitor cells after chemotherapy in AML and ALL and its relation to the rate of bone marrow regeneration after aplasia. *Br J Haematol* 1989; **72**: 21–7.

5. Reiffers J, Vezon G, Bernard Ph et al, Collection of circulating granulocyte–macrophage precursors in patients with acute nonlymphocytic leukemia. *Plasma Ther Transfus Technol* 1986; **7**: 93–5.

6. Reiffers J, Vezon G, Bernard Ph et al, Stem cell apheresis in patients with acute nonlymphocytic leukemia. *Plasma Ther Transfus Technol* 1988; **9**: 115–18.

7. Reiffers J, Peripheral blood stem cell transplantation in acute myeloid leukemia: the experience of the Bordeaux Group. *Stem Cells* 1985; **13**(Suppl 3): 19–22.

8. Cantin G, Marchand-Laroche D, Bouchard MM, Leblond PF, Blood-derived stem cell collection in acute nonlymphoblastic leukemia: predictive factors for a good yield. *Exp Hematol* 1989; **17**: 991–6.

9. To LB, Juttner CA, Peripheral blood stem cell autografting: a new therapeutic option for AML? *Br J Haematol* 1987; **66**: 285–8.

10. Tilly H, Vannier JP, Jean P et al, Daily evaluation of circulating granulocyte–monocyte progenitors during bone marrow recovery from induction therapy in acute leukemia. *Leuk Res* 1986; **10**: 353–6.

11. Gianni AM, Siena S, Bregni M et al, Granulocyte–macrophage colony-stimulating factor to harvest circulating hemopoietic stem

cells for auto-transplantation. *Lancet* 1989; **ii:** 580–5.

12. Socinski MA, Cannistra SA, Elias A et al, Granulocyte–macrophage colony stimulating factor expands the circulating hemopoietic progenitor cell compartment in man. *Lancet* 1988; **i:** 1194–8.

13. Ohno R, Tomonaga M, Kobayashi T et al, Effect of granulocyte colony stimulating factor after intensive induction therapy in relapsed or refractory acute leukemia: a randomized controlled study. *N Engl J Med* 1990; **323:** 871–6.

14. Lévy V, Rio B, Belhocine R et al, Autologous stem cell transplantation (APSCT) with G-CSF primed peripheral blood in acute myelogenous leukemia (AML) in first complete remission (CRI). *Blood* 1996; **88**(Suppl 1): 238b.

15. Reichle A, Hennemann B, Meidenbauer N et al, Peripheral blood stem cell transplantation (PBSCT) during consolidation treatment of de novo acute myelogenous leukemia. *Blood* 1996; **88**(Suppl 1): 287b.

16. Demirer T, Petersen FB, Bensinger WI et al, Autologous transplantation with peripheral blood stem cells collected after granulocyte colony-stimulating factor in patients with acute myelogenous leukemia. *Bone Marrow Transplant* 1996; **18:** 29–34.

17. Takaue Y, Kawano Y, Abe T et al, Collection and transplantation of peripheral blood stem cells in very small children weighing 20 kg or less. *Blood* 1995; **86:** 372–80.

18. Takaue Y, Peripheral blood stem cell autografts for the treatment of childhood cancer: a review of the Japanese experience. *J Hematother* 1993; **2:** 513–18.

19. Juttner CA, To LB, Haylock DN et al, Circulating autologous stem cells collected in very early remission from acute non-lymphoblastic leukemia produce prompt but incomplete hemopoietic reconstitution after high dose melphalan or supralethal chemoradiotherapy. *Br J Haematol* 1985; **61:** 739–45.

20. Castaigne S, Calvo F, Douay L et al, Successful haematopoietic reconstitution using autologous peripheral blood mononucleated cells in a patient with acute promyelocytic leukaemia. *Br J Haematol* 1986; **63:** 209–11.

21. Reiffers J, Bernard P, David B et al, Successful autologous transplantation with peripheral blood haemopoietic cells in a patient with acute leukaemia. *Exp Hematol* 1986; **14:** 312–15.

22. Reiffers J, Körbling M, Labopin M et al, Autologous blood stem cell transplantation versus autologous bone marrow transplantation for acute myeloid leukemia in first complete remission. *Int J Cell Clon* 1992; **10**(Suppl 1): 111–13.

23. Körbling M, Fliedner TM, Holle R et al, Autologous blood stem cell (ABSCT) versus purged bone marrow transplantation (pABMT) in standard risk AML: influence of source and cell composition of the autograft on hemopoietic reconstitution and disease-free survival. *Bone Marrow Transplant* 1991; **7:** 343–9.

24. To LB, Haylock DN, Dyson PG et al, An unusual pattern of hemopoietic reconstitution in patients with acute myeloid leukemia transplanted with autologous recovery phase peripheral blood. *Bone Marrow Transplant* 1990; **6:** 109–14.

25. Reiffers J, Marit G, Vezon G et al, Autologous blood stem cell grafting in hematological malignancies. Present status and future directions. *Transfus Sci* 1992; **13:** 399–405.

26. Dunbar CE, Cottler-Fox M, O'Shaughnessy JA et al, Retrovirally marked CD34-enriched peripheral blood and bone marrow cells contribute to long-term engraftment after autologous transplantation. *Blood* 1995; **85:** 3048–57.

27. Reiffers J, Castaigne S, Tilly H et al, Hematopoietic reconstitution after autologous blood stem cell transplantation: a report of 46 cases. *Plasma Ther Transfus Technol* 1987; **8:** 360–2.

28. Reiffers J, Faberes C, Boiron JM et al, Peripheral blood progenitor cell transplantation in 118 patients with hematological malignancies: analysis of factors affecting the rate of engraftment. *J Hematother* 1994; **3:** 185–91.

29. To LB, Dyson PG, Juttner CA, Cell-dose effect in circulating stem cell autografting. *Lancet* 1986; **ii:** 404–5.

30. Reiffers J, Boiron JM, Cony-Makhoul P et al, Peripheral blood stem cell transplantation in acute myeloid leukemia. In: *Acute Leukemias. VI: Prognostic Factors and Treatment Strategies* (Buchner T et al, eds). Berlin: Springer-Verlag, 1997: 438–42.

31. Schiller G, Miller T, Lee M et al, Transplantation of autologous peripheral blood progenitor cells procured after high-dose cytarabine/G-CSF-based consolidation for adults with acute myelogenous leukemia in first complete remission. *Blood* 1996; **88**(Suppl 1): 127a.

32. Spitzer G, Adkins D, Spencer V et al, Randomized study of growth factors post-peripheral-blood stem-cell transplant: neutrophil recovery is improved with modest clinical bene-

fit. *J Clin Oncol* 1994; **12:** 661–70.

33. To LB, Russell J, Moore S, Juttner CA, Residual leukemia cannot be detected in very early remission peripheral blood stem cell collections in acute non-lymphoblastic leukemia. *Leuk Res* 1987; **11:** 327–30.

34. Castagnola C, Bonfichi M, Colombo A et al, Acute nonlymphocytic leukemia: evidence of clonogenic cells in peripheral blood in early complete remission. *Acta Haematol* 1989; **82:** 210–12.

35. Nagafuji K, Harada M, Takamatsu Y et al, Evaluation of leukaemic contamination in peripheral blood stem cell harvests by reverse transcriptase polymerase chain reaction. *Br J Haematol* 1993; **85:** 578–83.

36. Craig JIO, Langlands K, Parker AC, Anthony RS, Molecular detection of tumor contamination in peripheral blood stem cell harvests. *Exp Hematol* 1994; **22:** 898–902.

37. Laporte JP, Gorin NC, Feuchtenbaum J et al, Relapse after autografting with peripheral blood stem cells [Letter]. *Lancet* 1987; **ii:** 1393.

38. Mehta J, Powles R, Shinghal S et al, Peripheral blood stem cells transplantation may result in increased relapse of acute myeloid leukaemia due to reinfusion of a higher number of malignant cells. *Bone Marrow Transplant* 1995; **15:** 652–3.

39. Sanz MA, de la Rubia J, Sanz GF et al, Busulfan plus cyclophosphamide followed by autologous blood stem-cell transplantation for patients with acute myeloblastic leukemia in first complete remission: a report from a single institution. *J Clin Oncol* 1993; **11:** 1661–7.

40. Reiffers J, Labopin M, Sanz M et al, The source of stem cells does not affect the outcome of patients undergoing autologous stem cell transplantation for acute myeloid leukemia in first remission. *Blood* 1996; **88**(Suppl 1): 684a.

41. Reiffers J, Stoppa AM, Attal M, Michallet M, Is there a place for blood stem cell transplantation for the younger adult patient with acute myelogenous leukemia? *J Clin Oncol* 1994; **12:** 1100–1.

42. Reiffers J, Incidence of relapse following blood stem cell transplantation for acute myeloid leukemia in first remission. *Bone Marrow Transplant* 1996; **18:** 899–900.

5.3

Lymphoma

Philip J Bierman and James O Armitage

CONTENTS • **Introduction** • **Transplantation for non-Hodgkin's lymphoma** • **Transplantation for Hodgkin's disease** • **Comparison of ABMT and PBSCT** • **Early transplantation** • **Preparative regimens** • **Future directions**

INTRODUCTION

A substantial proportion of patients with Hodgkin's disease and non-Hodgkin's lymphoma will relapse or fail to attain a complete remission with initial chemotherapy. Only a small percentage of these patients will be cured with conventional salvage chemotherapy regimens.[1–4] These results have led to the increasing use of high-dose therapy followed by autologous bone marrow transplantation (ABMT) for patients with relapsed and refractory lymphoma. This approach is based upon the steep dose–response curves exhibited by many chemotherapeutic agents against lymphoma.[5] ABMT allows escalation of chemotherapy and radiation doses severalfold over what would otherwise lead to lethal myelosuppression.

Reports dating back nearly 40 years document attempts at using ABMT to abrogate the effects of chemotherapy- or radiation-induced myelosuppression.[6–8] However, techniques for bone marrow harvesting and cryopreservation were not refined, and interest in the use of ABMT to treat lymphomas did not increase until reports from the National Cancer Institute documented apparent cures in refractory lymphoma patients following high-dose chemo-

therapy and reinfusion of cryopreserved autologous bone marrow.[9,10]

The first unsuccessful reports of transplantation using hematopoietic progenitors obtained from the peripheral blood of identical twins appeared nearly 20 years ago.[11,12] These reports were followed by successful reconstitution of hematopoiesis for patients with solid tumors and lymphoma.[13,14]

The use of ABMT and autologous peripheral blood stem cell transplantation (PBSCT) has increased rapidly. Approximately 5000 patients with non-Hodgkin's lymphoma and 2000 patients with Hodgkin's disease have been registered with the North American Autologous Blood and Marrow Transplant Registry. The use of peripheral blood as a rescue source has surpassed the use of autologous bone marrow. A survey of European transplant activity in 1995 reported that approximately 2200 autologous transplants had been performed for non-Hodgkin's lymphoma, and approximately 900 for Hodgkin's disease.[15] Although autologous bone marrow and peripheral blood stem cells were frequently combined, the use of autologous bone marrow as a sole source of hematopoietic rescue was extremely uncommon.

Improvements in institutional experience,

patient selection, and supportive care have led to striking decreases in transplant-related mortality and cost.[16] Transplantation is routinely being performed by community oncologists, and can be performed safely in the outpatient setting.[17] Several trials have investigated the role of autologous transplantation in elderly patients.[18–20] Although survival rates in elderly patients may be lower than in younger patients, transplantation for lymphomas can be safely performed on selected patients in their seventh decade, and these patients should not be excluded from transplantation because of age alone.

TRANSPLANTATION FOR NON-HODGKIN'S LYMPHOMA

Results of several series employing high-dose therapy with ABMT or PBSCT for non-Hodgkin's lymphoma have been reported (Table 5.3.1). Patients represented in these trials are heterogeneous with respect to histology and pretransplant prognostic factors. In addition, selection criteria, preparative regimens and supportive care protocols vary widely among individual institutions. Patients in these trials were primarily transplanted with autologous bone marrow, although peripheral blood stem cells were used more widely in later trials. Despite these differences, these reports demonstrate that high-dose therapy followed by ABMT or PBSCT can yield long-term disease-free survival in a substantial proportion of patients. Although early transplant-related mortality rates as high as 36% have been noted, mortality rates as low as 3% have been seen. Early transplant-related mortality is now approximately 5% at most institutions performing ABMT and PBSCT for non-Hodgkin's lymphoma.

Prognostic factors

Increasing experience with autologous transplantation for non-Hodgkin's lymphoma has led to the identification of prognostic factors that are predictive of transplant outcome. These prognostic factors are useful in determining suitability for transplantation as well as selecting patients who may benefit from trials of novel preparative regimens.

The most important variable related to transplant outcome concerns sensitivity to conventional chemotherapy administered prior to transplantation. This concept was demonstrated convincingly in one of the first large trials of ABMT for non-Hodgkin's lymphoma.[21] Patients were divided into three groups based upon their response to primary and salvage chemotherapy. The first group of patients had failed to enter complete remission with their initial chemotherapy regimen and had not responded to salvage chemotherapy (primary refractory). These patients had an extremely poor prognosis and none were projected to be alive one year after transplantation (Figure 5.3.1). The remaining patients had achieved a complete remission with initial chemotherapy and had subsequently relapsed. These patients could be further separated on the basis of responsiveness to conventional doses of salvage chemotherapy administered after relapse. Patients who responded to conventional salvage chemotherapy (sensitive relapse) had a 36% projected disease-free survival, as compared with 14% for patients who did not respond (resistant relapse; Figure 5.3.1). Subsequent reports have confirmed the importance of disease sensitivity as the most important prognostic variable associated with transplantation for non-Hodgkin's lymphoma.[22,25,26,28,30–35]

Another important prognostic factor for the outcome of autologous transplantation for non-Hodgkin's lymphoma relates to the extent of treatment prior to transplantation. At the University of Nebraska, patients who had received more than three conventional chemotherapy regimens prior to transplantation had inferior outcomes.[28] Other investigators have noted similar results,[24,31,33,35] and this has led to recommendations that transplantation be performed early after relapse, when patients are best able to tolerate the procedure and prior to develop-

Table 5.3.1 Results of autologous transplantation for intermediate-grade and high-grade non-Hodgkin's lymphoma

Rescue source	Ref	n	Median follow-up	Early mortality (%)	Outcome	Comments
BM	21	100	40 months	21	19% 3-year DFS	—
BM	22	46	32 months	9	60% 3-year DFS	Includes patients in first CR. Includes low-grade lymphomas
BM	23	68	5.3 years	21	16% DFS	Includes patients with mycosis fungoides and malignant histiocytosis
BM	24	101	26 months	21	11% 5-year EFS	Includes patients in first CR; includes low-grade lymphomas and Hodgkin's disease
BM	25	70	2.3 years	13	32% FFS	Includes patients in first CR; includes low-grade lymphomas
BM	26	44	13 months	3	24 (55%) CCR (12–57 months)	Includes low-grade lymphomas
BM	27	44	42 months	36	57% DFS	Includes low-grade lymphomas
BM, PB	28	158	21 months	NS	29% 3-year FFS	—
BM, PB	29	53	19 months	8	40% 3-year EFS	Includes low-grade lymphomas
BM, PB	30	78	NS	7	43% 3-year FFS	Includes patients in first CR
BM, PB	31	53	643 days	17	45% 2-year EFS	Includes patients in first CR; includes low-grade lymphomas and Hodgkin's disease
BM, PB	32	72	2.5 years	10	53% 3-year EFS	Includes patients in first CR; includes low-grade lymphomas
BM, PB	33	48	906 days	23	30% 3-year FFS	Includes patients in first CR
BM	34	107	29 months	7	35% 5-year PFS	—
BM, PB	35	221	2.4 years	10	46% 5-year EFS 52% 5-year EFS	Includes patients in first CR; includes low-grade lymphomas; EFS is calculated for patients receiving chemotherapy alone, or chemotherapy and total body irradiation, respectively

BM = bone marrow; PB = peripheral blood; DFS = disease-free survival; EFS = event-free survival; FFS = failure-free survival; CCR = continuous complete remission; PFS = progression-free-survival; NS = not stated; CR = complete remission.

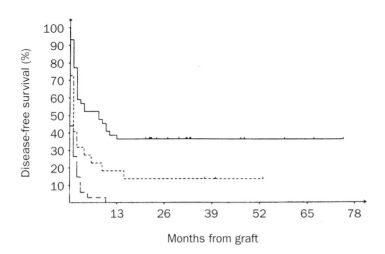

Figure 5.3.1 Actuarial three-year disease-free survival according to response to initial or salvage chemotherapy —————, patients with sensitive relapses; -----, patients with resistant relapse; ————, patients with no complete remission.

ing chemotherapy resistance. Other factors associated with adverse outcome include high lactic dehydrogenase (LDH) level at the time of transplant,[28,33] performance status[23,24] and high-grade histology.[22,24,30,31] The International Prognostic Index has become a widely used tool to predict prognosis with primary chemotherapy for patients with newly diagnosed non-Hodgkin's lymphoma.[36] This index, which uses age, stage, LDH level, performance status and number of extranodal sites of disease, can also be used to predict outcome following ABMT or PBSCT for non-Hodgkin's lymphoma.[37]

The presence of bulky disease prior to transplantation has also been associated with an adverse outcome.[28] Although the presence of bulky disease may simply be a surrogate for chemotherapy resistance, most investigators have attempted to use conventional chemotherapy to debulk patients prior to transplantation.[38] Rapoport et al reported that three-year event-free survival was 48% for non-Hodgkin's lymphoma patients transplanted with minimal disease, compared with 25% for patients with bulky disease ($p = 0.04$).[29] Some investigators have used pre-transplant involved-field radiation therapy to reduce tumor burden, although this has been associated with increased pulmonary toxicity.[26,27,33] Surgery has also been used to debulk patients prior to transplantation.[29] Selected patients, such as

those with low tumor burden, may benefit by proceeding directly to transplantation at relapse without additional conventional therapy. Mills et al[34] noted that progression-free survival was estimated at 59% in patients who were transplanted without additional conventional chemotherapy. However, investigators from Seattle reported that two-year event-free survival was estimated at 59% for patients who received pretransplant cytoreduction, compared with 38% for those who did not ($p = 0.41$).[31]

Some investigators have chosen to use involved-field consolidative radiation therapy following transplantation. It is difficult to evaluate the efficacy of this approach, although investigators from the University of Rochester Medical Center reported that projected event-free survival was 67% for patients receiving additional radiation therapy after transplant, as compared with 30% for other patients ($p = 0.05$).[29]

Comparison with conventional salvage chemotherapy

The results of transplantation for relapsed and refractory non-Hodgkin's lymphoma are superior to most reports of conventional-dose salvage chemotherapy (Table 5.3.1). Although it has been suggested that patients who proceed to transplantation may be highly selected,[39] recent trials provide additional evidence for the superiority of transplantation.

A retrospective analysis of 244 patients from the Groupe d'Etude des Lymphomes de l'Adulte (GELA) examined the outcome of patients with aggressive non-Hodgkin's lymphoma who had relapsed or progressed after receiving the LNH-84 chemotherapy regimen.[40] The median survival for patients treated with conventional salvage chemotherapy was 7 months and the four-year estimated overall survival was 14%. In contrast, the median survival for patients who were transplanted (autologous bone marrow, 39; allogeneic marrow, 4; autologous peripheral blood, 1) was 12 months, and overall survival was projected to be 33% ($p < 0.001$). A similar trial evaluating patients with relapsed childhood lymphoma showed that no patients achieved long-term survival with conventional salvage chemotherapy, although 27% of transplanted patients were alive and in remission four years after transplantation.[41]

The most convincing evidence for the superiority of transplantation for relapsed non-Hodgkin's lymphoma comes from the PARMA trial.[42] Patients with relapsed intermediate- and high-grade lymphoma who had responded to two cycles of conventional salvage chemotherapy with DHAP (dexamethasone, cytarabine, cisplatin) were randomized to receive four additional cycles of DHAP or to receive high-dose therapy with ABMT. Both groups also received post-transplant radiation therapy. The five-year event-free survival was 46% in transplanted patients, as compared with 12% in patients treated with conventional chemotherapy ($p = 0.001$). Overall survival rates were 53% and 32% respectively ($p = 0.038$; Figure 5.3.2). The economic advantages of transplantation for chemotherapy-sensitive relapsed non-Hodgkin's lymphoma have been demonstrated by additional analyses.[43]

Low-grade lymphoma

Although several phase II trials have been performed, there is relatively little experience with transplantation for low-grade lymphomas, as compared with more aggressive histological subtypes (Table 5.3.2). Results are difficult to interpret because of the heterogeneity of patients reported in these trials with respect to histological subtypes and pretransplant characteristics. In addition, a variety of autologous hematopoietic rescue sources have been used.

Results of transplantation for low-grade lymphomas suggest that disease sensitivity is also an important prognostic variable.[44,46,47,49] In addition, outcome is worse in extensively pretreated patients.[48,50,53] Patients transplanted after histological transformation have been reported

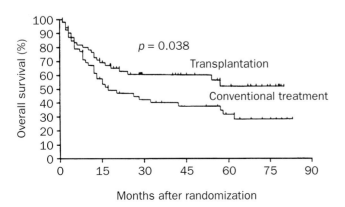

Figure 5.3.2 Kaplan–Meier curves for overall survival of patients in the transplantation and conventional treatment groups.

Table 5.3.2 Results of autologous transplantation for low-grade lymphoma

Rescue source	Ref	n	Early mortality (%)	Outcome	Comments
BM-P	44	51	2	47% 4-year DFS	Includes patients with small lymphocytic and diffuse intermediate histology
BM-P, BM-U	45	10	0	8 (80%) CCR (15–43 months)	Includes patients in first CR
BM-P, BM-U, PB	46	42	7	58% EFS	Includes patients with follicular large-cell histology
BM-P, BM-U	47	92	NS	52% PFS	—
BM-P	48	64	5	35 (55%) CCR (1–8 years)	Includes patients with follicular large-cell histology
BM-P, BM-U, PB	49	34	12	18% 2-year DFS	Includes patients with small lymphocytic histology
PB	50	60	8	53% 2-year FFS	Includes patients with follicular large-cell histology
PB	51, 52	48	4	76% 2-year DFS	Includes patients in first CR
BM-U, PB	53	100	8	44% 4-year FFS	—
BM-P	54	77	3	63% 3-year DFS	Includes patients in first CR

BM-P = purged bone marrow; BM-U = unpurged bone marrow; PB = peripheral blood; DFS = disease-free survival; CCR = continuous complete remission; EFS = event-free survival; PFS = progression-free survival; FFS = failure-free survival; NS = not stated; CR = complete remission to have inferior outcomes in some series,[47,50,55] although not in others.[30,44,56] Retrospective analyses have not demonstrated differences in outcome between ABMT and PBSCT among patients transplanted with low-grade lymphoma.[46,47,49,53]

Transplantation for low-grade lymphoma can be performed with minimal mortality, and long-term failure-free survival is possible (Table 5.3.2). However, these trials have generally shown a continuous pattern of treatment failure, similar to results observed following primary therapy for low-grade lymphoma. It is unclear whether patients are cured with this approach or whether survival is prolonged. Rohatiner et al[48] evaluated the results of purged ABMT in a subset of 41 patients with follicular lymphoma transplanted in second remission. Although freedom from recurrence was significantly better than historical controls, there was no significant difference in overall survival. Long-term follow-up will be required to evaluate the role of autologous transplantation for low-grade lymphoma, because of the long natural history of disease and because of late relapses following transplantation.[45,46,53]

Several trials have evaluated the role of autologous transplantation for low-grade lymphoma patients in first remission. Freedman et al[54] reported that three-year disease-free survival was 63% in 77 patients who were transplanted with purged autologous bone marrow after achieving a remission with CHOP (cyclophosphamide, doxorubicin, vincristine, prednisone) chemotherapy. The overall survival rate was 89%, suggesting that the natural history of disease may be altered, although a continuous pattern of relapse was noted and there was no evidence that patients are cured. Similar outcomes have been noted for other low-grade lymphoma patients transplanted in first remission, and it is not clear that such patients can be cured following ABMT/PBSCT.[52,57]

Phase II trials of allogeneic bone marrow transplantation for low-grade lymphoma are promising, although mortality rates are high and long-term follow-up will be required to determine whether patients are cured.[58]

TRANSPLANTATION FOR HODGKIN'S DISEASE

A large number of Phase II trials have evaluated the role of autologous transplantation for patients with relapsed and refractory Hodgkin's disease (Table 5.3.3). As for non-Hodgkin's lymphoma, it is difficult to compare one series with another due to differences in selection criteria, pretransplant prognostic factors and high-dose therapy regimens. However, these reports demonstrate that long-term disease-free survival can be achieved following either ABMT or PBSCT, and that transplantation can be performed with low mortality. However, late relapses have been identified following autologous transplantation for Hodgkin's disease, and prolonged follow-up is necessary.[60,61,66–68] The majority of patients in early reports were transplanted with autologous bone marrow, while peripheral blood stem cells have been used more commonly in later reports (Table 5.3.3).

Prognostic factors

Investigators at the MD Anderson Cancer Center and the University of Nebraska noted that median progression-free survival was 5.1 months for Hodgkin's disease patients who had failed at least two conventional chemotherapy regimens prior to transplantation, compared with 26.9 months for patients who were less heavily treated ($p = 0.019$).[72] Follow-up reports,[73,74] as well as others, have demonstrated that autologous transplantation is most likely to be successful if performed earlier in the course of disease.[68] However, Chopra et al[66] noted that progression-free survival was significantly better for patients transplanted in second or third relapse, compared with patients transplanted in first relapse. It was suggested that patients who had received several courses of therapy may have had more indolent disease.

Investigators from Vancouver developed a prognostic model based upon the presence of systemic symptoms at relapse, length of initial remission, and the presence of extranodal dis-

Table 5.3.3 Results of autologous transplantation for Hodgkin's disease

Rescue source	Reference	n	Median follow-up	Early mortality (%)	Outcome
BM	59	50	NS	4	12 (24%) CCR (9–32 months)
BM	60	26	3.8 years	23	27% PFS
BM	61	56	3.5 years	21	47% 5-year EFS
BM	26	35	13 months	3	16 (46%) CCR (10–52 months)
BM, PB	62	73	30 months	4	39% 4-year DFS
PB	63	25	67 months	NS	48% PFS
BM	64	47	40 months	17	50% DFS
BM, PB	29	47	2 years	17	49% 3-year EFS
BM, PB	65	58	2.3 years	5	64% PFS
BM	66	155	NS	10	50% 5-year DFS
BM, PB	67	128	77 months	9	25% 4-year FFS
BM, PB	68	85	28 months	8	58% 2-year EFS
BM, PB	69	62	NS	0	38% 3-year DFS
BM, PB	70	42	33 months	2	74% 2-year EFS
BM, PB	71	119	40 months	5	48% 4-year EFS

BM = bone marrow; PB = peripheral blood; CCR = continuous complete remission; PFS = progression-free-survival; EFS = event-free survival; DFS = disease-free survival; FFS = failure-free survival; NS = not stated.

ease at relapse for patients undergoing transplantation for Hodgkin's disease.[65] Progression-free survival at three years was inversely correlated with the number of adverse prognostic factors present. The presence of systemic symptoms at the time of transplant has been associated with inferior outcomes in other series.[69,71,75] The presence of extranodal disease at the time of transplant has also been associated with poor survival.[68] In addition, others have correlated the length of initial remission with outcome.[66,74,75]

Other prognostic factors associated with outcome following autologous transplantation for Hodgkin's disease include performance status,[60,61,67,70,76] sensitivity to chemotherapy,[66,75] absence of bulky disease[62,66,69] and LDH level.[70]

Most investigators administer conventional doses of chemotherapy to relapsed Hodgkin's disease patients prior to transplantation, in a manner similar to non-Hodgkin's lymphoma. Rapoport et al[29] noted that event-free survival was 70% at three years for Hodgkin's disease patients transplanted with minimal disease, compared with 15% for patients with bulky disease at the time of transplant ($p = 0.0001$). Crump et al[62] reported that disease-free survival was 68% for patients transplanted with no evidence of Hodgkin's disease, 26% for patients with non-bulky disease and 0% for those with bulky disease ($p = 0.0002$).

Selected Hodgkin's disease patients may benefit, however, by proceeding directly to transplant at the time of relapse without additional debulking therapy. Retrospective analyses have demonstrated that such patients may have outcomes significantly better than patients who receive debulking chemotherapy.[66,74] Other investigators have chosen to administer consolidative radiation therapy following transplantation for Hodgkin's disease. This approach may be able to convert patients with partial remission into durable remissions.[67] However, many patients cannot tolerate post-transplant radiation, and the benefits of this approach have been hard to evaluate.[62,66,77]

Comparison with conventional salvage chemotherapy

The best results of conventional salvage chemotherapy for Hodgkin's disease have been reported for patients after their first relapse, particularly when initial remission durations have exceeded one year.[3,4] The best results of autologous transplantation for Hodgkin's disease have been reported by Reece et al.[65] Progression-free survival was estimated to be 64% when patients with Hodgkin's disease were transplanted following relapse from their first chemotherapy regimen. When the initial remission duration was longer than one year, actuarial progression-free survival was 85%, while those with shorter remissions had progression-free survival estimated to be 48%. Comparable results have been reported from other investigations of autologous transplantation in Hodgkin's disease patients following first relapse.[63,66,68,74] Investigators from Stanford University compared the results of transplantation for Hodgkin's disease patients after first relapse with data from historical controls.[75] The four-year event-free survival for relapsed patients with short initial remissions was estimated to be 56% following transplantation, compared with 19% for historical controls ($p < 0.01$). Overall survival rates were 58% and 38% respectively ($p = 0.15$).

The only prospective trial comparing autologous transplantation and conventional salvage chemotherapy for Hodgkin's disease was conducted by the British National Lymphoma Investigation.[78] Patients with relapsed or refractory disease were randomized to receive conventional salvage chemotherapy with mini-BEAM (carmustine, etoposide, cytarabine, melphalan) or therapy with the same drugs administered at higher doses (BEAM) that required hematopoietic rescue. The probability of disease progression was lower in transplanted patients, and actuarial three-year event-free survival was 53%, compared with 10% for patients who received conventional salvage chemotherapy with mini-BEAM. There were no significant differences in overall survival, however (Figure 5.3.3).

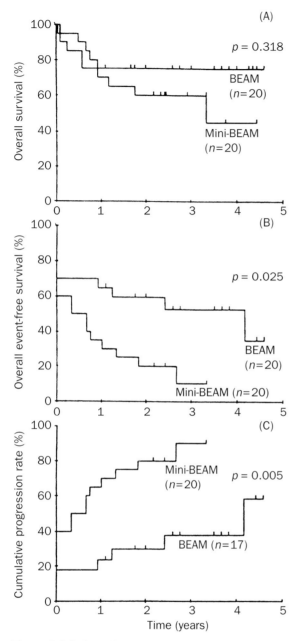

Figure 5.3.3 Overall survival (A), event-free survival (B) and cumulative progression rate (C) in BEAM plus ABMT and mini-BEAM groups.

The value of autologous transplantation for Hodgkin's disease can also be evaluated for patients who have primary refractory disease. Few patients who fail to enter complete remis-

sion with primary chemotherapy are cured with conventional salvage chemotherapy.[3,4] Reece et al[79] reported that actuarial progression-free survival was 42% in a cohort of Hodgkin's disease patients transplanted with disease that had persisted or progressed after primary chemotherapy. The Stanford group reported a four-year progression-free survival of 52% for patients who had failed initial therapy,[75] and similar results have been noted by other investigators.[63,64,66,68]

These results provide strong evidence for the use of ABMT or PBSCT for patients with primary refractory Hodgkin's disease and for those who relapse after an initial remission that is less than 12 months in duration. Failure-free survival rates following transplantation appear to be better than conventional salvage chemotherapy for patients with longer remissions, although it has been difficult to show advantages in overall survival. Although these patients may experience long-term survival with conventional salvage chemotherapy,[4] some physicians continue to recommend transplantation for all relapsed patients, regardless of initial remission duration.

COMPARISON OF ABMT AND PBSCT

The use of autologous peripheral blood progenitor cells instead of bone marrow has increased rapidly.[15] Many institutions are using peripheral blood stem cells exclusively for autologous transplantation. Many physicians and patients overlook the fact that the hematopoietic rescue product is supportive care that allows the use of higher doses of chemotherapy and radiation than would otherwise be possible. It is also overlooked that the main advantage of using peripheral blood stem cells is that this allows some patients, such as those with hypocellular marrow or marrow metastases, to receive high-dose therapy when this would otherwise be impossible.

Peripheral blood stem cells can be collected without general anesthesia, and sufficient cells can sometimes be obtained with a single apheresis.[80,81] It is also widely recognized that hematopoietic engraftment rates following PBSCT are significantly more rapid than following ABMT, although only two trials involving lymphoma patients have been prospective in nature (Table 5.3.4). The vast majority of trials have compared engraftment rates of mobilized peripheral blood stem cells with those of marrow collected in the steady state. A small amount of evidence suggests that autologous bone marrow that is collected after growth factor 'activation' may engraft as rapidly as mobilized peripheral blood stem cells.[90,91]

There may also be differences in immune reconstitution following ABMT and PBSCT for lymphoma. Such differences might explain reported differences in complication rates or relapse rates when ABMT and PBSCT have been compared. Roberts et al[92] examined reconstitution of $CD3^+$, $CD4^+$, $CD8^+$, $CD20^+$ and $CD56^+$ lymphocytes following ABMT and PBSCT. The pace of immune reconstitution following ABMT was generally midway between those of PBSCT and allogeneic bone marrow transplantation, although differences were not statistically significant. Few significant differences in immune reconstitution were observed between patients receiving autologous bone marrow and peripheral blood stem cells, although recipients of autologous bone marrow had significantly faster $CD20^+$ lymphocyte recovery. Scheid et al[93] noted that inducible natural killer (NK) activity and inducible lymphokine-activated killer (LAK) activity appeared within 10–14 days after PBSCT. Some patients showed higher LAK activity following transplantation than was present prior to receiving high-dose therapy, and it was suggested that this response might be exploited to decrease relapse rates following transplantation. Talmadge et al[94] compared immune reconstitution after ABMT and PBSCT for non-Hodgkin's lymphoma. Following PBSCT, it was noted that recovery of CD4 : CD8 lymphocyte ratios, NK cell numbers, and mitogen response were more rapid than the recovery after ABMT.

Many physicians feel that contaminating tumor cells in blood or bone marrow may con-tribute to relapse in patients undergoing autologous transplantation for lymphoma. This has led to the use of techniques to remove (purge) malignant cells from the autograft,[95] although retrospective analyses have failed to show a benefit from using purged bone marrow for patients undergoing transplantation for lymphoma.[24,25,27,96] Nevertheless, the use of peripheral blood stem cells may be preferred because of a lower incidence of tumor contamination than with the use of bone marrow.

In vitro culture studies have demonstrated that tumor cells can be cultured from approximately one-third of histologically normal bone marrow harvests of patients with intermediate- and high-grade non-Hodgkin's lymphoma, compared with 5–10% of peripheral blood stem cell collections.[97] Gribben et al[98] used polymerase chain reaction (PCR) to detect lymphoma cells in the bone marrow of 98% of patients undergoing bone marrow harvest prior to transplantation, while lymphoma cells were detectable in peripheral blood in 49% of patients. It was also shown that PCR-positive cells in the bone marrow are rapidly detectable in the circulation following marrow infusion. However, Negrin et al[99] noted that PCR was able to detect lymphoma cells in the peripheral blood in 86% of cases when lymphoma cells were detected in the bone marrow at the time of marrow harvest. Other investigators have shown that peripheral blood stem cell harvests are likely to contain malignant cells.[51,100,101]

Nevertheless, several indirect lines of evidence suggest that contaminating tumor cells may contribute to relapse, and support the preferential use of peripheral blood stem cells if they have less tumor contamination. Gene marking studies have demonstrated that transplanted tumor cells may contribute to relapse in some cases of acute and chronic myelogenous leukemia.[102,103] Early disseminated relapse following ABMT in some cases of non-Hodgkin's lymphoma also suggests that some relapses may result from reinfusion of malignant cells.[104,105] Gribben et al[106] reported results of purged ABMT in 114 non-Hodgkin's lymphoma patients who had tumor cells detectable by PCR prior to purging. After purging with

Table 5.3.4 Comparison of results of ABMT and PBSCT for lymphoma

Disease	Ref	Prospective	n	ABMT	PBSCT	p	Comments
HD and NHL	82	Yes	28	34% RFS	53% RFS	>0.7	PBSCT patients had more rapid engraftment and shorter hospital stays
HD and NHL	83	No	142	44% Rel/Prog	45% Rel/Prog		PBSCT patients had more rapid engraftment
NHL	28	No	158	23% 3-year FFS	40% 3-year FFS	0.014	Difference only significant in good-prognosis patients
HD	84	No	242	28% 4-year FFS	25% 4-year FFS	0.9	—
HD and NHL	85	No	41	11/19 CCR (12–40 months)	18/22 CCR (2–17 months)		—
HD	29	No	47	50% 3-year EFS	33% 3-year EFS	0.63	—
NHL			53	41% 3-year EFS	36% 3-year EFS	0.99	—
HD and NHL	86, 87	Yes	58	No differences in survival			PBSCT patients had more rapid engraftment, shorter hospital stays, less blood-product use and lower costs.
HD and NHL	88	No	153	45% 2-year EFS	36% 2-year EFS		Some PBSCT patients also received bone marrow; PBSCT patients had more rapid engraftment
HD	89	No (matched-pair analysis)	256	65% 4-year OS	53% 4-year OS	0.02	PBSCT patients had more rapid engraftment
NHL			454	57% 4-year OS	53% 4-year OS	0.41	—
NHL	35	No	221	60% 2-year OS	82% 2-year OS	<0.01	PBSCT patients had more rapid engraftment

ABMT = autologous bone marrow transplantation; PBSCT = peripheral blood stem cell transplantation; HD = Hodgkin's disease; NHL = non-Hodgkin's lymphoma; RFS = relapse-free survival; Rel/Prog = relapse or progression; FFS = failure-free survival; PFS = progression-free survival; CCR = continuous complete remission; EFS = event-free survival; OS = overall survival monoclonal antibodies and complement, 57 patients still had detectable tumor in their marrow, and 57 patients had no detectable tumor cells. At the time of median follow-up, 39% of patients transplanted with marrow that contained residual lymphoma cells had relapsed, compared with 5% of patients without detectable lymphoma cells ($p < 0.00001$). Sharp et al[107] have used an in vitro culture system and Southern analysis to detect lymphoma cells in the blood and bone marrow harvests of patients undergoing transplantation for non-Hodgkin's lymphoma. The five-year relapse-free survival rate was 57% for ABMT patients without detectable tumor cells in their marrow harvests, compared with 17% for patients whose harvests were histologically normal but contained tumor cells. The relapse-free survival rate was 64% for patients with histological evidence of lymphoma in their bone marrow, who were transplanted with peripheral blood stem cells.

Despite evidence supporting the possible role of relapse from infusion of malignant cells, the malignant potential of these cells remains uncertain. Haas et al[51] noted prolonged remissions in patients transplanted with peripheral blood stem cells that were PCR-positive, and also noted that a significant fraction of patients became PCR-negative between three and 16 months after transplantation.

Clinical results

Although peripheral blood stem cell collections may contain fewer malignant cells than bone marrow, the fundamental question is whether this has any impact on survival or whether differences in the rate of engraftment or immune reconstitution following ABMT or PBSCT influence transplant outcome. Several trials have compared the results of ABMT and PBSCT for patients with lymphoma (Table 5.3.4).

Three retrospective analyses have examined rescue source in cohorts that have contained both Hodgkin's disease and non-Hodgkin's lymphoma. Brice et al[83] noted that the median time to achieve an absolute neutrophil count (ANC) > 500/µl was 10 days earlier with PBSCT, and that platelet recovery occurred 8 days earlier than ABMT. Relapse rates were similar in each cohort. Similarly, Ager et al[85] noted that the median time to achieve an ANC > 500/µl was 11 days following PBSCT, as compared with 19 days in historical controls who received ABMT ($p < 0.0001$). Patients transplanted with peripheral blood stem cells required fewer days of hospitalization (median 21 days vs 28 days, $p < 0.001$), used fewer units of platelets (median 15 units vs 40 units, $p = 0.005$), and used less total parenteral nutrition (median 0 days vs 8 days, $p < 0.001$). It was estimated that savings were approximately £2370 for patients who were transplanted with peripheral blood stem cells. Eighty-two percent of patients undergoing PBSCT remained in remission 2–17 months after transplantation, compared with 58% of ABMT patients who remained in remission 12–40 months following transplantation. Brunvand et al[88] compared the outcome of 79 lymphoma patients undergoing ABMT and 74 patients undergoing PBSCT (18 received bone marrow with peripheral blood stem cells). Median time to neutrophil recovery occurred 4 days sooner in patients who received peripheral blood autografts ($p = 0.03$). In addition, the median time to achieve a self-sustaining platelet count greater than 20 000/µl was 24 days after bone marrow transplantation and 11 days after PBSCT ($p = 0.007$). Peripheral blood stem cell recipients also had a median of three fewer red blood cell transfusions ($p = 0.05$), 56 fewer units of platelets transfused ($p = 0.001$) and nine fewer days in hospital ($p = 0.0001$), compared with ABMT. Transplant-related mortality rates were 11% and 18% respectively ($p = 0.42$). An additional analysis examined 98 patients with non-Hodgkin's lymphoma who were transplanted with unpurged autologous bone marrow or peripheral blood stem cells (without additional bone marrow). Event-free survival at two years was estimated at 46% following ABMT, compared with 35% following PBSCT ($p = 0.53$).

The results of ABMT and PBSCT have been compared in cohorts containing a combination of Hodgkin's disease and non-Hodgkin's lymphoma in two prospective randomized trials.

The group from the University of Minnesota noted that lymphoma patients randomized to receive autologous peripheral blood stem cells reached an ANC > 500/µl a median of seven days earlier than autologous bone marrow recipients and that median hospital stays were seven days shorter.[82] No significant differences in relapse rate, overall survival or relapse-free survival were noted. A trial from six European centers also randomized lymphoma patients to transplantation with autologous bone marrow or peripheral blood stem cells.[86,87] Recipients of peripheral blood stem cells required a median of 16 days to recover platelets counts, compared with 23 days following ABMT ($p = 0.02$). Similarly, the median time to reach an ANC > 500/µl was 11 days and 14 days respectively ($p = 0.005$). Patients transplanted with peripheral blood stem cells required a median of two red blood cell transfusions, compared with three units following ABMT ($p = 0.002$). The median hospital stay was 17 days and 23 days respectively ($p = 0.002$), and estimated cost savings amounted to $13 521 (23%) for patients undergoing PBSCT. There were no significant differences in infectious or hemorrhagic episodes and no significant survival differences.

A retrospective analysis of non-Hodgkin's lymphoma patients from the University of Nebraska allowed a prognostic model to be developed based upon the extent of prior therapy, disease bulk, chemotherapy sensitivity and serum LDH level.[28] The three-year failure-free survival rates in poor-prognosis patients were similar in patients transplanted with autologous bone marrow or peripheral blood stem cells. However, among good-prognosis patients, actuarial failure-free survival was 70% following PBSCT, compared with 32% for recipients of autologous bone marrow ($p < 0.008$). A retrospective analysis of transplant results for patients with non-Hodgkin's lymphoma reported by Rapoport et al[29] noted that actuarial three-year event-free survival was 41% following ABMT, compared with 36% following PBSCT ($p = 0.99$). Investigators from Stanford also performed a retrospective analysis of transplant results for patients with non-Hodgkin's lymphoma.[35] Recipients of PBSCT

reached an ANC > 500/µl in 10 days, compared with 15 days following ABMT ($p < 0.001$). Similarly, the time to reach a platelet count greater than 25 000/µl was 16 days and 32 days respectively ($p < 0.001$). Overall survival at two years was estimated at 60% following ABMT, compared with 82% following PBSCT ($p < 0.01$). This difference was partly explained by higher transplant-related mortality following ABMT compared with PBSCT (13% vs 4%, respectively; $p = 0.05$).

The source of hematopoietic rescue has been analyzed in two retrospective series of Hodgkin's disease patients. At the University of Nebraska, four-year failure-free survival rates were 28% and 25% following ABMT and PBSCT respectively ($p = NS$).[84] Rapoport et al[29] performed a similar analysis, and noted that the actuarial event-free survival rates for Hodgkin's disease patients were 50% following ABMT, compared with 33% following PBSCT ($p = 0.63$).

A matched-pair analysis from the European Group for Blood and Marrow Transplantation has compared rescue source for lymphoma patients.[89] Recipients of peripheral blood stem cells had more rapid engraftment, although no

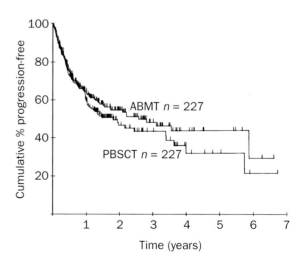

Figure 5.3.4 Progression-free survival of matched non-Hodgkin's lymphoma patients who received ABMT or PBSCT ($p = 0.2602$).

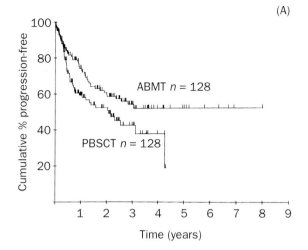

(A)

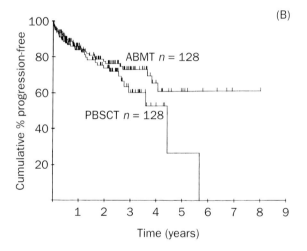

(B)

Figure 5.3.5 Progression-free survival ($p = 0.0082$) (A) and overall survival ($p = 0.0198$) (B) of matched Hodgkin's disease patients who received ABMT or PBSCT.

significant differences in early mortality rates were noted. The rescue source did not influence the rate of relapse or progression in non-Hodgkin's lymphoma patients. At four years progression-free survival was estimated at 44% following ABMT, as compared with 36% following PBSCT (Figure 5.3.4). Overall survival rates were not significantly different, either. Significant differences in outcome were noted

following transplantation for Hodgkin's disease, however. Progression-free survival rates at four years were estimated as 52% and 38% following ABMT and PBSCT respectively (Figure 5.3.5A). Similarly, overall survival rates were 65% and 53% respectively (Figure 5.3.5B).

Allogeneic transplantation

There is relatively little experience with allogeneic transplantation for non-Hodgkin's lymphoma compared with autologous transplantation.[15] Allogeneic transplantation eliminates the possibility of infusing malignant cells, and also has the potential advantage of a 'graft-versus-lymphoma effect' similar to the graft-versus-leukemia effect that is observed with allogeneic transplantation for acute and chronic leukemia.[108] However, disadvantages of allogeneic transplantation include the lack of donor availability for many patients as well as higher transplant-related mortality than autologous transplantation.

Investigators from Seattle found no significant differences in relapse rate or disease-free survival in a retrospective analysis of autologous, allogeneic and syngeneic transplantation in a cohort of patients with Hodgkin's disease and non-Hodgkin's lymphoma.[109] Jones et al[110] noted that the actuarial relapse rate was 46% following ABMT, compared with 18% following allogeneic transplantation in a cohort of patients with Hodgkin's disease and non-Hodgkin's lymphoma ($p = 0.02$). The lower relapse probability following allogeneic transplantation was offset by a 42% transplant-related mortality rate, and event-free survival rates were not statistically different. A similar analysis from Wayne State University noted that autologous transplantation for non-Hodgkin's lymphoma was associated with a 69% probability of disease progression, compared with 20% following allogeneic transplantation ($p = 0.001$).[111] They also noted no significant differences in progression-free survival, because of the high rate of transplant-related mortality that was associated with allogeneic transplantation. Similar findings were described in a case-controlled analysis of transplantation from the European Bone Marrow Transplant Group.[112] No significant differences in progression-free survival were noted among non-Hodgkin's lymphoma patients who received autologous or allogeneic marrow.

These results support the existence of a graft-versus-lymphoma effect, but they might also suggest that tumor contamination is responsible for a higher rate of relapse following autologous transplantation. Lower relapse rates in patients with chronic graft-versus-host disease also support a graft-versus-lymphoma effect.[111,112] A sufficiently large trial examining results of syngeneic transplantation for non-Hodgkin's lymphoma might resolve this issue.

Trials have also investigated the results of allogeneic bone marrow transplantation for patients with Hodgkin's disease. Investigators from Seattle found a lower relapse rate following allogeneic transplantation for Hodgkin's disease, but event-free survival rates were similar following autologous, allogeneic and syngeneic transplantation.[113] The International Bone Marrow Transplant Registry noted that disease-free survival at three years was estimated at 15% following allogeneic transplantation for Hodgkin's disease and that the probability of transplant-related mortality was 61%.[114] A case-matching study from the European Bone Marrow Transplant Registry noted that the four-year progression-free survival rates following autologous and allogeneic transplantation for Hodgkin's disease were 24% and 15% respectively.[115] Non-relapse mortality rates were 27% and 48% respectively.

Most institutions prefer autologous bone marrow or peripheral blood stem cells rather than allogeneic bone marrow for lymphoma. Nevertheless, most trials have shown similar survival rates. Lower relapse rates following allogeneic transplantation suggest that this approach may be used more frequently in the future if the mortality of allogeneic transplantation can be decreased.

EARLY TRANSPLANTATION

It is possible to identify newly diagnosed lymphoma patients who are less likely to be cured with primary chemotherapy than other patients.[36] These poor-prognosis patients are candidates for innovative treatment strategies such as the use of up-front transplantation as part of initial therapy. This strategy requires the ability to accurately identify poor-prognosis patients and the ability to perform transplantation with low mortality.

Several phase II trials of early transplantation for poor-prognosis non-Hodgkin's lymphoma have been performed (Table 5.3.5). These results demonstrate that early transplantation can be performed with low mortality and that results appear superior to historical controls. Nevertheless, the patients who proceed to early transplantation may be highly selected. Survival curves are often reported from the time of transplantation instead of the time of diagnosis, and it may be difficult to determine the number of poor-prognosis patients who were not able to come to transplantation. Some studies indicate that this may be a substantial fraction of patients.[118,125]

Prospective randomized trials have been performed to address the value of early transplantation for poor-prognosis non-Hodgkin's lymphoma patients. A GELA trial[129] randomized patients with intermediate- and high-grade non-Hodgkin's lymphoma in first complete remission to receive sequential conventional chemotherapy or to receive high-dose chemotherapy followed by ABMT. This initial report showed no benefit from early transplantation, although a trend in favor of improved disease-free survival was noted for poor-prognosis patients. An updated report of 541 randomized patients demonstrated that disease-free survival at five years is estimated as 59% for high-intermediate and high-risk groups randomized to high-dose therapy with ABMT, compared with 39% for patients who received sequential chemotherapy (Figure 5.3.6).[130] Overall survival rates were 65% and 52% respectively ($p = 0.06$).

The Milan Cancer Institute conducted a prospective trial in which poor-prognosis non-

Table 5.3.5 Results of non-randomized trials of autologous transplantation in first remission for poor-prognosis non-Hodgkin's lymphoma

n	Ref	Early mortality (%)	Outcome	Comments
14	116	0	11 (79%) CCR (31–71 months)	6 patients in CR at transplant; 8 patients in PR at transplant; survival significantly better than concurrent controls treated with chemotherapy alone
13	117	0	70% 4-year DFS	—
21	118	5	66% DFS	40 patients initially entered on trial
12	119	17	8 (67%) CCR (8–52 months)	Survival significantly better than historical controls treated with chemotherapy alone
9	120	0	6 (67%) CCR (12–113 months)	—
20	121	0	84% 13-months DFS	—
26	122	0	85% 28-month DFS	16 patients in CR at transplant; 10 patients in minimal disease state at transplant
28	123	0	83% EFS	Outcome includes 2 patients who relapsed prior to transplant
102	124	4	70% 5-year PFS	26 patients initially entered in trial
17	125	0	48% 3-year EFS	12 patients in CR at transplant; 4 patients in PR at transplant
16	126	0	100% DFS	
33	127	6	61% 2-year EFS	Survival significantly better than historical controls treated with chemotherapy alone
39	128	3	50% 32-months FFS	Outcome includes all 50 patients initially entered in trial

CR = complete remission; PR = partial remission; CCR = continuous complete remission; DFS = disease-free survival; EFS = event-free survival; PFS = progression-free survival.

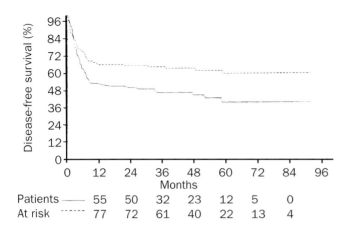

Figure 5.3.6 Estimated disease-free survival according to randomized consolidation procedure for high-intermediate and high-risk patients: —————, sequential chemotherapy (patients at risk, $n = 111$; five-year estimate, 39%); -----, autologous bone marrow transplantation (patients at risk, $n = 125$; five-year estimate, 59%). $p = 0.01$.

Hodgkin's lymphoma patients were randomized to receive MACOP-B chemotherapy[131] or a 60-day sequential regimen of debulking chemotherapy followed by high-dose chemotherapy with PBSCT.[132] Progression-free survival was projected to be 88% after the up-front transplantation regimen, compared with 41% following MACOP-B alone ($p = 0.0001$). Follow-up reports indicate that overall survival is significantly better with up-front high-dose chemotherapy.[133]

Slow response to initial chemotherapy for non-Hodgkin's lymphoma is also associated with a poor prognosis.[134] A Dutch trial randomized patients in partial remission after three cycles of CHOP (cyclophosphamide, doxorubicin, vincristine, prednisone) to receive five additional cycles of CHOP, or to receive one additional cycle of CHOP followed by high-dose chemotherapy and ABMT.[135] No significant differences in outcome were observed. An Italian trial randomized patients in partial remission after completion of two-thirds of primary therapy to treatment with conventional salvage chemotherapy, or to receive treatment with high-dose therapy followed by autologous transplantation.[136] Progression-free survival at 55 months was projected to be 73% in transplanted patients, compared with 52% for patients who received conventional salvage chemotherapy ($p = 0.3$). A non-randomized GELA trial noted that overall survival was 63%

for patients transplanted in first partial remission, compared with 46% for patients who received conventional salvage therapy ($p = 0.03$).[137]

There is limited experience with early transplantation for Hodgkin's disease. Carella et al[138] reported that event-free survival was 87% for poor-prognosis Hodgkin's disease patients transplanted in first complete remission, compared with 33% for patients who only received conventional chemotherapy. Moreau et al[139] reported that 16 patients with Hodgkin's disease transplanted in partial remission midway through primary therapy were alive and in remission between 8 and 52 months following transplantation. French registry data indicates that high-risk Hodgkin's disease patients transplanted in first complete remission had an actuarial seven-year event-free survival rate of 70%.[140]

PREPARATIVE REGIMENS

A wide variety of high-dose therapy regimens have been used prior to autologous transplantation for lymphoma. No prospective trials have conclusively demonstrated the superiority of any particular regimen. High-dose therapy regimens have often been grouped according to whether or not they contain total body irradiation (TBI). Retrospective analyses of several phase II trials have failed to demonstrate a survival advantage associated with the use of TBI-containing regimens.[21,24,25,28,47,50,53,68] Investigators from Stanford noted no survival advantage associated with a TBI-containing regimen in non-Hodgkin's lymphoma patients transplanted with autologous peripheral blood stem cells, although overall survival was superior in ABMT patients who received a TBI-containing regimen.[35] The use of TBI has been associated with increased pulmonary toxicity, especially in patients who have received prior chest irradiation,[24,60] and has also been associated with an increased risk of secondary myelodysplasia.[141]

A European Bone Marrow Transplant Registry survey noted that non-Hodgkin's lymphoma patients transplanted after receiving high-dose CBV (cyclophosphamide, carmustine, etoposide) had longer progression-free survival rates than patients who received high-dose BEAM (carmustine, etoposide, cytarabine, melphalan).[142] However, Hodgkin's disease patients had better outcomes with BEAM. Rapoport et al[29] noted that use of the high-dose BEAC (carmustine, etoposide, cytarabine, cyclophosphamide) regimen was associated with improved event-free survival for patients with Hodgkin's disease. Attempts at increasing drug doses in various regimens have often led to unacceptable toxicity.[27,143–145] The use of radiolabeled antibodies in combination with high-dose chemotherapy may result in improved preparative regimens for lymphoma.[146,147]

FUTURE DIRECTIONS

Long-term follow-up has identified an alarming incidence of myelodysplasia and secondary leukemia in patients undergoing ABMT and PBSCT for Hodgkin's disease and non-Hodgkin's lymphoma.[141,148–150] Continued observation is warranted to determine the ultimate role of transplantation, and to decrease long-term complications. Improvements in supportive care will continue to improve the safety and decrease the cost associated with transplantation.

Efforts to improve the results of transplantation will focus on clarifying the optimal patient groups for transplantation. Ongoing trials will refine the role of early transplantation for Hodgkin's disease and non-Hodgkin's lymphoma. In addition, ongoing trials will define the role of transplantation for low-grade lymphomas and other entities such as mantle cell lymphoma. It is hoped that improved preparative regimens will be developed, although this seems unlikely unless new drugs are introduced or agents are developed to protect against non-hematopoietic toxicity. It is hoped that the combination of radioactive antibodies and high-dose chemotherapy will improve the efficacy of preparative regimens.

There is continued interest in the use of additional therapy after transplantation to decrease relapse rates. Post-transplant therapy may consist of involved-field radiation, or even second transplants.[151] Ongoing trials are evaluating the role of monoclonal antibodies,[152] interferon,[153] interleukin-2[154–156] or cyclosporin following transplantation.[157]

REFERENCES

1. Armitage JO, Vose JM, Bierman PJ, Salvage therapy for patients with non-Hodgkin's lymphoma. *J Natl Cancer Inst Monogr* 1990; **10**: 39–43.

2. Rodriguez MA, Cabanillas FC, Velasquez W et al, Results of a salvage treatment program for relapsing lymphoma: MINE consolidated with ESHAP. *J Clin Oncol* 1995; **13**: 1734–41.

3. Longo DL, Duffey PL, Young RC et al, Conventional-dose salvage combination chemotherapy in patients relapsing with Hodgkin's disease after combination chemotherapy. The low probability for cure. *J Clin Oncol* 1992; **10**: 2101–8.

4. Bonfante V, Santoro A, Viviani S et al, Outcome of patients with Hodgkin's disease failing after

primary MOPP–ABVD. *J Clin Oncol* 1997; **15:** 528–34.

5. Frei E, Canellos GP, Dose: A critical factor in cancer chemotherapy. *Am J Med* 1980; **69:** 585–94.

6. McFarland W, Granville NB, Dameshek W, Autologous bone marrow infusion as an adjunct in therapy of malignant disease. *Blood* 1959; **14:** 503–21.

7. Clifford P, Clift RA, Duff JK, Nitrogen-mustard therapy combined with autologous marrow infusion. *Lancet* 1961; **i:** 687–90.

8. Kurnick NB, Autologous and isologous bone marrow storage and infusion in the treatment of myelo-suppression. *Transfusion* 1962; **2:** 178–87.

9. Appelbaum FR, Herzig GP, Ziegler JL et al, Successful engraftment of cryopreserved autologous bone marrow in patient with malignant lymphoma. *Blood* 1978; **52:** 85–95.

10. Applebaum FR, Deisseroth AB, Graw RG et al, Prolonged complete remission following high dose chemotherapy of Burkitt's lymphoma in relapse. *Cancer* 1978; **41:** 1059–63.

11. Hershko C, Ho WG, Gale RP, Cline MJ, Cure of aplastic anaemia in paroxysmal nocturnal hemoglobulinuria by marrow transfusion from identical twin: Failure of peripheral leucocyte transfusion to correct marrow aplasia. *Lancet* 1979; **i:** 945–7.

12. Abrams RA, Glaubiger D, Appelbaum FR, Deisseroth AB, Result of attempted hematopoietic reconstitution using isologous, peripheral blood mononuclear cells: A case report. *Blood* 1980; **56:** 516–20.

13. Körbling M, Döken B, Ho AD et al, Autologous transplantation of blood-derived hematopoietic stem cells after myeloablative therapy in a patient with Burkitt's lymphoma. *Blood* 1986; **67:** 529–32.

14. Kessinger A, Armitage JO, Landmark JD, Weisenburger DD, Reconstitution of human hematopoietic function with autologous cryopreserved circulating stem cells. *Exp Hematol* 1986; **14:** 192–6.

15. Gratwohl A, Hermans J, Baldomero H, Blood and marrow transplantation activity in Europe 1995. *Bone Marrow Transplant* 1997; **19:** 407–19.

16. Bennett CL, Armitage JL, Armitage GO et al, Costs of care and outcomes for high-dose therapy and autologous transplantation for lymphoid malignancies: Results from the University of Nebraska 1987 through 1991. *J Clin Oncol* 1995; **13:** 969–73.

17. Meisenberg BR, Miller WE, McMillan R et al, Outpatient high-dose chemotherapy with autologous stem-cell rescue for hematologic and nonhematologic malignancies. *J Clin Oncol* 1997; **15:** 11–17.

18. Miller CB, Piantadosi S, Vogelsang GB et al, Impact of age on outcome of patients with cancer undergoing autologous bone marrow transplant. *J Clin Oncol* 1996; **14:** 1327–32.

19. Lazarus HM, Horowitz MM, Nugent ML, Outcome of autotransplants in older adults. *Proc Am Soc Clin Oncol* 1996; **15:** 338.

20. Kusnierz-Glaz CR, Schlegel PG, Wong RM et al, Influence of age on the outcome of 500 autologous bone marrow transplant procedures for hematologic malignancies. *J Clin Oncol* 1997; **15:** 18–25.

21. Philip T, Armitage JO, Spitzer G et al, High-dose therapy and autologous bone marrow transplantation after failure of conventional chemotherapy in adults with intermediate-grade or high-grade non-Hodgkin's lymphoma. *N Engl J Med* 1987; **316:** 1493–8.

22. Colombat P, Gorin N-C, Lemonnier M-P et al, The role of autologous bone marrow transplantation in 46 adult patients with non-Hodgkin's lymphomas. *J Clin Oncol* 1990; **8:** 630–7.

23. Phillips GL, Fay JW, Herzig RH et al, The treatment of progressive non-Hodgkin's lymphoma with intensive chemoradiotherapy and autologous marrow transplantation. *Blood* 1990; **75:** 831–8.

24. Petersen FB, Appelbaum RF, Hill R et al, Autologous marrow transplantation for malignant lymphoma: A report of 101 cases from Seattle. *J Clin Oncol* 1990; **8:** 638–47.

25. Weisdorf DJ, Haake R, Miller WJ et al, Autologous bone marrow transplantation for progressive non-Hodgkin's lymphoma: clinical impact of immunophenotype and in vitro purging. *Bone Marrow Transplant* 1991; **8:** 135–42.

26. Lazarus HM, Crilley P, Ciobanu N et al, High-dose carmustine, etoposide, and cisplatin and autologous bone marrow transplantation for relapsed and refractory lymphoma. *J Clin Oncol* 1992; **10:** 1682–9.

27. Gulati S, Yahalom J, Acaba L et al, Treatment of patients with relapsed and resistant non-Hodgkin's lymphoma using total body irradiation, etoposide, and cyclophosphamide and autologous bone marrow transplantation. *J Clin Oncol* 1992; **10:** 936–41.

28. Vose JM, Anderson JR, Kessinger A et al, High-

dose chemotherapy and autologous hematopoietic stem-cell transplantation for aggressive non-Hodgkin's lymphoma. *J Clin Oncol* 1993; **11:** 1846–51.

29. Rapoport AP, Rowe JM, Kouides PA et al, One hundred autotransplants for relapsed or refractory Hodgkin's disease and lymphoma: Value of pretransplant disease status for predicting outcome. *J Clin Oncol* 1993; **11:** 2351–61.

30. Wheeler C, Strawderman M, Ayash L et al, Prognostic factors for treatment outcome in autotransplantation of intermediate-grade and high-grade non-Hodgkin's lymphoma with cyclophosphamide, carmustine, and etoposide. *J Clin Oncol* 1993; **11:** 1085–91.

31. Weaver CH, Petersen FB, Appelbaum FR et al, High-dose fractionated total-body irradiation, etoposide, and cyclophosphamide followed by autologous stem-cell support in patients with malignant lymphoma. *J Clin Oncol* 1994; **12:** 2559–66.

32. Horning SJ, Negrin RS, Chao NJ et al, Fractionated total-body irradiation, etoposide, and cyclophosphamide plus autografting in Hodgkin's disease and non-Hodgkin's lymphoma. *J Clin Oncol* 1994; **12:** 2552–8.

33. van Besien K, Tabocoff J, Rodriguez M et al, High-dose chemotherapy with BEAC regimen and autologous bone marrow transplantation for intermediate grade and immunoblastic lymphoma: durable complete remission, but a high rate of regimen-related toxicity. *Bone Marrow Transplant* 1995; **15:** 549–55.

34. Mills W, Chopra R, McMillan A et al, BEAM Chemotherapy and autologous bone marrow transplantation for patients with relapsed or refractory non-Hodgkin's lymphoma. *J Clin Oncol* 1995; **13:** 588–95.

35. Stockerl-Goldstein KE, Horning SF, Negrin RS et al, Influence of preparatory regimen and source of hematopoietic cells on outcome of autotransplantation for non-Hodgkin's lymphoma. *Biol Blood Marrow Transplant* 1996; **2:** 76–85.

36. The International Non-Hodgkin's Lymphoma Prognostic Factors Project: A predictive model for aggressive non-Hodgkin's lymphoma. *N Engl J Med* 1993; **329:** 987–94.

37. Moskowitz CH, Portlock CS, Simonaitis NA et al, The International Prognostic Index (IPI) predicts response and event free survival in an intent to treat autologous stem cell transplantation (ASCT) program for refractory and relapsed intermediate grade non-Hodgkin's lymphoma (IGL). *Proc Am Soc Clin Oncol* 1996; **15:** 415.

38. Press OW, Livingston R, Mortimer J et al, Treatment of relapsed non-Hodgkin's lymphomas with dexamethasone, high-dose cytarabine, and cisplatin before marrow transplantation. *J Clin Oncol* 1991; **9:** 423–31.

39. Surbone A, Armitage JO, Gale RP, Autotransplantations in lymphoma: Better therapy or healthier patients? *Ann Intern Med* 1991; **114:** 1059–60.

40. Bosly A, Coiffier B, Gisselbrecht C et al, Bone marrow transplantation prolongs survival after relapse in aggressive-lymphoma patients treated with the LNH-84 regimen. *J Clin Oncol* 1992; **10:** 1615–23.

41. Philip T, Hartmann O, Pinkerton R et al, Curability of relapsed childhood B-cell non-Hodgkin's lymphoma after intensive first line therapy: A report from the Société Francaise d'Oncologie Pédiatrique. *Blood* 1993; **81:** 2003–6.

42. Philip T, Guglielmi C, Hagenbeek A et al, Autologous bone marrow transplantation as compared with salvage chemotherapy in relapses of chemotherapy-sensitive non-Hodgkin's lymphoma. *N Engl J Med* 1995; **333:** 1540–5.

43. Messori A, Bonistalli L, Costantini M, Alterini R, Cost-effectiveness of autologous bone marrow transplantation in patients with relapsed non-Hodgkin's lymphoma. *Bone Marrow Transplant* 1997; **19:** 275–81.

44. Freedman AS, Ritz J, Neuberg D, Autologous bone marrow transplantation in 69 patients with a history of low-grade B-cell non-Hodgkin's lymphoma. *Blood* 1991; **77:** 2524–9.

45. Fouillard L, Gorin NC, Laporte JPh et al, Feasibility of autologous bone marrow transplantation for early consolidation of follicular non-Hodgkin's lymphoma. *Eur J Haematol* 1991; **46:** 279–84.

46. Colombat Ph, Donadio D, Fouillard L et al, Value of autologous bone marrow transplantation in follicular lymphoma: a France Autogreffe retrospective study of 42 patients. *Bone Marrow Transplant* 1994; **13:** 157–62.

47. Schouten HC, Colombat Ph, Verdonck LF et al, Autologous bone marrow transplantation for low-grade non-Hodgkin's lymphoma: The European Bone Marrow Transplant Group experience. *Ann Oncol* 1994; **5**(Suppl 2): S147–9.

48. Rohatiner AZS, Johnson PWM, Price CGA et al,

Myeloablative therapy with autologous bone marrow transplantation as consolidation therapy for recurrent follicular lymphoma. *J Clin Oncol* 1994; **12:** 1177–84.

49. Cervantes F, Shu XO, McGlave PB et al, Autologous bone marrow transplantation for non-transformed low-grade non-Hodgkin's lymphoma. *Bone Marrow Transplant* 1995; **16:** 387–92.

50. Bastion Y, Price P, Haioun C et al, Intensive therapy with peripheral blood progenitor cell transplantation in 60 patients with poor-prognosis follicular lymphoma. *Blood* 1995; **86:** 3257–62.

51. Haas R, Moos M, Karcher A et al, Sequential high-dose therapy with peripheral-blood progenitor-cell support in low-grade non-Hodgkin's lymphoma. *J Clin Oncol* 1994; **12:** 1685–92.

52. Haas R, Moos M, Möhle R et al, High-dose therapy with peripheral blood progenitor cell transplantation in low-grade non-Hodgkin's lymphoma. *Bone Marrow Transplant* 1996; **17:** 149–55.

53. Bierman PJ, Vose JM, Anderson JR et al, High-dose therapy with autologous hematopoietic rescue for follicular low-grade non-Hodgkin's lymphoma. *J Clin Oncol* 1997; **15:** 445–50.

54. Freedman AS, Gribben JG, Neuberg D et al, High-dose therapy and autologous bone marrow transplantation in patients with follicular lymphomas during first remission. *Blood* 1996; **88:** 2780–6.

55. Schouten HC, Bierman PJ, Vaughan WP et al, Autologous bone marrow transplantation in follicular non-Hodgkin's lymphoma before and after histologic transformation. *Blood* 1989; **74:** 2579–84.

56. Williams CD, Taghipour G, Lister TA et al, Chemosensitive transformed follicular non-Hodgkin's lymphoma (NHL) is a firm indication for high-dose therapy and autologous stem cell transplantation. *Blood* 1996; **88**(Suppl 1): 685a.

57. Morel P, Laporte JP, Noel MP et al, Autologous bone marrow transplantation as consolidation therapy may prolong remission in newly diagnosed high-risk follicular lymphoma: a pilot study of 34 cases. *Leukemia* 1995; **9:** 576–82.

58. van Besien KW, Mehra RC, Giralt SA et al, Allogeneic bone marrow transplantation for poor-prognosis lymphoma: Response, toxicity, and survival depend on disease histology. *Am J Med* 1996; **100:** 299–307.

59. Carella AM, Congiu AM, Gaozza E et al, High-dose chemotherapy with autologous bone marrow transplantation in 50 advanced resistant Hodgkin's disease patients: An Italian study group report. *J Clin Oncol* 1988; **6:** 1411–16.

60. Phillips GL, Wolff SN, Herzig RH et al, Treatment of progressive Hodgkin's disease with intensive chemoradiotherapy and autologous bone marrow transplantation. *Blood* 1989; **73:** 2086–92.

61. Reece DE, Barnett MJ, Connors JM et al, Intensive chemotherapy with cyclophosphamide, carmustine, and etoposide followed by autologous bone marrow transplantation for relapsed Hodgkin's disease. *J Clin Oncol* 1991; **9:** 1871–9.

62. Crump M, Smith AM, Brandwein J et al, High-dose etoposide and melphalan, and autologous bone marrow transplantation for patients with advanced Hodgkin's disease: Importance of disease status at transplant. *J Clin Oncol* 1993; **11:** 704–11.

63. Gianni AM, Siena S, Bregni M et al, High-dose sequential chemo-radiotherapy with peripheral blood progenitor cell support for relapsed or refractory Hodgkin's disease – A 6-year update. *Ann Oncol* 1993; **4:** 889–91.

64. Yahalom J, Gulati SC, Toia M et al, Accelerated hyperfractionated total-lymphoid irradiation, high-dose chemotherapy, and autologous bone marrow transplantation for refractory and relapsing patients with Hodgkin's disease. *J Clin Oncol* 1993; **11:** 1062–70.

65. Reece DE, Connors JM, Spinelli JJ et al, Intensive therapy with cyclophosphamide, carmustine, etoposide ± cisplatin, and autologous bone marrow transplantation for Hodgkin's disease in first relapse after combination chemotherapy. *Blood* 1994; **83:** 1193–9.

66. Chopra R, McMillan AK, Linch DC et al, The place of high-dose BEAM therapy and autologous bone marrow transplantation in poor-risk Hodgkin's disease. A single-center eight-year study of 155 patients. *Blood* 1993; **81:** 1137–45.

67. Bierman PJ, Bagin RG, Jagannath S et al, high dose chemotherapy followed by autologous hematopoietic rescue in Hodgkin's disease: Long term follow-up in 128 patients. *Ann Oncol* 1993; **4:** 767–73.

68. Nademanee A, O'Donnell MR, Snyder DS et al, High-dose chemotherapy with or without total body irradiation followed by autologous bone marrow and/or peripheral blood stem cell

transplantation for patients with relapsed and refractory Hodgkin's disease: Results in 85 patients with analysis of prognostic factors. *Blood* 1995; **85:** 1381–90.

69. Burns LJ, Daniels KA, McGlave PB et al, Autologous stem cell transplantation for refractory and relapsed Hodgkin's disease: factors predictive of prolonged survival. *Bone Marrow Transplant* 1995; **16:** 13–18.

70. Lumley MA, Milligan DW, Knechtli CJC et al, High lactate dehydrogenase level is associated with an adverse outlook in autografting for Hodgkin's disease. *Bone Marrow Transplant* 1996; **17:** 383–8.

71. Horning SJ, Chao NJ, Negrin RS et al, High-dose therapy and autologous hematopoietic progenitor cell transplantation for recurrent or refractory Hodgkin's disease: Analysis of the Stanford University results and prognostic indices. *Blood* 1997; **89:** 801–13.

72. Jagannath S, Armitage JO, Dicke KA et al, Prognostic factors for response and survival after high-dose cyclophosphamide, carmustine, and etoposide with autologous bone marrow transplantation for relapsed Hodgkin's disease. *J Clin Oncol* 1989; **7:** 179–85.

73. Armitage JO, Bierman PJ, Vose JM et al, Autologous bone marrow transplantation for patients with relapsed Hodgkin's disease. *Am J Med* 1991; **91:** 605–11.

74. Bierman PJ, Anderson JR, Freeman MB et al, High-dose chemotherapy followed by autologous hematopoietic rescue for Hodgkin's disease patients following first relapse after chemotherapy. *Ann Oncol* 1996; **7:** 151–6.

75. Yuen AR, Rosenberg SA, Hoppe RT et al, Comparison between conventional salvage therapy and high-dose therapy with autografting for recurrent or refractory Hodgkin's disease. *Blood* 1997; **89:** 814–22.

76. Spinolo JA, Jagannath S, Velásquez et al, Cisplatin–CBV with autologous bone marrow transplantation for relapsed Hodgkin's disease. *Leukemia Lymphoma* 1993; **9:** 71–7.

77. Poen JC, Hoppe RT, Horning SJ, High-dose therapy and autologous bone marrow transplantation for relapsed/refractory Hodgkin's disease: The impact of involved field radiotherapy on patterns of failure and survival. *Int J Radiat Oncol Biol Phys* 1996; **36:** 3–12.

78. Linch DC, Winfield D, Goldstone AH et al, Dose intensification with autologous bone-marrow transplantation in relapsed and resistant Hodgkin's disease: results of a BNLI randomised trial. *Lancet* 1993; **341:** 1051–4.

79. Reece DE, Barnett MJ, Shepherd JD et al, High-dose cyclophosphamide, carmustine (BCNU), and etoposide (VP16-213) with or without cisplatin (CBV ± P) and autologous transplantation for patients with Hodgkin's disease who fail to enter a complete remission after combination chemotherapy. *Blood* 1995; **86:** 451–6.

80. Pettengell R, Morgenstern GR, Woll PJ et al, Peripheral blood progenitor cell transplantation in lymphoma and leukemia using a single apheresis. *Blood* 1993; **82:** 3770–7.

81. Negrin RS, Kusnierz-Glaz CR, Still BJ et al, Transplantation of enriched and purged peripheral blood progenitor cells from a single apheresis product in patients with non-Hodgkin's lymphoma. *Blood* 1995; **85:** 3334–41.

82. Weisdorf D, Daniels K, Miller W et al, Bone marrow vs peripheral blood stem cells for autologous lymphoma transplantation: A prospective randomized trial. *Blood* 1993; **82**(Suppl 1): 444a.

83. Brice P, Marolleau JP, Pautier P et al, High dose chemotherapy and autologous stem cell transplantation for advanced lymphomas: comparison of bone marrow versus peripheral blood stem cell (PBSC) in 147 patients. *Br J Haematol* 1994; **87**(Suppl 1): 27.

84. Bierman P, Vose J, Anderson J et al, Comparison of autologous bone marrow transplantation (ABMT) with peripheral stem cell transplantation (PSCT) for patients with Hodgkin's disease. *Blood* 1993; **10**(Suppl 1): 445a.

85. Ager S, Scott MA, Mahendra P et al, Peripheral blood stem cell transplantation after high-dose therapy in patients with malignant lymphoma: a retrospective comparison with autologous bone marrow transplantation. *Bone Marrow Transplant* 1995; **16:** 79–83.

86. Schmitz N, Linch DC, Dreger P et al, Randomised trial of filgrastim-mobilised peripheral blood progenitor cell transplantation versus autologous bone-marrow transplantation in lymphoma patients. *Lancet* 1996; **347:** 353–7.

87. Smith TJ, Hillner BE, Schmitz N et al, Economic analysis of a randomized clinical trial to compare filgrastim-mobilized peripheral-blood progenitor-cell transplantation and autologous bone marrow transplantation in patients with Hodgkin's and non-Hodgkin's lymphoma. *J Clin Oncol* 1997; **15:** 5–10.

88. Brunvand MW, Bensinger WI, Soll E et al, High-dose fractionated total-body irradiation, etoposide and cyclophosphamide for treatment of malignant lymphoma: comparison of autologous bone marrow and peripheral blood stem cells. *Bone Marrow Transplant* 1996; **18:** 131–41.

89. Majolino I, Pearce R, Taghipour G, Goldstone AH, Peripheral-blood stem-cell transplantation versus autologous bone marrow transplantation in Hodgkin's and non-Hodgkin's lymphomas: A new matched-pair analysis of the European Group for Blood and Marrow Transplantation Registry Data. *J Clin Oncol* 1997; **15:** 509–17.

90. Janssen W, Smilee R, Elfenbein G, A prospective randomized trial comparing blood- and marrow-derived stem cells for hematopoietic replacement following high-dose chemotherapy. *J Hemother* 1995; **4:** 139–40.

91. Dicke KA, Hood DL, Arneson M et al, Effects of short-term in vivo administration of G-CSF on bone marrow prior to harvesting. *Exp Hematol* 1997; **25:** 34–8.

92. Roberts MM, To LB, Gillis et al, Immune reconstitution following peripheral blood stem cell transplantation, autologous bone marrow transplantation and allogeneic bone marrow transplantation. *Bone Marrow Transplant* 1993; **12:** 469–75.

93. Scheid C, Pettengel, R, Ghielmini M et al, Time-course of the recovery of cellular immune function after high-dose chemotherapy and peripheral blood progenitor cell transplantation for high-grade non-Hodgkin's lymphoma. *Bone Marrow Transplant* 1995; **15:** 901–6.

94. Talmadge JE, Reed E, Ino K et al, Rapid immunologic reconstitution following transplantation with mobilized peripheral blood stem cells as compared to bone marrow. *Bone Marrow Transplant* 1997; **19:** 161–72.

95. Rizzoli V, Carlo-Stella C, Stem cell purging: An intriguing dilemma. *Exp Hematol* 1995; **23:** 296–302.

96. Williams CD, Goldstone AH, Pearce R et al, Purging of bone marrow in autologous bone marrow transplantation for non-Hodgkin's lymphoma lymphoma: A case-matched comparison with unpurged cases by the European Blood and Marrow Transplant Lymphoma Registry. *J Clin Oncol* 1996; **14:** 2454–64.

97. Sharp JG, Mann S, Murphy B, Weekes C, Culture methods for the detection of minimal tumor contamination of hematopoietic harvests:

98. Gribben JG, Neuberg D, Barber M et al, Detection of residual lymphoma cells by polymerase chain reaction in peripheral blood is significantly less predictive for relapse than detection in bone marrow. *Blood* 1994; **83:** 3800–7.

99. Negrin RS, Pesando J, Detection of tumor cells in purged bone marrow and peripheral-blood mononuclear cells by polymerase chain reaction amplification of bcl-2 translocations. *J Clin Oncol* 1994; **12:** 1021–7.

100. Hardingham JE, Kotasek D, Sage RE et al, Molecular detection of residual lymphoma cells in peripheral blood stem cell harvests and following autologous transplantation. *Bone Marrow Transplant* 1993; **11:** 15–20.

101. McCann JC, Kanteti R, Shilepsky B et al, High degree of occult tumor contamination in bone marrow and peripheral blood stem cells of patients undergoing autologous transplantation for non-Hodgkin's lymphoma. *Biol Blood Marrow Transplant* 1996; **2:** 37–43.

102. Brenner MK, Rill DR, Moen RC, Gene-marking to trace origin of relapse after autologous bone-marrow transplantation. *Lancet* 1993; **341:** 85–6.

103. Deisseroth AB, Zu Z, Claxton D et al, Genetic marking shows that Ph⁺ cells present in autologous transplants of chronic myelogenous leukemia (CML) contribute to relapse after autologous bone marrow in CML. *Blood* 1994; **83:** 3068–76.

104. Vaughan WP, Weisenburger DD, Sanger et al, Early leukemic recurrence of non-Hodgkin's lymphoma after high-dose anti-neoplastic therapy with autologous marrow rescue. *Bone Marrow Transplant* 1987; **1:** 373–8.

105. Rossetti F, Deeg HJ, Hackman RC, Early pulmonary recurrence of non-Hodgkin's lymphoma after autologous marrow transplantation: evidence for reinfusion of lymphoma cells. *Bone Marrow Transplant* 1995; **15:** 429–32.

106. Gribben JG, Freedman AS, Neuberg D et al, Immunologic purging of marrow assessed by PCR before autologous bone marrow transplantation for B-cell lymphoma. *N Engl J Med* 1991; **325:** 1525–33.

107. Sharp JG, Kessinger A, Mann S et al, Outcome of high-dose therapy and autologous transplantation in non-Hodgkin's lymphoma based on the presence of tumor in the marrow or infused hematopoietic harvest. *J Clin Oncol* 1996; **14:** 214–19.

a review. *J Hematother* 1995; **4:** 141–8.

108. Butturini A, Bortin MM, Gale RP, Graft-versus-leukemia following bone marrow transplantation. *Bone Marrow Transplant* 1987; **2**: 233–42.

109. Appelbaum FR, Sullivan KM, Buckner CD et al, Treatment of malignant lymphoma in 100 patients with chemotherapy, total body irradiation, and marrow transplantation. *J Clin Oncol* 1987; **5**: 1340–7.

110. Jones RJ, Ambinder RF, Piantadosi S et al, Evidence of a graft-versus-lymphoma effect associated with allogeneic bone marrow transplantation. *Blood* 1991; **77**: 649–53.

111. Ratanatharathorn V, Uberti J, Karanes C et al, Prospective comparative trial of autologous versus allogeneic bone marrow transplantation in patients with non-Hodgkin's lymphoma. *Blood* 1994; **84**: 1050–5.

112. Chopra R, Goldstone AH, Pearce R et al, Autologous versus allogeneic bone marrow transplantation for non-Hodgkin's lymphoma: A case-controlled analysis of the European bone marrow transplant group registry data. *J Clin Oncol* 1992; **10**: 1690–5.

113. Anderson JE, Litzow MR, Appelbaum FR et al, Allogeneic, syngeneic, and autologous marrow transplantation for Hodgkin's disease: The 21-year Seattle experience. *J Clin Oncol* 1993; **11**: 2342.

114. Gajewski JL, Phillips GL, Sobocinski KA et al, Bone marrow transplants from HLA-identical siblings in advanced Hodgkin's disease. *J Clin Oncol* 1996; **14**: 572–8.

115. Milpied N, Fielding AK, Pearce RM et al, Allogeneic bone marrow transplant is not better than autologous transplant for patients with relapsed Hodgkin's disease. *J Clin Oncol* 1996; **14**: 1291–6.

116. Gulati SC, Shank B, Black P et al, Autologous bone marrow transplantation for patients with poor-prognosis lymphoma. *J Clin Oncol* 1988; **6**: 1303–13.

117. Milpied N, Ifrah N, Kuentz M et al, Bone marrow transplantation for adult poor prognosis lymphoblastic lymphoma in first complete remission. *Br J Haematol* 1989; **73**: 82–7.

118. Santini G, Congiu AM, Coser P et al, Autologous bone marrow transplantation for adult advanced stage lymphoblastic in first CR. A study of the NHLCSG. *Leukemia* 1991; **5**(Suppl 1): 42–5.

119. Baro J, Richard C, Calavia J et al, Autologous bone marrow transplantation as consolidation therapy for non-Hodgkin's lymphoma lym-phoma patients with poor prognostic features. *Bone Marrow Transplant* 1991; **8**: 283–9.

120. Verdonck LF, Dekker AW, de Gast GC et al, Autologous bone marrow transplantation for adult poor-risk lymphoblastic lymphoma in first remission. *J Clin Oncol* 1992; **10**: 644–6.

121. Nademanee A, Schmidt GM, O'Donnell MR et al, High-dose chemoradiotherapy followed by autologous bone marrow transplantation as consolidation therapy during first complete remission in adult patients with poor-risk aggressive lymphoma: A pilot study. *Blood* 1992; **80**: 1130–4.

122. Freedman AS, Takvorian T, Neuberg D et al, Autologous bone marrow transplantation in poor-prognosis intermediate-grade and high-grade B-cell non-Hodgkin's lymphoma in first remission: A pilot study. *J Clin Oncol* 1993; **11**: 931–6.

123. Jackson GH, Lennard AL, Taylor PRA et al, Autologous bone marrow transplantation in poor-risk high-grade non-Hodgkin's lymphoma in first complete remission. *Br J Cancer* 1994; **70**: 501–5.

124. Sweetenham JW, Proctor SJ, Blaise D et al, High-dose therapy and autologous bone marrow transplantation in first complete remission for adult patients with high-grade non-Hodgkin's lymphoma: The EBMT experience. *Ann Oncol* 1994; **5**(Suppl 2): S155–9.

125. Jost LM, Jacky E, Dommann-Scherrer C et al, Short-term weekly chemotherapy followed by high-dose therapy with autologous bone marrow transplantation for lymphoblastic and Burkitt's lymphomas in adult patients. *Ann Oncol* 1995; **6**: 445–51.

126. Fanin R, Silvestri F, Geromin A et al, Primary systemic CD30 (Ki-1)-positive anaplastic large cell lymphoma of the adult: Sequential intensive treatment with the F-MACHOP regimen ($\pm$radiotherapy) and autologous bone marrow transplantation. *Blood* 1996; **87**: 1243–8.

127. Pettengell R, Radford JA, Morgenstern GR et al, Survival benefit from high-dose therapy with autologous blood progenitor-cell transplantation in poor-prognosis non-Hodgkin's lymphoma. *J Clin Oncol* 1996; **14**: 586–92.

128. Vitolo U, Cortellazzo S, Liberati AM et al, Intensified and high-dose chemotherapy with granulocyte colony-stimulating factor and autologous stem-cell transplantation support as first-line therapy in high-risk diffuse large-cell lymphoma. *J Clin Oncol* 1997; **15**: 491–8.

129. Haioun C, Lepage E, Gisselbrecht C et al, Comparison of autologous bone marrow transplantation with sequential chemotherapy for intermediate-grade and high-grade non-Hodgkin's lymphoma in first complete remission: A study of 464 patients. *J Clin Oncol* 1994; **12:** 2543–51.

130. Haioun C, Lepage E, Gisselbrecht C et al, Benefit of autologous bone marrow transplantation over sequential chemotherapy in poor-risk aggressive non-Hodgkin's lymphoma: Updated results of the prospective study LNH87-2. *J Clin Oncol* 1997; **15:** 1131–7.

131. Klimo P, Connors JM, Updated clinical experience with MACOP-B. *Semin Hematol* 1987; **24**(Suppl 1): 26–34.

132. Gianni AM, Bregni M, Siena S et al, 5-year update of the Milan Cancer Institute randomized trial of high-dose sequential (HDS) vs MACOP-B therapy for diffuse large-cell lymphomas. *Proc Am Soc Clin Oncol* 1994; **13:** 373.

133. Gianni AM, Bregni M, Siena S et al, Is high-dose better than standard-dose chemotherapy as initial treatment of poor-rise large-cell lymphomas? A critical analysis from available randomized trials. *Ann Oncol* 1996; **7**(Suppl 3): 12.

134. Haq R, Sawka CA, Franssen E et al, Significance of a partial or slow response to front-line chemotherapy in the management of intermediate-grade or high-grade non-Hodgkin's lymphoma: A literature review. *J Clin Oncol* 1994; **12:** 1074–84.

135. Verdonck LF, van Putten WLJ, Hagenbeek A et al, Comparison of CHOP chemotherapy with autologous bone marrow transplantation for slowly responding patients with aggressive non-Hodgkin's lymphoma. *N Engl J Med* 1995; **332:** 1045–51.

136. Martelli M, Vignetti M, Zinzani PL et al, High-dose chemotherapy followed by autologous bone marrow transplantation versus dexamethasone, cisplatin, and cytarabine in aggressive non-Hodgkin's lymphoma with partial response to front-line chemotherapy: A prospective randomized Italian multicenter study. *J Clin Oncol* 1996; **14:** 534–42.

137. Haioun C, Lepage E, Gisselbrecht C et al, Autologous transplantation versus conventional salvage therapy in aggressive non-Hodgkin's lymphoma (NHL) partially responding to first line chemotherapy. A study of 96 patients enrolled in the LNH87-2 protocol. *Blood* 1995; **86**(Suppl 1): 211a.

138. Carella AM, Carlier P, Congiu A et al, Autologous bone marrow transplantation as adjuvant treatment for high-risk Hodgkin's disease in first complete remission after MOPP/ABVD protocol. *Bone Marrow Transplant* 1991; **8:** 99–103.

139. Moreau P, Milpied N, Mechinaud-Lacroix F et al, Early intensive therapy with autotransplantation for high-risk Hodgkin's disease. *Leukemia Lymphoma* 1993; **12:** 51–8.

140. Moreau P, Fleury J, Bouabdallah R et al, Early intensive therapy with autologous stem cell transplantation (ASCT) in high-risk Hodgkin's disease (HD): Report of 158 cases from the French Registry (SFGM). *Blood* 1996; **88**(Suppl 1): 486a.

141. Darrington DL, Vose JM, Anderson JR et al, Incidence and characterization of secondary myelodysplastic syndrome and acute myelogenous leukemia following high-dose chemoradiotherapy and autologous stem-cell transplantation for lymphoid malignancies. *J Clin Oncol* 1994; **12:** 2527–34.

142. Fielding AK, Philip T, Carella A et al, Autologous bone marrow transplantation for lymphomas – A 15 year European Bone Marrow Transplant Registry (EBMT) experience of 3325 patients. *Blood* 1994; **84**(Suppl 1): 536a.

143. Mills W, Strang J, Goldstone AH et al, Dose intensification of etoposide in the BEAM ABMT protocol for malignant lymphoma. *Leukemia Lymphoma* 1995; **17:** 263–70.

144. Wheeler C, Antin JH, Churchill WH et al, Cyclophosphamide, carmustine, and etoposide with autologous bone marrow transplantation in refractory Hodgkin's disease and non-Hodgkin's lymphoma: A dose finding study. *J Clin Oncol* 1990; **8:** 648–56.

145. Weaver CH, Appelbaum FR, Petersen FB et al, High-dose cyclophosphamide, carmustine, and etoposide followed by autologous bone marrow transplantation in patients with lymphoid malignancies who have received dose-limiting radiation therapy. *J Clin Oncol* 1993; **11:** 1329.

146. Bierman PJ, Vose JM, Leichner PK et al, Yttrium 90-labeled antiferritin followed by high-dose chemotherapy and autologous bone marrow transplantation for poor-prognosis Hodgkin's disease. *J Clin Oncol* 1993; **11:** 698–703.

147. Press OW, Eary JF, Appelbaum FR et al, Radiolabeled-antibody therapy of B-cell lymphoma with autologous bone marrow support. *N Engl J Med* 1993; **329:** 1219–24.

148. Miller JS, Arthur DC, Litz CE et al, Myelodysplastic syndrome after autologous bone marrow transplantation: An additional late complication of curative cancer therapy. *Blood* 1994; **83:** 3780–6.

149. Traweek ST, Slovak ML, Nademanee AP et al, Clonal karyotypic hematopoietic cell abnormalities occurring after autologous bone marrow transplantation for Hodgkin's disease and non-Hodgkin's lymphoma. *Blood* 1994; **84:** 957–63.

150. Bhatia S, Ramsay N, Steinbuch M et al, Malignant neoplasms following bone marrow transplantation. *Blood* 1995; **87:** 3633–9.

151. Ahmed T, Lake DE, Beer M et al, Single and double autotransplants for relapsing/refractory Hodgkin's disease: results of two consecutive trials. *Bone Marrow Transplant* 1997; **19:** 449–54.

152. Grossbard ML, Gribben JG, Freedman AS et al, Adjuvant immunotoxin therapy with anti-B4-blocked ricin after autologous bone marrow transplantation for patients with B-cell non-Hodgkin's lymphoma. *Blood* 1993; **81:** 2263–71.

153. Schenkein DP, Dixon P, Desforges JF et al, Phase I/II study of cyclophosphamide, carboplatin, and etoposide and autologous hematopoietic stem-cell transplantation with posttransplant interferon alfa-2b for patients with lymphoma and Hodgkin's disease. *J Clin Oncol* 1994; **12:** 2423–31.

154. Verma UN, Areman E, Dickerson SA et al, Interleukin-2 activation of chemotherapy and growth factor-mobilized peripheral blood stem cells for generation of cytotoxic effectors. *Bone Marrow Transplant* 1995; **15:** 199–206.

155. Benyunes MC, Higuchi C, York A et al, Immunotherapy with interleukin 2 with or without lymphokine-activated killer cells after autologous bone marrow transplantation for malignant lymphoma: a feasibility trial. *Bone Marrow Transplant* 1995; **16:** 283–8.

156. Robinson N, Benyunes MC, Thompson JA et al, Interleukin-2 after autologous stem cell transplantation for hematologic malignancy: a phase I/II study. *Bone Marrow Transplant* 1997; **19:** 435–42.

157. Gryn J, Johnson E, Goldman N et al, The treatment of relapsed or refractory intermediate grade non-Hodgkin's lymphoma with autologous bone marrow transplantation followed by cyclosporine and interferon. *Bone Marrow Transplant* 1997; **19:** 221–6.

5.4

Myeloma

Nikhil C Munshi, Sundar Jagannath, Guido Tricot and Bart Barlogie

CONTENTS • Introduction • Hematopoietic stem cell source • Stem cell purging • Conditioning regimen • Importance of transplant timing • Transplantation in newly diagnosed patients • Refractory and relapsed patients • Prognostic factors • Transplantation in patients with renal failure • Transplantation in older patients • Myelodysplastic syndrome following transplantation myeloma • Summary

INTRODUCTION

Multiple myeloma is a B-cell malignancy that still remains incurable with standard-dose chemotherapy. For the past 30 years, standard dose regimens, such as melphalan and prednisone or combinations containing Adriamycin and other alkylating agents, have produced objective responses (>50% reduction in myeloma production) in 50–60% of patients. Complete responses (CR) are achieved in only 5% of the patients, defined by normal bone marrow and absence of monoclonal protein in the blood and urine. The median response duration does not exceed 18 months, while median survival is 30–36 months.[1–5] The low incidence of CR with standard induction chemotherapy suggests a marked drug resistance, even in newly diagnosed multiple myeloma, that is possibly acquired during a prolonged subclinical course of the disease during which complex karyotypic aberrations and multiple gene deletions and mutations occur.[6]

These observations prompted evaluation of dose intensity as a means of overcoming drug resistance. A pilot study by the late Tim McElwain and his colleagues at the Royal Marsdon Hospital evaluated high-dose melphalan ($140\,mg/m^2$), and achieved CRs in patients who were refractory to standard-dose treatment.[7] This initial study was performed without bone-marrow support. Subsequently, even higher melphalan doses ($200\,mg/m^2$) or chemoradiotherapy with melphalan ($140\,mg/m^2$) and total body irradiation were used, initially with autologous bone-marrow support and, more recently, with peripheral blood stem cell (PBSC) support.[8–13]

High-dose chemotherapy presents a unique challenge in patients with multiple myeloma who are older (median age at diagnosis, 65 years), and frequently have renal disorder or multi-organ dysfunctions due to amyloid and light-chain deposits. Moreover, extensive prior alkylating agent therapy with its ensuing damage to the hematopoietic stem cells makes peripheral blood stem cell collections difficult. We summarize here the current state of the art in autotransplants for myeloma, and discuss the variables and prognostic factors related to high-dose chemotherapy and future treatment options.

HEMATOPOIETIC STEM CELL SOURCE

Bone marrow was used as a source of stem cells in earlier studies of high-dose chemotherapy in

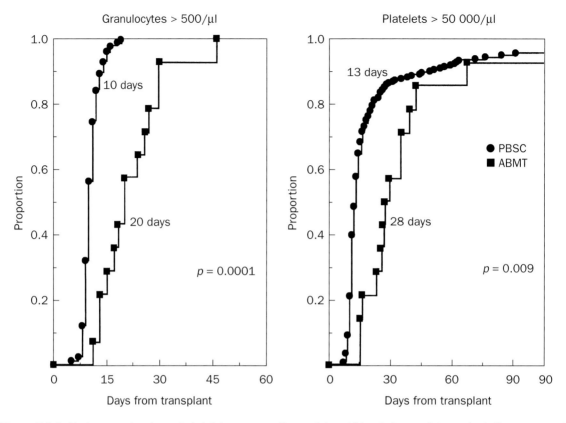

Figure 5.4.1 Faster granulocyte and platelet recovery after peripheral blood stem cell transplantation compared with bone-marrow transplantation in myeloma patients with less than 1 year of prior therapy.

patients with myeloma. However, more recent studies have used mobilized PBSC because this provides faster engraftment.[14] Myeloma patients with less than one year of prior therapy had faster granulocyte and platelet recovery after PBSC transplants compared with bone-marrow autografts (Figure 5.4.1). In a study to identify favorable variables for rapid engraftment in 225 patients with multiple myeloma undergoing PBSC transplant,[15] a highly significant correlation was observed between the number of CD34$^+$ cells/kg infused and recovery of both granulocyte and platelet counts (Figure 5.4.2). Sufficient quantities of CD34$^+$ cells required for tandem transplant were easily obtained in patients who had short exposure to standard chemotherapy (91%), while satisfac-

tory PBSC collections were obtained in only 28% of patients who had more than 24 months of prior chemotherapy. In a randomized study of 44 multiple myeloma patients, PBSC mobilization with granulocyte colony-stimulating factor (G-CSF) alone was compared with high-dose cytoxan plus G-CSF. Although patients receiving high-dose cytoxan with G-CSF had more CD34$^+$ cells collected, an adequate number of cells for two transplants was collected in the group receiving G-CSF alone.[16] However, toxicity was significantly reduced and the duration of the collection phase was shorter in the latter group. The engraftment kinetics and toxicities after the first and second transplant were similar in both the groups.

The duration of prior chemotherapy, espe-

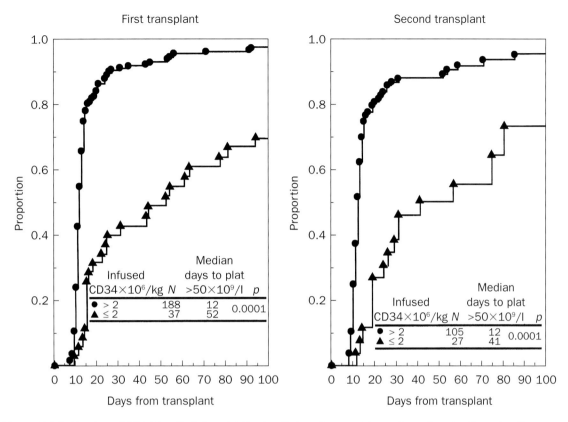

Figure 5.4.2 Number of CD34$^+$ cells infused following first and second transplantation significantly affects platelet recovery.

cially with stem cell damaging agents (melphalan, BCNU and cyclophosphamide), along with radiation to bone marrow-containing areas significantly affects the ability to procure adequate quantities of peripheral blood stem cells and the engraftment kinetics post transplant[15] (Figure 5.4.3). In patients with limited prior therapy ($\leq$12 months), mobilization with high-dose G-CSF[10–16] does provide adequate PBSC for the safe conduct of tandem transplants. However, in patients who have undergone more than 12 months of prior therapy, collection of CD34$^+$ cells is adequate in only one-third. Addition of stem cell factor has been shown to improve mobilization in this group.[17] The optimal method for PBSC mobilization is still under

investigation in this group of patients.

Differential mobilization of myeloma cells and normal hematopoietic stem cells has been described after treatment with cyclophosphamide and granulocyte–macrophage colony-stimulating factor (GM-CSF).[18] The highest proportions of hematopoietic progenitor cells are collected during the first 3 days of leukapheresis, while peak levels of myeloma cells are present on the subsequent days. In addition, during the last days of collection, mobilized tumor cells show a higher labelling index and a more immature phenotype (CD19$^+$). This differential mobilization can be exploited by performing large-volume leukophereses so that collection can be completed within 3 days.

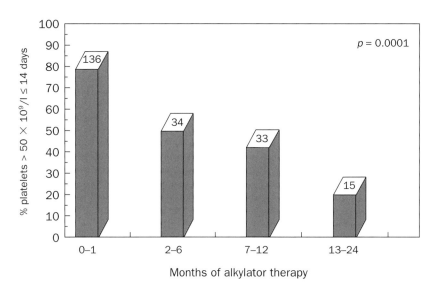

Figure 5.4.3 Effect of prior alkylating agent therapy on platelet recovery following autologous transplantation represented by percentage of patients recovering their platelet count above 50×10^9/litre in 14 days post transplantation.

STEM CELL PURGING

Tumor cell contamination of autologous bone marrow or PBSC collection is universally observed. In earlier studies, it was hypothesized that contamination with up to 30% plasma cells in the bone marrow may not significantly affect outcome, because most of these myeloma cells are extremely slowly proliferating.[19] Gene marking studies performed in patients with acute leukemia and neuroblastoma, suggest that relapses are at least partially related to infusion of tumor cells.[20] In the absence of confirmative gene marking results in myeloma, various attempts have been made to purge autografts of myeloma cells and immature B cells prior to clinical use. A relatively small degree of PBSC contamination can now be readily assessed by the CDR III PCR technology.[21] Using this method, virtually all mobilized unsorted PBSC preparations show myeloma cells in quantities from less than 0.01 to more than 10%.[22,23] After flow sorting of CD34+, Thy1+, Lin− cells, no evidence of myeloma cell contamination was observed, based on flow cytometric and PCR analysis. A quantitative PCR technique for the CDR III region showed a depletion of clonal B cells by 2.7–7.3 logs.[22–25]

An alternative negative selection method of bone-marrow purging has been studied in small number of patients. One group used a monoclonal antibody cocktail containing CD10 (common acute lymphoblastic leukemia antigen), CD20 (a pan B-cell antigen) and PCA-1, which detects a plasma cell-associated antigen. Following addition of complement to the marrow samples with these antibodies, bone-marrow samples, which previously contained up to 10% plasma cells, were devoid of cells bearing this antigen as measured by flow cytometry.[26] A separate group used peanut agglutinin (PNA) and anti-CD19 antibody bound to magnetized microspheres to deplete the bone marrow of B cells.[27] The early follow-up results from these studies have not revealed any significant advantage in responses or survival, but consistently shows a delay in engraftment post transplantation.

CONDITIONING REGIMEN

The preparative regimens that are most commonly used for multiple myeloma are melphalan ($200 \, \text{mg}/\text{m}^2$), melphalan ($140 \, \text{mg}/\text{m}^2$) with total body irradiation, or a combination of busulfan and cyclophosphamide. The pharmacological characteristics of melphalan, with its predominant myelotoxicity and metabolism independent of renal function, are ideal for multiple myeloma patients, who commonly have renal function abnormalities. Melphalan seems to be superior to thiotepa when given with total body irradiation (TBI), achieving longer relapse-free and overall survival duration.[28] Busulfan combined with cyclophosphamide, thiotepa or TBI induces occasional responses in patients relapsing after high-dose melphalan.[29–34] A combination regimen containing high-dose carboplatin with etoposide and cytoxan or a combination with CBV (cyclophosphamide, BCMU (carmustine), VP-16 (etoposide)) has been investigated in resistant patients with occasional responses noted.[9,35,36]

IMPORTANCE OF TRANSPLANT TIMING

An important question concerning autologous transplantation concerns the ideal timing of the transplantation. In order to obtain high-quality hematopoietic stem cells, it is very clear that they should be collected early in the course of the disease to avoid hematopoietic stem cell damage from the standard alkylating agent therapy.[15] Most larger studies have established that the complete response rate with autotransplants in refractory myeloma is, at best, 15–20%, compared with 40–50% in newly diagnosed patients. This information suggests that early institution of high-dose therapy may overcome the relative resistance of myeloma cells observed with standard therapy. Delay in high-dose chemotherapy and transplantation may lead to increased resistance, as well as further genetic changes resulting in more aggressive disease. A definitive answer to the question of when to transplant can only be obtained through a prospective randomized study of early versus late transplantation. An ongoing Intergroup trial in the United States should provide an answer, since patients are randomized to standard therapy or up-front high-dose therapy, and patients relapsing on standard therapy will receive high-dose therapy as salvage treatment.

TRANSPLANTATION IN NEWLY DIAGNOSED PATIENTS

As high-dose chemotherapy and PBSC transplant trials reported by various centers differ markedly in the characteristics of patients, disease stage, treatment regimen and supportive care, we first report on our large single-institution study in newly diagnosed patients.

A phase II study was initiated in August 1990, evaluating a regimen combining all therapeutic modalities available at the time in an effort to achieve the maximum cytoreduction in newly diagnosed patients with multiple myeloma.[37] The treatment schema, termed 'total therapy', is shown in Figure 5.4.4. 'Total therapy' applies intensive remission induction with three non-cross-resistant regimens prior to two cycles of myeloablative therapy with hematopoietic stem cell support. All newly diagnosed myeloma patients aged under the age of 70 years with no or at the most one cycle of standard chemotherapy were eligible. The VAD (vincristine, Adriamycin and dexamethasone) regimen was used for remission induction because of a marked and speedy tumor cell kill without damage to stem cells; VAD was followed by high-dose cyclophosphamide and GM-CSF for stem cell collection; EDAP (etoposide, dexamethasone, cytosine arabinoside and cisplatin) regimen was administered subsequently to target the more immature tumor cell compartment. This was followed by two autologous transplantations intended to be administered within 6 months of each other. The preparative regimen for the first autotransplant was melphalan at 200 mg/m^2. For the second transplant, the same regimen was given to responding patients. Those achieving less than a partial response received melphalan at 140 mg/m^2 plus TBI (1125 cGy in nine fractions with maximum lung dose < 800 cGy), and nonresponders under the age of 56 years with a matched sibling donor were offered an allogeneic transplant. Following two autotransplants and a complete hematological recovery, patients were offered interferon-α at 3 MU/m^2, three times a week, as maintenance.

A total of 231 newly diagnosed multiple

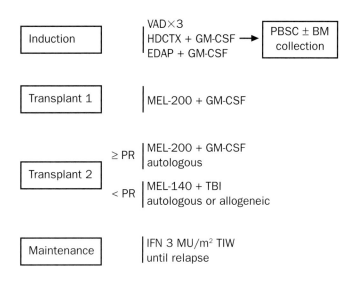

Figure 5.4.4 Treatment schema of 'total therapy'.
VAD = vincristine, Adriamycin, dexamethasone;
EDAP = etoposide, dexamethasone, cytosine arabinoside, cisplatin;
MEL = melphalan;
IFN = interferon; HDCTX = high-dose cytoxan.

myeloma patients with a median age of 51 years (range 21–70 years) were entered on this study. The patient population characteristics showed that approximately half the patients had poor prognostic criteria with elevated β_2-microglobulin, C-reactive protein (CRP) and stage III disease (Table 5.4.1).

Partial response (PR) and complete response (CR) rates increased progressively as patients completed the different phases of the treatment plan. The $\geq$PR and CR rates after induction-therapy were 69% and 14% respectively; after

the first high-dose melphalan these were 82% and 30% respectively, and after the second transplant they were 95% and 48%. With an intent-to-treat approach, the true CR rate was 37%. At the median follow-up of 37 months, event-free survival (EFS) and overall survival (OS) were 43 and 62, months respectively. The OS, EFS and relapse rate in the first 123 patients are shown in Figure 5.4.5. The median duration of cytopenia (neutropenia $< 500/\text{ml}$ and platelets $< 50\,000/\text{ml}$) is shown in Table 5.4.2. Treatment-related mortality in the first 12 months on the study was 4%. The results of the previously untreated patients on 'total therapy' were compared with those in patients treated with standard therapy on various SWOG studies.[38] From 1123 patients, 116 pair-mates were selected and matched for age, β_2-microglobulin and serum creatinine, the most important prognostic variables in patients, receiving standard chemotherapy. Using an-intent-to-treat approach, 'total therapy' was superior to standard treatment, resulting in a higher $\geq$PR rate (86% vs 52%; $p = 0.0001$) and longer median duration of EFS (49 vs 22 months; $p = 0.0001$) and OS ($\geq$62 vs 48 months; $p = 0.01$), with a projected five-year EFS of 36% vs 19% and OS of 61% vs 39% (Figure 5.4.6).

Table 5.4.1 Characteristics of 231 newly diagnosed patients entered on 'total therapy' program

Parameter	Percentage
Age > 50 years	51
Stage III	53
β_2-microglobulin $\geq$ 3 mg/l	55
One course of prior therapy	33

Median follow-up of alive patients = 37 months.

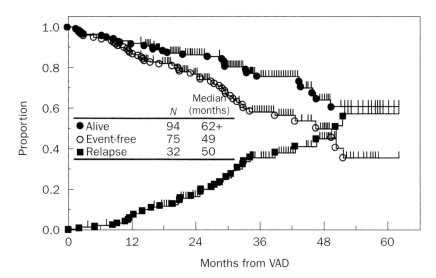

Figure 5.4.5 Overall and event-free survival and relapse analysis of 123 newly diagnosed patients with multiple myeloma treated with 'total therapy' regimen. VAD = vincristine, Adriamycin, dexamethasone.

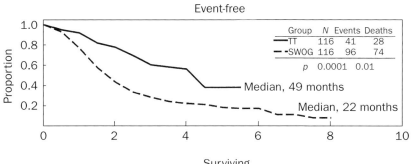

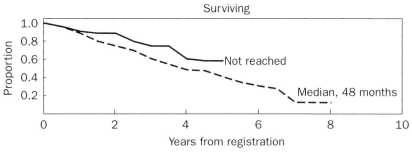

Figure 5.4.6 Newly diagnosed patients with myeloma treated on 'total therapy' regimen (TT) had superior overall and event-free survival compared with closely matched pair-mates treated with standard dose therapy according to SWOG protocols.

The same question of the superiority of high-dose chemotherapy with autologous PBSC transplant versus standard chemotherapy was investigated in a prospective randomized trial by a French Intergroup study on myeloma.[39] Newly diagnosed patients ($n = 200$) under the age of 65 years with multiple myeloma were enrolled on this study and randomly assigned to receive either conventional therapy with VMCP (vincristine, melphalan, cyclophosphamide, prednisone) or high-dose therapy with a single autologous bone-marrow transplant.

Table 5.4.2 Median duration of cytopenia (absolute granulocyte <500/μl and platelets <50 000/μl) during each phase of 'total therapy' regimen

Regimen[a]	n	Granulocytes <500/μl	Platelets <50 000/μl
HDXTX	218	8	3
EDAP	203	6	7
Tx-1 (MEL 200)	195	6	7
Tx-2[b]			
MEL 200	121	6	7
Other	29	6	8

[a] HDCTX = high-dose cytoxan; EDAP = etoposide, dexamethasone, cytosine arabinoside, cisplatin; MEL = melphalan; TX = transplant.
[b] Excludes 11 allotransplants and 3 matched unrelated donor (MUD) transplants.

The treatment schema and responses are shown in Figure 5.4.7. The reported response rate (≥50% reduction in myeloma protein) on the standard therapy arm was 57% (5% CR), while in the high-dose therapy arm 81% of the patients achieved PR (22% CR) ($p < 0.001$). The high-dose chemotherapy arm showed significant improvement in the EFS and OS, with projected five-year EFS at 28% and OS at 52% compared with 10% and 12% respectively for the standard-therapy arm (Figure 5.4.8). The same group of researchers is currently investigating the efficacy of one versus two transplants. Our results with a much higher CR rate and longer EFS seem to indicate that tandem transplants are superior while not associated with a higher transplant-related mortality.

Other institutions have studied the use of high-dose chemotherapy with autologous bone-marrow transplantation (ABMT) in myeloma. Cunningham et al[40] treated 63 newly diagnosed patients with melphalan 140 mg/m² without bone-marrow support, achieving an 82% response rate with 32% CR. The treatment-related mortality was 14%. At a median follow-up of 74 months (range 63–100 months), 43% patients were alive, with a median survival duration of 47 months.[40] A subsequent study tested melphalan 200 mg/m² and methylprednisolone 1.5 g daily for 5 days with autologous bone marrow rescue in 53 patients previously treated with cycles of VAMP (vincristine, Adriamycin and methylprednisolone) and showing responsive disease. The early mortality was considerably lower (2%), mainly due to the stem cell support, while the CR rate increased to 75%.[40] Bensinger et al[41] studied 63 previously treated patients with high-dose chemotherapy consisting of busulfan, melphalan with or without TBI followed by bone marrow or PBSC support. Of 48 evaluable patients, 19 (40%) achieved a CR. Early mortality was high at 25%, and the probability of three-year EFS and OS was 17% and 42% respectively. The high early mortality rate was probably due to the intensity of the preparative regimen. Harousseau et al[42] studied intensive induction chemotherapy followed by ABMT and/or PBSC transplantation. The study shows a 37% CR and 46% PR rate with 4% early deaths. With a median follow-up of 35 months, the median time to treatment failure was 22 months and the median overall survival was 46 months. Schiller et al[25] purified CD34+ cells from PBSC collected after intermediate-dose

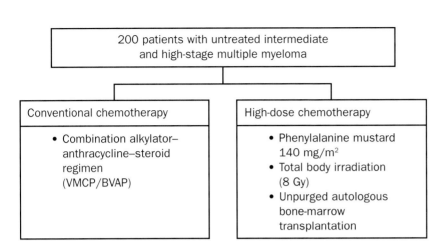

Figure 5.4.7 Treatment schema and responses in the French Intergroup study (Phase III, 1995) randomizing newly diagnosed myeloma patients between standard-dose therapy versus single high-dose chemotherapy with autologous transplantation. The complete responses are significantly superior in the high-dose therapy compared with the standard-therapy arm.

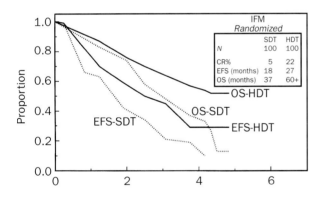

Figure 5.4.8 Superior overall survival (OS) and event-free survival (EFS) in patients undergoing high-dose chemotherapy (HDT) compared with standard-dose therapy (SDT) in the randomized French Intergroup study.

cyclophosphamide and G-CSF.[25] Using patient-specific CDR 3 primers, polymerase chain reaction was positive in 8 of 14 apheresis products; $CD34^+$ cell selection resulted in a 2.7–4.5 log reduction in myeloma cell contamination, and residual tumor cell contamination was detected in only 3 patient products. In this study, 37 patients were treated with busulfan (14 mg/kg) and cyclophosphamide (120 mg/kg). The median time to neutrophil and platelet recovery was 12 days. Patients receiving fewer than

2×10^6 $CD34^+$ cells had significantly slower engraftment kinetics. Of 34 evaluable patients, 5 (15%) achieved a CR and 82% $\geqslant$PR. Treatment-related mortality was 8%.

Björkstrand et al[43] investigated whether molecular remission occurred after autotransplants. Fifteen patients underwent tandem transplants with melphalan 200 mg/m[2] for the first transplant, and melphalan 140 mg/m[2] and TBI for the second transplant. Of the 15 patients, 8 achieved a CR. Five of these patients were stud-

Table 5.4.3 Phase II autotransplant studies for multiple myeloma

Regimen	Transplant	Authors	Prior chemotherapy	Responsive only	n	Median age (years)	Follow-up years	ED (%)	CR (%)	EFS	OS
										Median years	
MEL 200	ABMT	Cunningham et al[40]	−	+	53	52	2.6	2	75	2	6.7
MEL-TBI	AMBT purged	Anderson et al[26]	±|	+	52	49	NA	2	40	2.6	4.2
BU-CY ± TBI	PBSC ABMT	Bensinger et al[41]	+	−	63	51	NA	25	30	0.8	2.8
MEL ± TBI	PBSC ABMT	EBMTR	+	−	207	49	NA	4	46	2.4	2.7
MEL-TBI	PBSC	Reiffers et al[11]	±|	−	73	54	2	3	45	2	4.5
TBI-CC	PBSC	Fermand et al[46]	±|	−	63	44	7.5	11	20	3.6	6.4
MEL-TBI	PBSC ABMT	Harousseau et al[48]	−	−	133	52	3	4	37	2	3.8
MEL 200 × 2	PBSC	Arkansas	−	−	231	51	3	2	37	3.6	5.2

Key: MEL = melphalan; BU = busulphan; CY = cyclophosphamide; TBI = total body irradiation; CC = combination chemotherapy; ABMT = autologous bone marrow transplantation; PBSC = peripheral blood stem cells; ED = early death; CR = complete response; EFS = event-free survival; OS = overall survival; NA = not applicable.

ied by PCR analysis of the clonal immunoglobulin gene rearrangement; 4 of the 5 patients were reportedly negative up to 33 months for the myeloma-specific clone. Various other studies with more than 50 patients are presented in Table 5.4.3.[26,40,41,44–47] Keeping in mind the variability in stringently defining CR, and the variability in duration of prior treatments, between 20% and 40% of patients achieved CR, and OS varied between 2.7 and 6.7 years. The treatment-related mortality was 2–10%, which is similar to the mortality rate observed with standard-dose therapy during the first year. These studies confirm the feasibility, safety and efficacy of high-dose chemotherapy with autologous stem cell transplantation.

REFRACTORY AND RELAPSED PATIENTS

High-dose chemotherapy with ABMT or PBSC transplantation, in fact, was initially studied in a pilot protocol in patients with refractory myeloma prior to its evaluation in newly diagnosed patients. Harousseau et al[48] treated 44 refractory/relapsed multiple myeloma patients with melphalan 140 mg/m^2, with PBSC support. The CR rate in this study was 21%, with 66% patients achieving $\geq$PR. The median overall survival was 17 months in this group. Vesole et al[14] reported on 135 patients with advanced refractory myeloma treated with high-dose chemotherapy, with or without autologous transplantation. Initially, 47 patients were treated with melphalan at 90–100 mg/m^2 without autotransplants; 21 patients were treated with melphalan 140 mg/m^2 or thiotepa 750 mg/m^2 plus TBI and ABMT; and 67 patients were treated with melphalan 200 mg/m^2 with PBSC and ABMT plus GM-CSF. In a multivariate analysis, a tandem transplant using melphalan 200 mg/m^2 was one of the most important favorable variables in achieving a median duration of EFS and OS of 21 and 43+ months respectively. Patients with primary unresponsive disease (not responding to standard induction therapy) had superior outcome to patients with resistant relapse (relapsing after initial response), with EFS of 37 versus 17 months ($p = 0.0004$) and OS

of 43+ versus 21 months ($p = 0.0003$) respectively. Less than 1 year of prior therapy was the only significant parameter associated with a higher CR rate. The study shows improvement in response rates and EFS and OS in patients relapsing after prior chemotherapy with increasing melphalan dose.

PROGNOSTIC FACTORS

Various prognostic variables have been studied in 496 consecutive patients with multiple myeloma enrolled in clinical trials of tandem transplants with PBSC support, of which 470 have completed the first autotransplants with melphalan 200 mg/m^2, and 363 (73%) have completed the second transplant with melphalan 200 mg/m^2 (40%), melphalan 140 mg/m^2 with TBI (17%) or other combination (16%).[49] In this large group of patients, a CR was achieved in 36%, and the median duration of EFS and OS after transplant was 26 and 41 months respectively. Less than 12 months of prior therapy, and low β_2-microglobulin ($\leq$2.5 mg/l) and CRP ($\leq$0.4 mg/dl) were the most significant standard parameters associated with prolonged EFS and OS. When cytogenetics were included, 11q abnormalities and/or complete or partial deletion of chromosome 13 emerged as a dominant negative feature for both EFS and OS (Table 5.4.4 and Figure 5.4.9). In addition to these pretransplant parameters, attainment of a CR and application of two transplants within 6 months significantly extended EFS and OS. In the study by Bensinger et al,[41] multivariate analysis showed that increased β_2-microglobulin (>2.5 mg/l), two different regimens of standard therapy or eight cycles of treatment prior to transplantation, time to transplant longer than three years from diagnosis, and prior radiation therapy were all associated with adverse outcome.

TRANSPLANTATION IN PATIENTS WITH RENAL FAILURE

Approximately 20% of patients with multiple myeloma have renal insufficiency, one-half of

Table 5.4.4 Multivariate analysis of prognostic variables with and without inclusion of cytogenetics in 470 patients with myeloma undergoing high-dose chemotherapy with autologous transplantation

Without cytogenetics

Favorable	EFS	Favorable	OS
CRP ≤0.4 mg/dl	0.0001	B2M ≤2.5 mg/l	0.0001
B2M ≤2.5 mg/l	0.0001	CRP ≤0.4 mg/dl	0.0001
Sensitive	0.0008	Sensitive	0.0004
≤12 months prior treatment	0.006	Non-IgA	0.04
Non-IgA	0.007	LDH ≤190 IU/l	0.1
LDH ≤190 IU/l	0.2	Creatinine ≤2.0 mg/l	0.3

With cytogenetics

Favorable	EFS	Favorable	OS
No 11/13	0.0001	No 11/13	0.0001
B2M ≤2.5 mg/l	0.0001	B2M ≤2.5 mg/l	0.0001
≤12 months prior treatment	0.0001	CRP ≤0.4 mg/dl	0.0006
CRP ≤0.4 mg/dl	0.0005	Sensitive	0.002
Sensitive	0.03	≤12 months prior treatment	0.03
Non-IgA	0.04	Creatinine ≤2.0 mg/l	0.05

Key: CRP = C-reactive protein; B2M = β_2-microglobulin; LDH = lactate dehydrogenase.

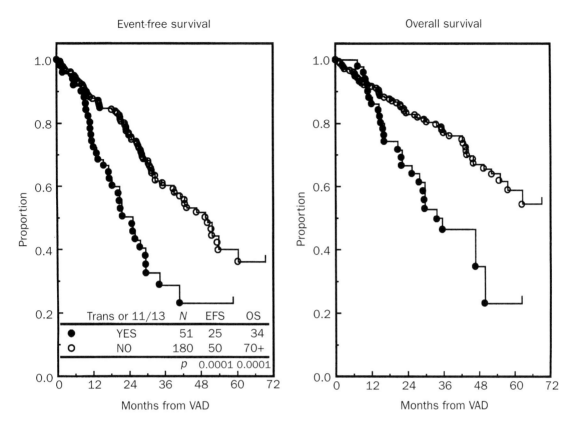

Figure 5.4.9 Presence of cytogenetic abnormality; translocation of 11q or 13q or deletion of chromosome 13 adversely affects overall survival (OS) and event-free survival (EFS).

whom recover their renal function following correction of hypercalcemia, improved hydration or following chemotherapy.[50] Melphalan[51] and busulfan,[29] both active agents in myeloma, are pharmacokinetically independent of renal function, allowing high-dose administration without dose modification in patients with impaired renal functions. At the University of Arkansas for Medical Sciences, we have treated 20 patients with severe renal insufficiency (creatinine clearance < 40 ml/min), including 5 patients on chronic hemodialysis, with melphalan at 200 mg/m^2 over a period of 2 days followed by PBSC rescue. Pharmacokinetic studies in the patients with renal failure did not show any impact on median half-life, area under the curve and clearance of melphalan compared

with patients who have normal renal function. Renal insufficiency also did not affect post-transplant engraftment, transfusion requirements or incidence of mucositis or overall survival. However, the patients with renal insufficiency required longer hospitalization due to prolonged mucositis and anorexia. This study shows the feasibility and safety of high-dose melphalan followed by PBSC transplantation in patients with myeloma and renal insufficiency.

TRANSPLANTATION IN OLDER PATIENTS

Multiple myeloma is a malignancy typically of older patients, with a median age of 65 years.[52] The 'total therapy' study included patients up to 70 years of age. In a separate study, we have explored the feasibility of high-dose chemotherapy with PBSC support in patients over 70 years of age. Twenty-three patients aged over 70 years (median age 72 years; range 71–78 years) were treated with melphalan 200 mg/m^2 ($n = 11$) or melphalan 140 mg/m^2 ($n = 12$) with PBSC support.[53] Additionally 6 patients also received a second high-dose chemotherapy cycle with PBSC support. Treatment-related mortality was 9%; CR was achieved in 17% of the patients, and EFS and OS were 9 and 23 months respectively. All 7 patients with albumin > 3.5 mg/dl and lactate dehydrogenase < 190 U/litre (favorable variables) are alive with the median follow-up of 45+ months.

MYELODYSPLASTIC SYNDROME FOLLOWING TRANSPLANTATION IN MYELOMA

Treatment-related myelodysplastic syndrome (MDS) and acute myeloid leukemia (AML) are well recognized complications following alkylating agent therapy. These complications have also been reported after high-dose alkylating agent therapy with PBSC support in patients with lymphoma. However, since all these patients had received multiple courses of standard therapy with alkylating agents, it is still not clear whether treatment-related AML/MDS is related to the standard chemotherapy or to the high-dose chemotherapy and radiotherapy in conjunction with transplant. To address this issue, Govindarajan et al[54] have studied 188 patients with myeloma undergoing high-dose melphalan followed by PBSC rescue: 71 patients were newly diagnosed while 117

patients had received standard-dose therapy prior to entry on high-dose therapy treatment. The median duration of pretransplant therapy in the newly diagnosed group was 7.6 months, which was significantly shorter than the 24 months in the previously treated group. In this study, 7 patients in the previously treated group (6%) developed MDS, compared with none in the newly diagnosed group. This finding suggests that prolonged standard-dose alkylating agent therapy may be responsible for development of secondary MDS, rather than the autotransplant-supported myeloablative regimen. It re-emphasizes the need to avoid stem-cell-damaging alkylating agent therapy prior to transplantation – not only to optimize PBSC collection, but also to prevent treatment-related MDS/AML.

SUMMARY

Dose intensification has an important role in the management of multiple myeloma. High-dose chemotherapy with PBSC support has been shown to have a beneficial effect on response rates as well as EFS and OS, as demonstrated in a randomized trial and in a large pair-mate analysis. Tandem transplantation appears to further improve the response rates and survival. For the safe conduct of two autologous PBSC transplants, complete avoidance of alkylating therapy prior to PBSC collection is important. Positive stem-cell selection with CD34$^+$ cells and post-transplant manipulation to eradicate minimal residual disease with immunological approaches are under investigation to further improve current therapy.

REFERENCES

1. Alexanian R, Dimopoulos M, The treatment of multiple myeloma. *N Engl J Med* 1994; **330:** 484–9.
2. Barlogie B, Alexanian R, Biology and therapy of multiple myeloma. *Acta Haematologica* 1987; **78**(Suppl 1): 171–4.
3. Barlogie B, Smith L, Alexanian R, Effective treatment of advanced multiple myeloma refractory to alkylating agents. *N Engl J Med* 1984; **310:** 1353–6.
4. Boccadoro M, Marmont F, Tribalto M et al, Multiple myeloma: Vmcp/Vbap alternating combination chemotherapy is not superior to melphalan and prednisone even in high-risk patients. *J Clin Oncol* 1991; **9:** 444–8.
5. Salmon SE, Tesch D, Crowley J et al, Chemotherapy is superior to sequential hemibody irradiation for remission consolidation in MM: a SWOG study. *J Clin Oncol* 1990; **8:** 1575–84.
6. Barlogie B, Hoover R, Epstein J, Multiple myeloma – recent developments in molecular and cellular biology. *Curr Top Microbiol Immunol* 1995; **194:** 37–41.
7. McElwain T, Powles R, High-dose intravenous melphalan for plasma-cell leukemia and myeloma. *Lancet* 1983; **i:** 822–4.
8. McElwain TJ, Selby PJ, Gore ME et al, High-dose chemotherapy and autologous bone marrow transplantation for myeloma. *Eur J Haematol* 1989; **51**(Suppl): 152–6.
9. Fermand JP, Levy Y, Gerota J et al, Treatment of aggressive multiple myeloma by high-dose chemotherapy and total body irradiation followed by blood stem cells autologous graft. *Blood* 1989; **73:** 20–3.
10. Gore ME, Selby PJ, Viner C et al, Intensive treatment of multiple myeloma and criteria for complete remission. *Lancet* 1989; **ii:** 879–82.
11. Reiffers J, Marit G, Boiron JM, Autologous blood stem cell transplantation in high-risk multiple myeloma [Letter]. *Br J Haematol* 1989; **72:** 296–7.
12. Harousseau JL, Milpied N, Garand R, Bourhis JH, High dose melphalan and autologous bone marrow transplantation in high risk myeloma [Letter]. *Br J Haematol* 1987; **67:** 493.
13. Barlogie B, Hall R, Zander A et al, high-dose melphalan with autologous bone marrow transplantation for multiple myeloma. *Blood* 1986; **67:** 1298–301.
14. Vesole DH, Barlogie B, Jagannath S et al, High-dose therapy for refractory multiple myeloma: improved prognosis with better supportive care and double transplants. *Blood* 1994; **84:** 950–6.
15. Tricot G, Jagannath S, Vessole D et al, Peripheral blood stem cell transplants for multiple myeloma: identification of favorable variables for rapid engraftment in 225 patients. *Blood* 1995; **85:** 588–96.
16. Desikan KR, Jagannath S, Siegel D et al, Post-transplant engraftment kinetics and toxicities in multiple myeloma (MM) patients are comparable following mobilization of PBSC with G-CSF with or without high dose cyclophosphamide (HD CTX). *Blood* 1996; **88**(Suppl 1): 679a.
17. Tricot G, Jagannath S, Desikan KR et al, Superior mobilization of peripheral blood progenitor cells (PBSC) with r-metHuSCF (SCF) and r-metHuG-CSF (filgrastim) in heavily pretreated multiple myeloma (MM) patients. *Blood* 1996; **88**(Suppl 1): 388a.
18. Gazitt Y, Tian E, Barlogie B et al, Differential mobilization of myeloma cells and normal hematopoietic stem cells in multiple myeloma after treatment with cyclophosphamide and granulocyte–macrophage colony-stimulating factor. *Blood* 1996; **87:** 805–11.
19. Jagannath S, Barlogie B, Dicke K et al, Autologous bone marrow transplantation in multiple myeloma: identification of prognostic factors. *Blood* 1990; **76:** 1860–6.
20. Brenner MK, Rill DR, Moen RC et al, Gene-marking to trace origin of relapse after autologous bone-marrow transplantation. *Lancet* 1993; **341:** 85–6.
21. Billadeau D, Blackstadt M, Greipp P et al, Analysis of B-lymphoid malignancies using allele specific PCR: a technique for sequential quantitation of residual disease. *Blood* 1991; **78:** 3021–9.
22. Gazitt Y, Reading CC, Hoffman R et al, Purified CD34$^+$ Lin$^-$ Thy$^+$ stem cells do not contain clonal myeloma cells. *Blood* 1995; **86:** 381–9.
23. Lemoli RM, Fortuna A, Motta MR et al, Concomitant mobilization of plasma cells and hematopoietic progenitors into peripheral blood of multiple myeloma patients: positive selection and transplantation of enriched CD34$^+$ cells to remove circulating tumor cells. *Blood* 1996; **87:** 1625–34.
24. Vescio RA, Hong CH, Cao J et al, The hematopoietic stem cell antigen, CD34, is not expressed on the malignant cells in multiple myeloma. *Blood* 1994; **84:** 3283–90.
25. Schiller G, Vescio R, Freytes C et al,

Transplantation of CD34$^+$ peripheral blood progenitor cells after high-dose chemotherapy for patients with advanced multiple myeloma. *Blood* 1995; **86:** 390–7.

26. Anderson KC, Andersen J, Soiffer R et al, Monoclonal antibody-purged bone marrow transplantation therapy for multiple myeloma. *Blood* 1993; **82:** 2568–76.

27. Rhodes EG, Baker PK, Rhodes JM et al, Autologous bone marrow transplantation for myeloma patients using PNA- and CD19-purged marrow rescue. *Bone Marrow Transplant* 1994; **13:** 795–9.

28. Jagannath S, Barlogie B, Autologous bone marrow transplantation for multiple myeloma. *Hematol–Oncol Clin North Am* 1992; **6:** 437–49.

29. Mansi J, da Costa F, Viner C et al, High-dose busulfan in patients with myeloma. *J Clin Oncol* 1992; **10:** 1569–73.

30. Reece DE, Barnett MJ, Connors JM et al, Treatment of multiple myeloma with intensive chemotherapy followed by autologous BMT using marrow purged with 4-hydroperoxycyclophosphamide. *Bone Marrow Transplant* 1993; **11:** 139–46.

31. Tribalto M, Papa G, Coppetelli U et al, Treatment of multiple myeloma with autologous blood stem cell transplantation. Preliminary results of an Italian multicentric pilot study. *Int Artificial Organs* 1993; **16**(Suppl 5): 51–6.

32. Alegre A, Lamana M, Arranz R et al, Busulfan and melphalan as conditioning regimen for autologous peripheral blood stem cell transplantation in multiple myeloma. *Br J Haematol* 1995; **91:** 380–6.

33. Phillips GL, Shepherd JD, Barnett MJ et al, Busulfan, cyclophosphamide, and melphalan conditioning for autologous bone marrow transplantation in hematologic malignancy. *J Clin Oncol* 1991; **9:** 1880–8.

34. Dimopoulos MA, Alexanian R, Przepiorka D et al, Thiotepa, busulfan, and cyclophosphamide: a new preparative regimen for autologous marrow or blood stem cell transplantation in high-risk multiple myeloma. *Blood* 1993; **82:** 2324–8.

35. Adkins DR, Salzman D, Boldt D et al, Phase I trial of dacarbazine with cyclophosphamide, carmustine, etoposide, and autologous stem-cell transplantation in patients with lymphoma and multiple myeloma. *J Clin Oncol* 1994; **12:** 1890–901.

36. Ventura GJ, Barlogie B, Hester JP et al, High dose cyclophosphamide, BCNU and VP-16 with autologous blood stem cell support for refrac-

tory multiple myeloma. *Bone Marrow Transplant* 1990; **5:** 265–8.

37. Jagannath S, Tricot G, Vesole D et al, Total therapy with tandem transplants for 231 newly diagnosed patients with multiple myeloma. *Blood* 1996; **88**(Suppl 1): 685a.

38. Barlogie B, Jagannath S, Vesole D et al, Superiority of tandem autologous transplantation over standard therapy for previously untreated multiple myeloma. *Blood* 1997; **89:** 1789–93.

39. Attal M, Harousseau JL, Stoppa AM et al, A prospective, randomized trial of autologous bone marrow transplantation and chemotherapy in multiple myeloma. Intergroupe Français du Myelome. *N Engl J Med* 1996; **335:** 91–7.

40. Cunningham D, Paz-Ares L, Milan S et al, High-dose melphalan and autologous bone marrow transplantation as consolidation in previously untreated myeloma. *J Clin Oncol* 1994; **12:** 759–63.

41. Bensinger WI, Rowley SD, Demirer T et al, High-dose therapy followed by autologous hematopoietic stem-cell infusion for patients with multiple myeloma. *J Clin Oncol* 1996; **14:** 1447–56.

42. Harousseau JL, Attal M, Divine M et al, Autologous stem cell transplantation after first remission induction treatment in multiple myeloma. A report of the French Registry on Autologous Transplantation in Multiple Myeloma. *Stem Cells* 1995; **13**(Suppl 2): 132–9.

43. Björkstrand B, Ljungman P, Bird JM et al, Double high-dose chemoradiotherapy with autologous stem cell transplantation can induce molecular remissions in multiple myeloma. *Bone Marrow Transplant* 1995; **15:** 367–71.

44. Cunningham D, Paz-Ares L, Gore ME et al, High-dose melphalan for multiple myeloma: long-term follow-up data. *J Clin Oncol* 1994; **12:** 764–8.

45. Marit G, Faberes C, Pico JL et al, Autologous peripheral-blood progenitor-cell support following high-dose chemotherapy or chemoradiotherapy in patients with high-risk multiple myeloma. *J Clin Oncol* 1996; **14:** 1306–13.

46. Fermand JP, Ravaud P, Chevret S et al, High-dose therapy and autologous blood stem cell transplantation in multiple myeloma: preliminary results of a randomized trial involving 167 patients. *Stem Cells* 1995; **13**(Suppl 2): 156–9.

47. Björkstrand B, Ljungman P, Bird JM et al, Autologous stem cell transplantation in multiple myeloma: results of the European Group for

Bone Marrow Transplantation. *Stem Cells* 1995; **13**(Suppl 2): 140–6.

48. Harousseau JL, Milpied N, Laporte JP et al, Double-intensive therapy in high-risk multiple myeloma. *Blood* 1992; **79**: 2827–33.

49. Vesole DH, Tricot G, Jagannath S et al, Autotransplants in multiple myeloma: what have we learned? *Blood* 1996; **88**: 838–47.

50. Barlogie B, Alexanian R, Jagannath S, Plasma cell dyscrasias. *J Am Med Assoc* 1992; **268**: 2946–51.

51. Tricot G, Alberts DS, Johnson C et al, Safety of autotransplants with high-dose melphalan in renal failure: a pharmacokinetic and toxicity study. *Clin Cancer Res* 1996; **2**: 947–52.

52. Kyle RA, Multiple myeloma: review of 869 cases. *Mayo Clin Proc* 1975; **50**: 2940.

53. Siegel D, Jagannath S, Desikan KR et al, Feasibility of high dose chemotherapy with peripheral blood stem cell support for multiple myeloma patients over age of 70. *Blood* 1996; **88**(Suppl 1): 130a.

54. Govindarajan R, Jagannath S, Flick JT et al, Preceding standard therapy is the likely cause of MDS after autotransplants for multiple myeloma. *Br J Haematol* 1996; **95**: 782–6.

5.5

High-dose chemotherapy in solid tumours: Breast cancer

Robert CF Leonard

CONTENTS • **Introduction** • **Breast cancer: the clinical challenge** • **Dose intensity: laboratory and theoretical models** • **Clinical studies of intensity within the standard range: adjuvant chemotherapy** • **Studies of dose variations: metastatic disease** • **Adjuvant high-dose chemotherapy** • **High-dose chemotherapy for metastatic disease**

INTRODUCTION

The common solid cancers for which high-dose chemotherapy has been used or for which trials are ongoing include small-cell lung cancer, ovarian cancer, teratoma and above all breast cancer. The dominance of breast cancer is such that this chapter will focus almost exclusively on that disease and will rely on it as a paradigm for many of the issues surrounding the technology, toxicity and cost of this approach, even if the outcomes are disease-specific.

The interest in small-cell lung cancer is in any case largely historical – and a lesson in the too-early and uncritical application of high-dose chemotherapy in a disease of older patients that is certainly more drug-resistant than we realized in the early 1980s when these high-dose programmes began in earnest.

BREAST CANCER: THE CLINICAL CHALLENGE

Most patients present with what appears to be localized breast cancer, and, despite careful clinical, biochemical and radiological assessment, have no evidence of secondary tumours.

However, many of these women will ultimately die from secondary breast cancer, and the current accepted paradigm is that breast cancer presents as a systemic disease in many cases, with the micrometastatic disease being present at diagnosis. This concept has important implications for increasing the curability by elimination of the putative microscopic secondary disease at the time of initial presentation.

The most important prognostic factor for patients who present with apparently localized disease is the status of the axillary lymph nodes. If the nodes are not involved, local and standard adjuvant systemic therapy is curative in approximately 70% or more of cases, but for patients with lymph node metastases the prognosis is poor, and it deteriorates progressively as the node numbers increase.[1] Probably between 60% and 80% of women with four or more lymph nodes involved will eventually develop overt metastases.

In 1969 Cooper and colleagues, in a paper never published in more than abstract form,[2] reported that chemotherapy could also profoundly influence the outcome of advanced breast cancer. In the subsequent 25 years a variety of clinical trials were performed that failed to show a major benefit from chemotherapy for advanced disease in terms of survival gain. Even used in the adjuvant setting, chemotherapy did not show clear survival gains, with different trials showing diverse results. Eventually the overview analyses combining the results of individual randomized trials (at the last analysis including an aggregate of some 75 000 women) clearly showed for the first time that adjuvant systemic chemotherapy does reduce the death rate from breast cancer up to 10 years following treatment.[3] It is now accepted that combination chemotherapy in standard doses must work by destroying the hypothetical micrometastatic disease.[4]

The management of hormone-insensitive advanced disease has long been an area of controversy, with a balance being sought between optimizing cancer control against side-effects of chemotherapy. Recent developments in medical technology have encouraged a limited amount of experimentation with infusional chemotherapy, as well as exploiting the properties of growth factors to enhance the anticancer effect by increasing drug doses.

DOSE INTENSITY: LABORATORY AND THEORETICAL MODELS

The relationship between drug dose and cell kill of cancer cell lines or human tumour xenografts in experimental models follows a complex sigmoid curve. There is at lowest drug doses a threshold to be reached to achieve any effect (the lag phase), then a linear phase and finally a plateau. The tumour response during the linear phase, especially when using alkylating agents, is steep and logarithmic.[4–8] Reducing doses in this phase will result in failure to eradicate the cancer. In animal models, this may not be reflected in the complete response pattern, which may remain deceptively high, but will emerge as ultimate relapse in place of cure. These results were observed in a series of experiments performed by Skipper and colleagues using the Ridgeway osteosarcoma tumour in rodents.[6,7] Thus the two-drug combination of cyclophosphamide and melphalan was capable of producing 100% cures at one

dose level, whereas a further reduction of dose produced 10% complete response and 0% cure.[7] These observations are not lost on the clinician who recognizes a clear enough relationship in similar proportions between CR rate and cure, with the best results for both being in testicular cancer, intermediate results being obtained for lymphomas, and a low CR rate of around 10% with no cure being seen in the majority of 'sensitive' solid cancers such as advanced breast cancer. Studies of primary systemic therapy of breast cancer provide valuable insights into the same system, where a very high rate of clinical complete response is not reflected by the pathological response rate, and resulting long-term cure may be confined only to the small subset of pathological responders.[9]

A further point of importance translating into clinical studies is the observation in vitro of the occurrence of spontaneous mutations at around 1 per 10^6 to 1 per 10^7 cells.[8] This makes a case for the use of more than one cytotoxic agent with a different mode of action to minimize the risk of somatic mutation-associated cross-resistance. The interest in exploiting high-dose chemotherapy therefore emanates from a variety of clinical and laboratory experiments.

The classical model for demonstrating a dose–response effect from chemotherapy was developed by Skipper and Schabel using the murine L1210 leukaemia cell line. This was reproduced when human cell lines became available, and results from studies on tumour cell lines, including the MCF 7 breast cancer cell line, mimic the results of the L1210 leukaemic mode. Thus Skipper and Frei have shown that in vitro many alkylating agents when escalated linearly demonstrate a logarithmic cell kill against MCF 7.[10–14] These results are often quoted as the laboratory rationale that underpins the logic of true dose intensification in the adjuvant setting, where micrometastases are thought to be the closest clinical analogue of the in vitro experiment.[11] It follows that increasing the cytotoxic drug dose in a sensitive system will increase the cure rate, and demonstrable logarithmic increments in cell kill are observed after doubling the dose. Finally, in vitro, breast cancer cell lines, like other cancer cell lines, routinely show an absence of cross-resistance between alkylating agents, justifying their combination, especially where, for most alkylating agents, the second-organ toxicities differ and the main toxicity remains bone marrow.

CLINICAL STUDIES OF INTENSITY WITHIN THE STANDARD RANGE: ADJUVANT CHEMOTHERAPY

With the recognition that therapy could affect outcome, clinicians immediately began to address the question of a dose effect – at first retrospectively. Hryniuk and colleagues, in a flawed but very influential review of published trials,[15] and Bonadonna, in a retrospective analysis of his adjuvant CMF trial,[16] claimed to show a relationship between applied dose and survival.[17] These analyses seemed to support the interpretation of the laboratory studies by Skipper, Frei and colleagues. Subsequently, however, dose–response studies were performed in randomized clinical trials, and have shown somewhat conflicting results.

It is very difficult to mimic the laboratory experiments in the clinic. Thus Hryniuk's retrospective dose-intensity analysis of several trials, both in an adjuvant setting and in advanced breast cancer, estimated the delivered dose per unit time (mg/m^2 per week) for each drug in a combination chemotherapy schedule, and compared that dose rate against an arbitrary standard dose intensity. Unfortunately, owing to variations in schedule design, many of the chosen examples studied either had extra drugs added or had drugs excluded. Also, assumptions not justified by our knowledge of drug action or by observed effects in the laboratory (for example, unlike alkylating agents, antimetabolites demonstrate far less or no dose–response effects against cell lines) gave average dose intensity for a given combination regimen that gave equal weight to the impact of halving cyclophosphamide as that of halving methotrexate. Significantly, no regard was paid to potentially important schedule effects, which are probably very important for agents such as 5-fluorouracil.[18]

Despite theoretical problems, when this sort of analysis was applied to breast cancer trials, the correlation between calculated relative dose intensity and outcome was impressive, providing support for the idea that actual dose delivered impacts on the response rate and survival of this relatively chemosensitive cancer.

A critical rebuttal of the Hryniuk and Bonadonna analyses, however, by Gelman and Henderson demands caution in interpretation of such retrospective analyses.[4]

STUDIES OF DOSE VARIATIONS: METASTATIC DISEASE

A relationship between dose, schedule and outcome might be expected to be more important in the adjuvant setting than in advanced disease, where, for a number of reasons (mainly to do with drug access and tumour biology), the clinical equivalent of the cell-line/drug log-linear dose relationship is much less likely to obtain.

Whilst trials have been conducted in adjuvant therapy of breast cancer, the more difficult and unsatisfactory field of treatment has been in the management of metastatic disease with chemotherapy. Currently the disease is regarded as a uniformly fatal condition – albeit one with a widely variable course and speed of progression – and therefore is treated with chemotherapy in a palliative mode. It is nevertheless a relatively responsive tumour, and in a large unselected series of metastatic breast cancer patients reviewed by Eddy[19] the overall response rate from chemotherapy is between 13% and 83%, with complete remissions occurring in less than 10% (mostly of limited duration between 3 and 17.5 months). However, chemotherapy probably does improve the survival of breast cancer by a few months, although the overall survival is poor, at between 18 and 24 months from presentation with secondary disease. Limited to the cases where hormonal therapy has failed or is deemed inappropriate, the survival from commencement of chemotherapy is much poorer, at around 12 months according to a large series of patients from an audit at Guy's Hospital.[20] Many patients who commence chemotherapy have a relatively short survival – either because they have tumours with a more aggressive natural history or because, by the time chemotherapy is commenced, they have already failed one or more endocrine manoeuvres. The main aims of chemotherapy for metastatic disease are therefore to maintain or restore the quality of life following improvement of cancer symptoms balanced against the side-effects of chemotherapy. This is thus essentially an area where one tries to improve the therapeutic index of drugs.

To improve the present results of chemotherapy, it is necessary to develop new potent drugs, or, in palliative designs, drugs with a better therapeutic index. The taxoids may represent a real advance in this area of therapy. A further option is to experiment with dose intensification in an effort to improve the response rate and disease control and to extend the survival within the limits of accepted tolerability. Amongst these new approaches, high-dose chemotherapy, as in the adjuvant setting, has been made possible – first, by the introduction of autologous bone marrow transplantation supported by colony-stimulating factor (CSF) therapy, and, more recently, by the use of CSFs to develop stem-cell-supported dose intensification.

Is there any evidence from studies of dose intensity within the standard range that dose intensification might usefully be examined in metastatic breast cancer? Unfortunately, despite the positive interpretation of retrospective data by Hryniuk, the results of subsequent prospective randomized trials have been conflicting. The most positive interpretation of these outcomes may be summarized as follows.

- The studies are all on a small scale, and small advantages are likely to be missed.
- Results in metastatic disease are compromised by the problems of patient fitness, drug access, and prior chemotherapy (including adjuvant therapy inducing resistance).

- Metastatic tumour cell growth characteristics, which obey Gompertzian rules of a falling growth fraction, are inherently less responsive and, in contrast to the adjuvant micrometastatic situation, do not show log-linear kill.
- Compared against dose ranges observed and attainable in the laboratory, the dose range within the standard clinical schedules is unrealistically small and unlikely to show important effects.
- As previously argued, many of the drugs used to treat breast cancer do not exhibit clear dose–response relationships, even in the idealized conditions of the in vitro experiment.
- In the published data, few papers discuss the given doses of drugs as opposed to intended doses.
- It is highly probable that pharmacological effects produce important variability in the actual level of drug present, regardless of the received dose.
- In nearly all advanced disease and adjuvant studies, the question being addressed within the standard dose range was 'Can we reduce dose safely?'.

These rationalizations, coupled with encouraging experience of tolerance and safety from using dose-intensive regimens in leukaemia and lymphoma treatment, led many investigators to conclude that the results of standard-dose chemotherapy in metastatic breast cancer at least did not disprove a dose–response effect and that the data, although flawed, could in some studies be seen to indicate a slight association between dose and positive outcome, even in terms of quality of life![21] Again a note of uncertainty in the interpretation is implied by the possibility that in the lower-intensity arm of the trial quoted, the dose was below an acceptable 'threshold' level for useful effect, and so was not a true test of dose intensity as many would interpret it.

With the gradual acquisition of skill in managing complications of marrow suppression and the availability of new cytokines, many have concluded that the way to test fairly the concept of dose intensity to match the laboratory results was to resort to autologous marrow and more recently peripheral blood progenitor cell support, escalating alkylating agents by 5–10 fold above standard doses.

ADJUVANT HIGH-DOSE CHEMOTHERAPY

Experimental models suggest an invariable and inverse relationship between size of tumour and curability with cytotoxic agents. Thus chemotherapy that can produce substantial but non-eradicative cytoreduction in patients with overt metastases might nevertheless cure patients at an earlier stage harbouring a far smaller tumour burden. Clinical research seems to confirm these predictions, since conventional-dose chemotherapy reduces relapse and prolongs survival in stage II disease far more impressively than in stage IV disease. However, the results of adjuvant therapy are still unsatisfactory – particularly for patients with extensive axillary lymph node involvement. A lot of work has been conducted looking at various pathological and biological parameters predicting outcome.[22,23] However, there is still no individual feature that matches the information available from simply obtaining and counting the number of pathologically involved lymph nodes in the axilla at the time of primary surgery. Based on this, we have a very good definition of relapse rates and survival in relation to node number. As a result, a series of survival cures may be plotted against nodal status. No node-positive groups achieve better than 80% survival at 5 years, but the worst groups (particularly those with more than 10 involved lymph nodes) show completely inadequate survival (<50%) at 5 years.

The overview analysis of adjuvant therapy of breast cancer points to benefit from both endocrine therapy and chemotherapy. There is still a debate as to whether chemotherapy exerts its benefit for premenopausal patients through secondary ovarian suppression, but only one trial has ever directly addressed this question. The Scottish Group combined with Guy's Hospital tested ovarian ablation against chemotherapy, and the overall results published in the *Lancet* in 1993 suggested an equivalent effect, with no discernible overall benefit for one or the other treatment.[24] However, interestingly, a subgroup analysis according to oestrogen-receptor status exactly fitted the hypothesis that patients with oestrogen-receptor-positive tumours gained more from ovarian suppression, whereas those with oestrogen-receptor-negative tumours gained benefit from chemotherapy. This suggests that biologically separate subgroups require tailored adjuvant therapy.

Within clinical research, the partial success of adjuvant chemotherapy in the treatment of breast cancer together with clinically meaningful dose–response effects in advanced disease provides a clinical rationale for studying very high-dose chemotherapy in patients with a high risk in early-stage disease. Two interesting studies show encouraging preliminary results in single-arm studies of high-dose chemotherapy in patients with breast cancer involving 10 or more axillary lymph nodes.[25,26]

Peters treated patients with at least 10 positive lymph nodes with a regimen comprising cyclophosphamide, Adriamycin and 5-FU over four successive conventional courses followed by a single consolidation course comprising high-dose carmustine (BCNU), cyclophosphamide and cisplatin (the CBP regimen). This had been developed from the experience of treating metastatic breast cancer with a different induction but similar high-dose regimen producing a high overall response rate and an impressive 'tail' on the survival curve, with some patients with metastatic disease going into unmaintained remission beyond 10 years. In the adjuvant trial, all patients received autologous bone marrow rescue (ABMR), and in later recruits ABMR was supplemented by granulocyte colony-stimulating factor (G-CSF)-mobilized peripheral blood progenitor cells (PBPC). With a median follow-up of 3.3 years, 72% of patients remained free of relapse. Compared against this, matched controls from the Cancer and Leukaemic Group B had relapse-free survival at 3.3 years for around

35%. Interestingly, many of the relapses that occurred in Peters' study were locoregional and affected patients who were recruited prior to the institution of a policy of routine chest-wall irradiation. However, randomized trials have now been commenced on the background of encouraging outcomes from phase II trials where the outcomes have been compared against historical controls.

In a further development of intensive chemotherapy, Gianni and colleagues examined a sequence of doxorubicin followed by high doses of cyclophosphamide, methotrexate, cisplatin and melphalan. PBPC were harvested following the cyclophosphamide course to rescue the melphalan high-dose therapy. Relapse-free survival at 5 years in this group of patients with at least 10 positive lymph nodes was 50%, which again is well above what would be predicted for this high-risk group of patients. Thus the data from Duke University and from Milan both indicate very high relapse-free survival rates at 3 and 5 years, which are clearly superior to those of 'matched' controls.

However, these preliminary study results have not yet been substantiated. Prospective randomized trials must therefore be performed. The outcomes in terms of survival from systemic therapy with standard-dose chemotherapy in high-risk (multiple-node-positive) adjuvant disease are simply too poor not to test such promising approaches. The safety factors involved have changed the applicability of high-dose therapy such that, whereas 10 years ago up to 25% of patients were dying from complications of dose intensification, the figures are now well under 5% and possibly under 3%.[27] The result is that at least four European trials have commenced or are about to commence testing dose intensification, and there is one very large trial that is further ahead in North America. Within the next 3–5 years, we shall begin to get clear indications as to whether or not there is true benefit from this approach.

Since the pragmatic experiments with autologous bone marrow rescue at the beginning of the 1980s, the area of dose-intensification research in the clinic has become much more widely practised, particularly for the haematological malignancies. Since then, we have collectively learned lessons about lethal complications, including 'second-organ toxicity'. With increasing confidence in controlling complications of therapy, clinicians are now beginning to discover the potential benefits for this sort of approach in chemosensitive solid cancers, including breast cancer.

The evidence in favour of micrometastases being a common problem in 'localized' breast cancer is thus overwhelming, and is substantiated by the ongoing studies of immunomicrodetection with anti-epithelial monoclonal antibodies and by some investigators' ability to culture tumour cells from bone marrow.[28] These studies indicate an increasing level of risk of marrow involvement as the risk factors rise in relation to the primary tumour. This means that between 30% and 50% of bone marrows may have detectable disease, depending on the clinical stage of the tumour at presentation. Studies are currently underway to determine the importance of marrow or PBPC contamination by tumour and to develop methods to deplete or eliminate the tumour population either by 'negative' selection with drugs or antibody against tumour or positive selection of the progenitor cells with antibody to the CD34 antigen.[29]

HIGH-DOSE CHEMOTHERAPY FOR METASTATIC DISEASE

The initial studies of very high-dose chemotherapy in advanced breast cancer were part of a programme of testing the concept of high-dose treatment in a variety of non-haematological malignancies. Frei, Peters and colleagues at the Dana Farber Cancer Institute led this research using autologous bone marrow to support patients during recovery from escalating multiple alkylating agent chemotherapy given to patients with advanced refractory solid cancers. This was based on firm pharmacological principles (see above), but the problems of acquired or inherent chemoresistance soon became apparent, as did the problem of acute and often lethal treatment-induced toxicity. Amongst the positive outcomes of such approaches, however, the relative responsiveness of breast cancer became apparent.[12]

Eder and colleagues showed that 50% of selected patients with metastatic disease could achieve objective responses, with 25% achieving temporary complete responses.[12] Subsequent clinical trials indicated that in metastatic breast cancer high-dose chemotherapy is feasible and produces an objective response in 70–90% of tumours, with 30–80% in apparent complete response – many converted by the high-dose therapy from induction regimens where the complete response rate is around 10%.[12]

Studies in patients with newly diagnosed metastatic disease or in continuing objective response to induction chemotherapy could achieve CR rates in excess of 50%, with 25% of these complete responders durable beyond 5 years.[19]

The reason that the highest response rates are seen in patients who have demonstrated an objective response to the induction chemotherapy is clearly because they have been selected as having chemosensitive tumours. This experience appears to mimic the experience with the haematological malignancies, including lymphomas, where reduction of the tumour burden by remission-induction chemotherapy is now emerging as the best strategy.

The toxicity found in the earlier experiments was extremely high, with up to 25% immediate or early treatment-associated mortality.[19] However, with improved haemopoietic support, morbidity and mortality has been substantially reduced. For some agents, such as cyclophosphamide, cytokines alone can provide adequate rescue without the need for bone marrow or stem cell autografts. The latter technique, replacing bone marrow autografting, has not yet been used widely or for long enough to assess its relative benefits and disbenefits in breast cancer treatment as compared with bone marrow autografting; however, the early experience in terms of acute outcome looks very promising.

Several studies in metastatic breast cancer have demonstrated the ability of high-dose chemotherapy to increase complete response rates, converting from partial response achieved in induction therapy. This is important, because the achievement of high complete response rates could represent the first step toward curative treatment in this setting. The duration of response in high-dose therapy varies from 6 to 20 months, and survival rates at 1 and 2 years are between 45% and 65%. These results from non-randomized trials do not indicate prolonged survival for high-dose chemotherapy for all patients, but some are alive and free of disease at 5–10 years, which is suggestive of a very significant antitumour effect that is not seen with conventional chemotherapy.[12]

However, the very uncontrolled nature of the studies, with variable selection criteria and a variety of treatments involved, makes it impossible to evaluate the true impact of high-dose chemotherapy outside randomized clinical trials. It is difficult to assess whether one regimen is superior to the other, and the underexplored area of patient selection is particularly germane to the metastatic breast cancer population, where the natural history of the disease is so extraordinarily variable. This is a subject that deserves far greater attention. Even allowing for the fact that most American trials have focused on the treatment of hormone-insensitive disease, any experienced clinician is nevertheless only too aware of the wide range in the natural history of metastatic disease. In some patients the survival is measured in weeks from first recurrence, whereas for others the survival may even extend beyond a decade of tolerable life with secondary cancer. These variations were sharply illustrated by the data from Guy's Hospital in their 1993 report of an audit of some 790 patients managed by chemotherapy for recurrent disease.[20] Similar points emerge from Eddy's sceptical analysis of the outcomes of intensive therapy for advanced disease based on small uncontrolled phase II trials.[19]

Developed from clinical and laboratory experience, most of the high-dose regimens are based on intensive alkylating combinations that are very effective theoretically and have also been shown to be practically applicable. Theoretically, it is important that alkylating agents should be considered after induction with antimetabolites and anthracyclines, because the multidrug resistance phenotype germane to the drugs in the induction regimen is not thought to be relevant to the alkylating agent affect. The most widely used regimen has been the cyclophosphamide, thiotepa, carboplatin regimen (CTCb) developed at the Dana Farber Cancer Institute. In 29 cases of advanced breast cancer, an 80% response rate was seen, with only one toxic death.[12] The tolerance of high-dose chemotherapy has been improved with better support expertise, use of growth factors and particularly by the supplementation or replacement of ABMR by PBPC.

Results for late phase II studies have shown that PBPC following high-dose chemotherapy gives an earlier reconstitution both of neutrophils and particularly and rather surprisingly of blood platelets compared with ABMR. The lower number of platelet transfusions required and the shorter period of hospital stay is now beginning to show economic as well as toxicity benefits for patients.

Finally, in view of the very poor results in the long-term outcome for stage II inoperable disease, there seems to be a good case to examine intensified treatment.

The last two years have provided studies that challenge many assumptions from both the pro and anti camps concerning high-dose chemotherapy. First, Bezwoda's flawed and small trial showed unequivocal benefit for tandem high-dose therapy compared against a rather idiosyncratic standard regimen.[30] Then Peters and colleagues published a study showing that although high-dose chemotherapy in first remission provided a clearly superior disease-free survival to standard-dose therapy, the overall survival was enhanced in the group who had high-dose chemotherapy in first relapse, i.e. as rescue therapy! Possibly the high-dose treatment in the first-remission group had poorer salvage because of diminished marrow tolerance, few patients in either group achieving curative cytoreduction.[31]

The MD Anderson group has produced two studies, one so far in abstract form only, that suggest two things:

- Conventional chemotherapy can be made to look as good as high-dose therapy if the results of anthracycline therapy are examined only in patients whose presentation features would have made them suitable for high-dose treatment according to the institution's own selection criteria.[32]
- Conventional anthracycline chemotherapy can be associated with many years of disease-free survival and probably cure.[33]

The challenge of the latter data is that the proportion is very small (only 3% of some 1600 individuals), but the unanswered questions are: How does one recognize them except by therapeutic trial, and could the proportion cured be higher if intensive chemotherapy were used judiciously in selected chemosensitive individuals?

Finally, in their review of North American practice, Antmann and colleagues showed that most high-dose chemotherapy in USA and Canada is in breast cancer – and has been for several years.[27]

There are still no trials that demand this approach as standard therapy, and yet the number of patients in randomized trials in the USA are only a tiny percentage of all those receiving intensive chemotherapy.

We may rue the day that we forget the lessons of history. For a large part of this century, it was taken as self-evident that increasingly radical surgery must improve the outcome for patients. Too many years passed before an alternative paradigm was accepted. The current model may also prove to be mistaken. The surgical hubris of the acolytes of Halsted is being replaced by the medical hubris of the transplanters. Those of us actively pursuing the goal of maximizing the benefits of chemotherapy for breast cancer sufferers must remain our own most severe critics.

REFERENCES

1. Carter CC, Allen C, Hensen DE, Relation of tumour size and lymph node to status of survival in 24,470 breast cancer cases. *Cancer* 1989; **63:** 181–7.
2. Cooper RG, Combination chemotherapy in hormone resistant breast cancer. *Proc Am Assoc Cancer Res* 1969; **10:** 15.
3. Early Breast Cancer Trialists' Collaborative Group, Systemic treatment of early breast cancer by hormonal, cytotoxic or immune therapy: 133 randomised trials involving 31000 recurrences and 24000 deaths among 75000 women. *Lancet* 1992; **339:** 1–5, 71–85.
4. Henderson IC, Harris J, Kinne DW et al, Cancer of the breast. In: *Cancer: Principles and Practice of Oncology,* 3rd edn (DeVita VT, Hellman S, Rosenberg SA, eds). Philadelphia: JB Lippincott, 1989: 1197–268.
5. Skipper HE, Critical variables in the design of combination chemotherapy regimens to be used alone or in adjuvant setting. *Neoadjuvant Chemotherapy. Colloque INSERM* 1986; **137:** 11–12.
6. Skipper H, Schabel F, Wilcox WS, Experimental evaluation of potential anticancer agents No 12. On the criteria and kinetics associated with 'curability' of experimental leukaemia. *Cancer Chemother Rep* 1964; **35:** 1–111.
7. Skipper H, Schabel F, Mellet J, Implications of biochemical, cytokinetic, pharmacologic and toxicological relationships in the design of optimal therapeutic schedules. *Cancer Chemother Rep* 1950; **5:** 431–50.
8. Norton L, Simon R, The Norton–Simon hypothesis revisited. *Cancer Treat Rep* 1986; **70:** 163–9.
9. Cameron DA, Anderson EDC, Levack P et al, Primary systemic therapy for operable breast cancer – 10 year survival data after chemotherapy and hormone therapy. *Br J Cancer* 1997; **76:** 1099–105.
10. Skipper H, Data and analyses having to do with the influence of dose intensity and duration of treatment (single drug combinations) on lethal toxicity and therapeutic response of experimental neoplasms. *Southern Research Institute, Birmingham Booklets* 13 (1986) and 2–13 (1987).
11. DeVita VT, Principles of chemotherapy. In: *Cancer: Principles and Practice of Oncology*, 3rd edn (DeVita VT, Hellman S, Rosenberg SA, eds). Philadelphia: JB Lippincott, 1989: 276–96.
12. Antman K, Dose-intensive chemotherapy in breast cancer. In: *High Dose Cancer Therapy. Pharmacology, Haemopoietins, Stem Cells* (Armitage J, Antman K, eds). Baltimore: Williams and Wilkins, 1992: 702–18.
13. Teicher B, Cucchi C, Lee J et al, Alkylating agents. Studies of cross resistance patterns in human tumor cell lines. *Cancer Res* 1987; **46:** 4379–83.
14. Teicher BA, Holden SA, Cucchi CA et al, Combination thiotepa and cyclophosphamide in vitro and in vivo. *Cancer Res* 1988; **48:** 94–100.
15. Hryniuk W, Levine MN, Analysis of dose intensity of adjuvant chemotherapy trials in stage II breast cancer. *J Clin Oncol* 1986; **4:** 1162–70.
16. Bonadonna G, Valagussa P, Dose response effect of adjuvant chemotherapy in breast cancer. *N Engl J Med* 1981; **304:** 10–15.
17. Cooper RG, Holland JF, Glidewell O, Adjuvant chemotherapy of breast cancer. *Cancer* 1979; **44:** 893–8.
18. Leonard RCF, 5-fluorouracil. In: *Therapeutic Drugs* (Dollery C, ed). Edinburgh: Churchill Livingstone, 1991: F68–F74.
19. Eddy DM, High-dose chemotherapy with autologous bone marrow transplantation for the treatment of metastatic breast cancer. *J Clin Oncol* 1992; **10:** 657–70.
20. Gregory W, Smith P, Richards MA et al, Chemotherapy of advanced breast cancer: outcome and prognostic factors. *Br J Cancer* 1993; **68:** 988–95.
21. Tannock I et al, A randomised trial of 2 dose levels of cyclophosphamide and methotrexate in 5-FU for chemotherapy in patients with metastatic breast cancer. *J Clin Oncol* 1988; **6:** 1366–87.
22. Leonard RCF, Tumour markers of prognosis (Editorial). *J Clin Oncol* 1991; **97:** 1102–4.
23. Clark G, Sledge GW, Osborne CK et al, Survival from first recurrence: the relative importance of prognostic factors in 1015 breast cancer patients. *J Clin Oncol* 1987; **5:** 55–61.
24. The Scottish Breast Cancer Trials and Guy's Hospital Breast Groups. Adjuvant ovarian ablation versus CMF chemotherapy in premenopausal women with pathological stage II breast carcinoma – The Scottish Trial. *Lancet* 1993; **341:** 1293–8.
25. Gianni A, Valagussa P, Bonaodonna G et al, Growth factor supported high dose sequential adjuvant chemotherapy in breast cancer with more than 10 nodes. *Proc Am Soc Clin Oncol* 1993; **11:** 60.

26. Peters W, Vredenburgh J, Shpall E et al, High-dose chemotherapy and autologous bone marrow support as consolidation after standard-dose adjuvant therapy for high risk primary breast cancer. *J Clin Oncol* 1993; **11:** 1132–43.

27. Antman K, Rawlings IA, Vaughan WP et al, High dose chemotherapy with autologous hemopoietic stem cell support for breast cancer in North America. *J Clin Oncol* 1997; **15:** 1870–9.

28. Ross A, Cooper V, Lazarus H et al, Detection and viability of tumour cells in peripheral blood stem cell collections from breast cancer patients using immunocytochemical and clonogenic assay techniques. *Blood* 1993; **82:** 2605–10.

29. Shpall E, Jones R, Bearman S, Transplantation of enriched CD34 positive autologous marrow into breast cancer patients following high dose chemotherapy; influence of CD34 positive peripheral blood progenitors and growth factors on engraftment. *J Clin Oncol* 1994; **12:** 228–36.

30. Bezwoda WR, Seymour L, Dansey RD, High dose chemotherapy with hemopoietic rescue as primary treatment for metastatic breast cancer. A randomized trial. *J Clin Oncol* 1995; **13:** 2483–9.

31. Peters WB, Jones RB, Vredenburgh JJ et al, A large prospective randomised trial of high dose combination alkylating agent (CPB) with autologous cellular support (ABMS) as consolidation for patients with metastatic breast cancer achieving complete remission after intensive doxorubicin-based induction therapy (AFM). *Proc Am Soc Clin Oncol* 1995; **14:** 121 (Abst 149).

32. Rahman Z, Frye D, Buzdar A, Hortobagyi G, A retrospective analysis to evaluate the impact of selection processes for high dose chemotherapy (HDCT) on the outcome of patients (PT) with metastatic breast cancer (MBC). *Proc Am Soc Clin Oncol* 1995; **14:** 95 (Abst 78).

33. Greenberg PAC, Hortobagyi GN, Smith TL et al, Long-term follow-up of patients with complete remission following combination chemotherapy for metastatic breast cancer. *J Clin Oncol* 1996; **14:** 2197–205.

6

Haematopoietic recovery following transplantation

Ruth Pettengell

CONTENTS • **Introduction** • **Blood stem cell populations** • **Stromal requirements for haematopoiesis** • **Sources of cells for haematopoietic transplantation** • **Cell numbers required for engraftment** • **Failure to engraft** • **Immune reconstitution** • **Conclusions**

INTRODUCTION

In fetal life, haematopoiesis first appears in the yolk sac.[1,2] Subsequently the liver, spleen and finally the bone marrow are colonized.[3,4] In the fetus, stem cells move between these haematopoietic organs by circulating in the blood. In adult life, the bone marrow and circulating stem cell pools are in dynamic equilibrium, with over 98% of all committed progenitor cells in the marrow at any one time[5] and very few stem cells circulating in the blood. The presence of homing receptors on haematopoietic stem cells (HSC) facilitates reconstitution of the bone marrow from the blood following myeloablative therapy and haematopoietic progenitor cell reinfusion. Successful engraftment requires not only adequate numbers and quality of HSC but also appropriate localization of these cells within the bone marrow microenvironment. Under normal conditions, the majority of the haematopoietic stem cells are quiescent in the G0 phase of the cell cycle. The small proportion of these cells that are replicating give rise to all of the haemopoietic cells.[6–8] It has been reasoned that this proliferative inactivity allows time to repair DNA damage, thus conserving and maintaining the genetic integrity of this important population.[9] These stem cells must be capable of extensive and perhaps indefinite self-renewal to maintain a continuing supply of progeny that proliferate and differentiate into committed lineage-specific blood progenitors, which in turn undergo further proliferation and differentiation (to produce morphologically recognizable precursors), before they finally mature into functional cells that are released to circulate in the peripheral blood.

BLOOD STEM CELL POPULATIONS

Haematopoietic progenitor cell (HPC) transplantation is used to restore normal haematopoiesis following myeloablative chemoradiotherapy. This requires both lineage-committed progenitors, to effect early engraftment, and primitive progenitors, to effect long-term reconstitution. Karyotyping of recipients after sex-mismatched allogeneic bone marrow transplantation in humans has proved that donor cells are indeed responsible for long-term engraftment. Retroviral gene-marking techniques have been used in children undergoing autologous bone marrow rescue to show that cells of both myeloid and lymphoid lineages were derived from a common precursor and that such cells are capable of sustained haematopoietic reconstitution over 18 months.[10] Sex-mismatched allogeneic transplantation using mobilized blood stem cells is expected to confirm that functional blood stem cells can also be collected from the peripheral blood at apheresis.

Although lineage-committed progenitors are readily detected by in vitro cloning assays, there is no method that positively identifies the most primitive totipotent haematopoietic stem cells (Chapter 2). Primitive pluripotent cells are required for durable haematopoietic reconstitution after myeloablative therapy. Both primitive and lineage-committed progenitor cells are present within the CD34$^+$ cell population of marrow and blood, which constitutes 1–5% of cells in adult bone marrow. It is important to note that different haematopoietic products may contain different proportions of early and late progenitors. Thus high numbers of CD34$^+$ cells in the haematopoietic product may not necessarily imply the presence of high numbers of cells with stem cell phenotype.[11,12] It can therefore be misleading to measure a single progenitor cell subpopulation, such as colony-forming units granulocyte–macrophage (CFU-GM) or CD34$^+$ cells, when assessing the transplantation potential of HSC. For example, in newly diagnosed patients with breast cancer receiving chemotherapy with granulocyte colony-stimulating factor (G-CSF), CD34$^+$ cell numbers increased following successive cycles of combination chemotherapy, but numbers of CFU-GM and more particularly long-term culture-initiating cells (LTC-IC) fell significantly.[11,12] This lack of correlation is even more evident in heavily pretreated patients. In this group of patients, expansion in culture may be normal for 1–2 weeks and then fall to baseline by 3 weeks, suggesting a deficit of early precursors including LTC-IC that generate secondary progenitors at later stages of the culture.[13]

One of the controversies surrounding the repopulating capacities of stem cells is whether primitive progenitors are capable of short-term and long-term repopulation after transplantation. Long-term haematopoietic reconstitution is a function of primitive, non-clonogenic cells and generally correlates poorly with CFU-GM numbers. Some murine studies suggest that cells capable of producing short- and long-term engraftment are separable,[14] whereas other studies demonstrate that purified stem cells alone can produce physiologically relevant numbers of mature cells very early.[15] In man, it has been generally assumed that the rapid engraftment obtained following autograft of mobilized blood stem cells (BSC) is attributable to the high proportion of clonogenic cells administered, or to some phenotypic characteristic that accompanies their ability to be mobilized. Indirect evidence for this comes from bone marrow autografts treated with 4-hydroperoxycylophosphanide (4HC) to purge malignant cells, which depletes clonogenic progenitors to undetectable levels but maintains LTC-IC numbers.[16] Such products engraft but slightly slower than unpurged marrow.[17] The finding that chronic myeloid leukaemia (CML) patients reinfused with >95% Ph$^+$ clonogenic cells and 95% Ph$^-$ LTC-IC have >95% Ph$^-$ cells at 1–6 months post autograft provides further evidence that the role of LTC-IC in short-term engraftment is small.[18] Sutherland et al[19] were unable to show any significant correlation between the LTC-IC content in the graft and numbers of CFC or CD34$^+$ cells or with the speed of engraftment in a series of 21 patients with a variety of malignancies. However the patients who had very delayed (>5 weeks) blood count recoveries were also those who had very low numbers of LTC-IC in their autografts.[18] Similarly, LTC-IC numbers correlated with platelet recovery and the time to normalize the blood count, but not with time to neutrophil recovery in a paediatric study.[20]

The maturation pathway of individual haemopoietic clones can vary in length.[21] The number of divisions that the haematopoietic repopulating cells must undergo to reconstitute the marrow is inversely related to the number reinfused, and may have implications for telomere loss and senescence.[22] Chromosomes have repetitive non-coding sequences at their ends (telomeres) that protect against replicative loss and chromosomal integrity. In addition, telomeres have important functions during mitosis. At each cell division, there is incomplete replication of the 3' termini by DNA polymerase, leading to telomere shortening.[23–25] In normal life, peripheral leukocyte telomeres shorten by approximately 9 bp per year. Senescence is associated with telomere shortening, and occurs in somatic cells after 30–75 population doublings – the 'Hayflick limit'.[23] In cultures of fetal, neonatal and adult human haematopoietic cells, 40–50 telomere base pairs are lost during cell division.[24] Telomerase is a ribonucleoprotein that can add telomeric repeats to the chromosome ends. It is not expressed in somatic cells except for stem cell populations. In haematopoietic cells, telomerase is repressed in quiescent stem cells (CD34$^+$ CD38$^-$); it is activated upon cell proliferation, expansion, cell cycle entry and progression into the progenitor compartment (CD34$^+$CD38$^-$); and it is repressed again upon further differentiation (CD34$^-$).[26,27] Telomerase activity in haematopoietic cells reduces – but does not prevent – telomere shortening during proliferation. In the setting of clinical HSC transplantation, if the haematopoietic stem cells have proliferated extensively prior to transplantation and few are engrafted, then they may reach they Hayflick limit, leading to delayed marrow failure. One of the attractions of umbilical cord blood as a source of BSC for transplantation is that the replicative limit will take longer to reach. There is evidence that fetal liver has even greater regenerative capacity than adult HSC.[22,28,29]

STROMAL REQUIREMENTS FOR HAEMATOPOIESIS

Surprisingly little is known about the precise cellular and molecular effects of high-dose chemotherapy on the bone marrow microenvironment. Soluble factors, stromal cells and the extracellular matrix are critical elements of the bone marrow stroma; they provide a structural framework and a responsive physiological environment, both of which are essential for haematopoiesis. Stromal cells comprise a variety of cell types, including fibroblasts, endothe-lial cells and adipocytes.[30] Distinct stromal cell lines can be isolated that support the growth of early and late haematopoietic progenitors, and it is postulated that these form niches within bone marrow where the microenvironment supports different cell lineages.[31] The stromal cells and matrix proteins supply secreted haematopoietic growth factors and an adhesive microenvironment that maintains both high local growth factor concentrations and cell-to-cell contact. Fibronectin promotes cell proliferation by selective adhesion processes, whereas glycosaminoglycans specifically retain and deliver growth factors. Fibrinogen and its D-fragment potentiate the effect of interleukin-3 (IL-3) on early haematopoietic cells.[32] Direct contact between the HSC and stroma is needed for the survival of human repopulating cells. Some LTC-IC subsets and progenitors, however, can survive when separated from the stroma by a semipermeable membrane.[33,34]

Successful haemopoietic engraftment depends not only on the quality of the infused cells, but also on the recipient stroma. In heavily pretreated patients, the bone marrow stroma may have been damaged by prior chemotherapy and radiotherapy, the conditioning regimen, and the underlying disease. If this is the case, marrow regeneration will be jeopardized – no matter what the number or source of the haemopoietic progenitors used for transplantation. Following myeloablation and reinfusion of allogeneic bone marrow, several studies[35,36] have shown that the haematopoietic cells are of graft origin but the stroma remains of recipient type. The stromal cells are exposed to the myeloablative regime, and the final recovery of haematopoiesis can be limited by the degree of stromal injury.[37] For example, busulphan causes permanent damage to both the primitive stem cell compartment and the haemopoietic microenvironment of the marrow, impairing the ability of mice to mobilize progenitor cells.[38] Long-term marrow damage occurs even after conventional chemotherapy. When designing chemotherapy regimens, it is important to be aware of their effects on bone marrow, in addition to antitumour effects. The effects of radiotherapy have been elegantly demonstrated by

Schick et al,[39] who showed by magnetic resonance imaging and proton spectroscopy that intensively irradiated areas of marrow are not involved in marrow reconstitution. In addition, these authors suggest that marrow inhomogeneity on magnetic resonance imaging predicts for delayed haematological recovery.

SOURCES OF CELLS FOR HAEMATOPOIETIC TRANSPLANTATION

Bone marrow

Until recently, aspirated bone marrow was the preferred source of stem cells for haematopoietic reconstitution following myeloablative therapy. This has the advantage of supplying the full range of haematopoietic and stromal cells. Engraftment is generally accepted as $\geq 0.5 \times 10^9$/litre neutrophils in the peripheral blood. Neutrophil recovery following bone marrow transplantation takes between 8 and 30 days, and depends on the underlying disease, the preparative regimen, the bone marrow source (allogeneic or autologous) and the regimen used to treat graft-versus-host disease (GVHD). Platelet ($\geq 20 \times 10^9$/litre) and red cell (reticulocytes >1.55%) engraftment usually follow neutrophil recovery. Although the median day of platelet recovery occurs soon after neutrophil recovery, the distribution is skewed and can extend to beyond 100 days. In uncomplicated transplants, reticulocyte counts peak around day 40. No correlation has been shown between the number of nucleated marrow cells reinfused and the duration of neutropenia. Haemopoietic growth factors can shorten early neutropenia following bone marrow transplantation. In a phase III trial of G-CSF in 315 patients following bone marrow transplantation, the time to neutrophil recovery above 0.5×10^9/litre was reduced from 20 to 14 days in both autograft and allograft recipients receiving G-CSF.[40] These patients had fewer days of infection, required fewer antibiotics and spent less time in hospital. Clinical and culture-proven infection rates were similar in the two groups. Since the haemopoietic growth factors

do not reduce the period of absolute neutropenia (neutrophils < 0.1×10^9/litre), this is unsurprising. Neither G-CSF nor GM-CSF affect platelet recovery times. It is hoped that thrombopoietin (megakaryocyte growth and development factor) will reduce platelet recovery times and transfusion requirements.

Attempts to improve the yield of specific haematopoietic subpopulations by priming bone marrow donors with 5-fluorouracil (5-FU)[41] or cytokines have met with limited success.[42,43] Pretreatment with haematopoietic cytokines prior to bone marrow collection increases the numbers of lineage-restricted progenitors that are obtained, but the time to haemopoietic engraftment of platelets is unchanged.[44]

Autologous blood stem cells

For autologous transplantation, mobilized HSC collected by apheresis have now almost completely superseded bone marrow. In early studies, blood stem cells were collected during steady-state haematopoiesis, and demonstrated engraftment kinetics similar to those of cryopreserved bone marrow, except for a moderate risk of delayed or failed platelet recovery. Subsequently the use of interventions to 'mobilize' or increase the number of circulating blood stem cells and progenitors prior to collection have demonstrated markedly improved results. Comparative studies have shown that mobilized blood stem cells lead to earlier recovery of neutrophil and platelet counts than bone marrow transplantation, leading to reduced hospital stays and costs. In patients with solid tumours ($n = 47$), those randomized to BSC transplantation achieved 0.5×10^9 granulocytes/litre at median day 10 and 20×10^9 platelets/litre at day 10, whereas those receiving bone marrow took 11 and 17 days respectively.[45] In patients with lymphoma ($n = 58$), those randomized to BSC transplantation achieved 0.5×10^9 granulocytes/litre at median day 11 (9–38) and 20×10^9/litre platelets at day 16 (8–52), whereas those receiving bone marrow took 14 (9–25) and 23 (13–56) days respectively.[46] Significantly fewer red cell and platelet transfusions were required in the BSC group, and the hospital stay was reduced from 23 to 17 days, with consequent economic savings.[47] Indeed these savings exceed the cost of BSC mobilization and collection.

Although exogenous haematopoietic growth factors can accelerate neutrophil recovery following autologous BSC transplantation,[48] it is unclear to what extent this reduces morbidity when adequate numbers of CD34[+] cells are administered.[49] In view of the outpouring of endogenous growth factors after myelotoxic treatment, it is perhaps surprising that treatment with exogenous G-CSF or GM-CSF has any further effect.

Transplantation of enriched CD34[+] cells from bone marrow or from peripheral blood has demonstrated that both primitive and lineage-committed progenitor populations reside in the CD34[+] fraction.[50,51] Engraftment of neutrophils to 0.5×10^9 by day 12 and platelets to 20×10^9 by day 13 is comparable to unseparated mononuclear cell populations.[52,53]

Whilst there is little doubt that use of mobilized blood stem cells leads to more rapid engraftment than bone marrow and to reduced morbidity, there is less evidence that this has altered the risk of transplant-related mortality. It is also unknown whether the use of BSC has changed the risk of relapse. In a recent study that examined factors predicting morbidity following blood stem cell transplantation (BSCT), patients transplanted with BSC had a lower incidence of pulmonary dysfunction (20 vs 40%, $p = 0.006$) and liver dysfunction (4 vs 14%, $p = 0.05$) than patients receiving bone marrow.[54]

Although most experience has been gained with single myeloablative treatments and BSC transplantation, an increasing number of centres are performing multiple transplant procedures and using BSC to support dose-intensive submyeloablative chemotherapy. In most published studies, BSC are collected before starting the dose-intensive treatment, and are stored in aliquots. This has the advantage of ensuring that the haematopoietic cells are not damaged by the treatment, but damage to the marrow stroma may still delay re-engraftment in later cycles[55] and has the disadvantage that each aliquot carries the same risk of malignant contamination. The observation that peripheral blood contains high numbers of BSC following mobilization, and that leukapheresis is a relatively inefficient process, led us to examine the use of unprocessed whole blood as a source of BSC.[56] We have shown that adequate cell numbers for transplantation are present in 1 litre of blood.[56–58] BSC can be stored in leukapheresis products or whole blood for up to 72 hours at 4°C with comparable viability to cryopreserved products.[59] The use of BSC in unprocessed whole blood is an economical way of supporting multicyclic dose-intensive chemotherapy.

Allogeneic blood stem cells

Because blood stem cells contain 10-fold more T cells than bone marrow, there has been concern that their use might worsen GVHD, and as a result, the use of allogeneic BSC has lagged behind that of blood stem cells for autologous transplantation. Early studies of unselected allogeneic blood stem cells mobilized by G-CSF suggest that they result in more rapid engraftment than is obtained with allogeneic marrow, and do not cause an obvious increase in the incidence of acute GVHD (see Chapter 10). Following allogeneic BSC transplantation, recovery of granulocytes to $0.1–0.5 \times 10^9$/litre is seen in approximately 15 and 20 days respectively, and platelet independence can be expected in 14 days with a wide range.[60] If methotrexate is used in GVHD prophylaxis, recovery is delayed by about 4 days. Where CD34[+] selection has been used to reduce T-cell numbers in the graft, rapid engraftment is still observed, with no obvious increase in the incidence of graft failure, but no reduction in GVHD has been observed. However, this has yet to be tested in randomized trials.

Human umbilical cord blood

There has been increasing interest in the use of stem cells from human umbilical cord blood for transplantation (Chapter 11). The limited number of blood stem cells that can be obtained from a single human umbilical cord is a potential disadvantage of this cell source. A relationship between the dose of infused cells and the time to myeloid recovery was reported in unrelated human umbilical cord blood recipients. In this patient group, recovery to neutrophils to 0.5×10^9/litre was seen at 22 (14–37) days, platelets to 20×10^9/litre at 56 (35–89) days and red cells at 55 (32–90) days.[61,62] Only 12 patients weighing more than 40 kg have been transplanted, and of these only 5 are adults.[62] The International Cord Blood Transplant registry, however, found no such correlation in recipients of placental blood from related donors.[63] Techniques to expand stem and progenitor cell populations ex vivo might circumvent this problem in the future.

CELL NUMBERS REQUIRED FOR ENGRAFTMENT

Undoubtedly, the number of HSC reinfused following myeloablative therapy influences the time to haematopoietic recovery.[60,64] The minimum number of HSC required for haematopoietic reconstitution after myeloablation has not been determined. This is partly due to the incompleteness of the information available on the composition of the haematopoietic product obtained after various BSC mobilizing regimens and partly due to heterogeneity of patient populations. Different laboratories use a variety of reagents and methods for the bioassay of CFC and estimation of CD34$^+$ cells, so assays performed in different laboratories are never directly comparable. As a result, it is difficult to compare results from different studies. Any recommendations must be pragmatic and give a wide margin of safety.

Each transplant centre will adopt a threshold BSC number for autologous and allogeneic transplantation that takes into account the characteristics of the local patient population, and the mobilizing regimens and methods of apheresis and cryopreservation that are used. Ideally, this threshold should be validated using a range of progenitor assays to assess early and late progenitors. Once established, such assays may not be routinely required – indeed, a simple surrogate such as mononuclear cell or CD34$^+$ cell number can be used.[48,65] It is, however, important to stress that any change in the mobilization, collection or treatment protocol will require that the threshold be revalidated using formal haematopoietic assays. Caution is required in extrapolating from present practice to numbers of cells that will be required following any manipulation such as CD34$^+$ cell selection, purging or ex vivo expansion, or any change in the storage conditions.

Conventionally $\geqslant 3 \times 10^8$/kg mononuclear cells have been recommended for allogeneic bone marrow transplantation and $\geqslant 1 \times 10^8$/kg mononuclear cells for autologous bone marrow transplantation. Guidelines for adequate bone marrow harvests have not been expressed in terms of progenitor cells subsets, so the studies discussed below refer to BSC.

The numbers and types of BSC available for reinfusion will depend on the number of apheresis procedures and the success of mobilization, which in turn depends on the protocol used, the age of the donor, prior marrow disease and treatment history (Chapters 3 and 4). During progenitor mobilization, it is necessary to use surrogate markers of engraftment potential. Various parameters have been used to define an adequate BSC harvest, including numbers of nucleated and mononuclear cells, weight-adjusted mononuclear cells (MNC), CFU-GM, LTC-IC and CD34$^+$ cells. Interestingly, estimation of CFU-megakaryocytes is no better than CFU-GM in predicting time to platelet recovery.[66] Both CD34$^+$ cell and CFU-GM numbers have been shown to predict time to engraftment, but the CD34$^+$ cell number is gaining in popularity, probably because it can be standardized and performed rapidly.

A number of centres have established threshold doses appropriate to their own practice but it is difficult to compare these. Local preferences and priorities will determine the incidence of slow engraftment that is acceptable. The Milan group have defined their optimum dose of BSC as the number that allows 95% of patients to recover to 0.5×10^9 neutrophils/litre in 11 days and 50×10^9 platelets/litre in 14 days.[67] As a result, their harvest threshold is 8×10^6 CD34$^+$ cells/kg and 50×10^4 CFU-GM/kg. For autologous transplantation, most authors recommend $(1–5) \times 10^6$ CD34$^+$ cells/kg or $(1–5) \times 10^5$ CFU-GM cells/kg.[19,68–70] Similar cell numbers are required for allogeneic and autologous transplantation, although some authors advocate using a higher threshold dose for allogeneic BSCT.[71] As with autologous blood stem cell transplantation, the rapidity of engraftment and transplant-related morbidity can be related to the numbers of committed progenitor cells reinfused,[69,72] but no correlation between CD34$^+$ cell dose and engraftment was seen when a threshold of 2.5×10^6 CD34$^+$ selected cells/kg was used.[73] LTC-IC are rarely measured, but we and others have found a threshold of 2×10^4 LTC-IC/kg to be safe.[74,75] More recently, Breems et al[76] demonstrated that less than 5×10^3 LTC-IC/kg denoted poor stem cell quality.

In a Seattle series of 243 autologous procedures, there was no significant difference in neutrophil recovery times for patients receiving more than 2.5×10^6 CD34$^+$ cells/kg, but patients receiving less had delayed engraftment.[77] In contrast, higher numbers of CD34$^+$ cells led to more rapid platelet engraftment. Favourable features for high CD34$^+$ yields were a diagnosis of breast cancer, absence of bone marrow involvement, fewer cycles of prior chemotherapy and no prior radiotherapy. Age was not important.[77] Of 52 patients with lymphoma and solid tumours reported by Schwartzberg et al,[78] all 4 patients with slow engraftment had received less than 2×10^6 CD34$^+$ cells/kg. Zimmerman et al[79] studied 30 patients who received high-dose therapy for breast cancer. A cell dose less than 0.75×10^6/kg and a threshold of 2×10^6/kg were suggested for rapid engraftment. In a further study, 7 of 42 lymphoma patients who received less than 1×10^6 CD34$^+$/kg cells were slow to engraft.[48] As a result, this group identified 2.5×10^6 CD34$^+$ cells/kg as the threshold for transplantation.

Patients who require multiple aphereses to achieve a threshold yield engraft more slowly than patients achieving the same cell dose at a single apheresis.[48,80] The collection of a low total of progenitor cells even after multiple aphereses also bodes ill for rapid engraftment. Not surprisingly, therefore, patients requiring two or more mobilization procedures versus one to achieve the threshold also experience slower platelet recovery.[70] The implication is that poor mobilization in terms of progenitor cell quantity is also indicative of poor progenitor cell quality.

Although suboptimal doses of CD34$^+$ progenitor cells are associated with failure to engraft, supra-optimal doses do not lead to ever earlier engraftment. Granulocyte and platelet count recovery appear to require a minimum of 8 days. Ex vivo expansion strategies are being explored in the belief that relatively mature cells are responsible for early engraftment and that if sufficiently high numbers of committed progenitors are given, the period of pancytopenia following myeloablative chemotherapy might be reduced further (Chapter 6). Although it is tempting to speculate that use of non-cryopreserved BSC in apheresis product or whole blood will contain a wider range of maturing cells, leading to earlier engraftment, there are no data to support this. However, early engraftment is not a feature of the use of non-cryopreserved bone marrow for allogeneic transplantation.

FAILURE TO ENGRAFT

Mobilization chemotherapy, cytokine regimens, age, marrow disease, prior radiotherapy and chemotherapy affect the number of haematopoietic cells available for collection, with marked consequences on the time to engraft and graft stability. Graft failure occurs in 1–35% of all bone marrow recipients.[81] Failure of engraftment is defined as failure to achieve an absolute neutrophil count (ANC) $\geqslant 0.5 \times 10^9$/litre by day 20 after haemopoietic cell rescue or a sustained fall in ANC to $\leqslant 0.5 \times 10^9$/litre or of platelets to $\leqslant 20 \times 10^9$/litre for at least one week after the initial engraftment and before 100 days. Inadequate numbers of progenitors reinfused can lead to slow engraftment, whereas late graft failure can indicate poor stem cell levels or damage to bone marrow stroma. Although threshold values have been established, a proportion of patients who receive cell doses above them have slow engraftment. This is likely to be due to the quality of the progenitor cells or to the proportion of (as yet poorly defined) subsets of such cells responsible for rapid engraftment.

In numerous multivariate analyses of factors predicting BSC yields and engraftment, the most consistent adverse factor is treatment history. Both chemotherapy and radiotherapy have been shown to impact adversely on BSC mobilization, yield and engraftment. In one study, each cycle of prior chemotherapy on average reduced harvest yields by 0.2×10^6 CD34$^+$ cells/kg and large-field radiotherapy by 1.8×10^6 CD34$^+$ cells/kg.[80] In some studies, the effect of the number of prior chemotherapy regimens on neutrophil engraftment was independent of the log dose of infused CFU-GM, suggesting that the relationship was not a reflection of impaired stem cell mobilization, but rather of damage to the haematopoietic microenvironment. There is a particularly high incidence of long-term engraftment failure in patients with metastatic involvement of the bone marrow who have been heavily pre-treated.[82,83]

Certain drugs are known to be particularly damaging. Carmustine (BCNU), lomustine (methyl-CCNU), cisplatin, chlorambucil and melphalan are toxic to early stem cells, whereas agents such as cytosine arabinoside, vincristine and hydroxyurea probably have less effect.[48,68,84] Previous exposure to such drugs can result in stromal damage or damage to repopulating cells. Long-term marrow damage can be masked by compensatory mechanisms, which include expansion of the active bone marrow space, increased cycling of stem and progenitor cells and shortening of cell cycle times, leading to near-normal numbers of mature cells in the peripheral blood. This can lead to near-normal numbers of CD34$^+$ cells and CFU-GM in the presence of seriously reduced early progenitor numbers.[11,85]

The high-dose therapy regimen also affects engraftment times. Not all myeloablative regimens are equal. For example, recovery is faster following total body irradiation than after chemotherapy.[60,70]

The heterogeneity of patient populations makes comparisons between different centres difficult. Failure to engraft is more common in certain diagnostic groups, such as CML, but this may largely reflect stromal damage due to intensive prior chemoradiotherapy. Following allogeneic transplantation, graft rejection, GVHD and the anti-GVHD regimen can delay engraftment. Hepatic veno-occlusive disease can also contribute.[86] Disease relapse may present as failure to engraft, and must be suspected in any patient with otherwise unexplained cytopenia. Older patients are more likely to have problems engrafting. In practice, the commonest cause of delayed engraftment is probably infection. Bacterial, fungal and herpes simplex infections can delay haematopoietic recovery, whereas cytomegalovirus, *Pneumocystis carinii*, herpes zoster and other unusual infections are more likely to contribute to secondary graft failure. Bacterial infections predominate due to the lack of phagocytes. A direct relation has been demonstrated between the duration of neutropenia $<0.5 \times 10^9$ and $<0.1 \times 10^9$/litre and risk of infection.[87]

Thrombocytopenia, however, remains one of the critical problems that must be managed after myeloablative therapy and HSC rescue. With routine platelet transfusions, serious bleeding is unusual, and recovery is prompt in the absence of significant transplant complications. However, the administration of platelets is not without risk and is a costly practice. Thrombopoietic growth factors will soon be licensed for use in this patient group, but the relative cost of using them is not yet known. Two recent studies have examined risk factors for delayed platelet recovery after autologous and allogeneic transplantation. In a single-centre study of 1468 patients,[88] diagnosis (acute myeloid leukaemia versus primary breast cancer, non-Hodgkin's lymphoma, Hodgkin's disease, acute lymphocytic leukaemia and multiple myeloma) and source of stem cells (bone marrow versus peripheral blood) were strong predictors of delayed platelet recovery. Other risk factors identified in the multivariate analysis were infection prior to platelet recovery and seropositivity for cytomegalovirus. In a multicentre study including 789 patients from 18 centres, risk factors for delayed platelet recovery after BSC rescue that were identified in the multivariate analyses were low CD34[+] cell numbers reinfused, low platelet counts prior to transplantation, fever during the first 15 days, veno-occlusive disease of the liver, previous radiation therapy and the diagnosis at the time of transplantation.[89] In this study, cytomegalovirus seropositivity was not significantly associated with delayed platelet recovery.

Following allogeneic transplantation, the median time to platelet recovery was 21 days (range 7–98 days, Table 6.1).[88] Risk factors for delayed platelet recovery identified in the multivariate analysis were CML versus other diagnoses (including primary AML, ALL, myelodysplastic syndrome, multiple myeloma

and aplastic anaemia), source of bone marrow (HLA-matched unrelated donor (URD) versus HLA-matched related donor), GVHD, methotrexate for GVHD prophylaxis, infection, gender and age. The multicentre study identified veno-occlusive disease and T-cell depletion as additional risk factors.[89] Secondary failure of platelet engraftment was seen in 10% of autologous and 21% of allogeneic transplants. The estimated average 60-day cost per patient for platelet support was US$3500 for autologous BPC transplantations and US$9000 for allogeneic bone marrow transplantations.

IMMUNE RECONSTITUTION

In contrast to haematological recovery after autologous and allogeneic transplantations, immune reconstitution is slower and more difficult to document. Myeloablative therapy causes

---

Table 6.1 Platelet recovery by type of transplant and diagnostic group (adapted from Nash et al[88])

Transplant type	n	Conditional probability of platelet recovery[a]		Platelet recovery[b] (median day)	Platelet transfusions[c] (mean number)
		Day 35	Day 60–100		
Autologous	523				2.9
Other diagnoses (BSC)	224	0.85	0.90	10 (6–67)	1.3
AML (BSC)	23	0.74	0.79	14 (6–35)	1.8
Other diagnoses (BM)	208	0.56	0.76	24 (3–95)	4.0
AML (BM)	68	0.22	0.39	38 (12–87)	5.2
Allogeneic	945				2.0
CML (RD)	185	0.89	0.96	20 (7–75)	1.3
Other diagnoses (RD)	290	0.78	0.93	21 (9–70)	2.0
CML (RD)	161	0.78	0.91	22 (10–98)	2.1
Other diagnoses (URD)	309	0.61	0.88	21 (10–98)	2.6

[a] The probability of platelet recovery at day 35 or day 60 (autologous recipients) or 100 (allogeneic recipients) for patients alive and relapse-free.
[b] Median day to platelet recovery in patients who were alive and engrafted before relapse or before day 100.
[c] Mean number of platelet transfusion events per evaluable patient per week.
Key: BSC = blood stem cell; AML = acute myeloid leukaemia; BM = bone marrow; CML = chronic myeloid leukaemia; RD = related donor; URD = unrelated donor.

a profound immune paresis that can take over 12 months to recover. This is manifest as low phagocyte numbers, abnormal T-lymphocyte subsets and impaired immunoglobulin synthesis.[90] Although steady-state numbers may appear reasonable, there is a severely impaired ability to mount a functional immune response. Recovery is, however, faster following BSC than bone marrow transplantation. Seventeen-fold more helper and memory T cells are found in BSC than bone marrow.[91] The ratio of T cells to progenitors, and the distribution of T-cell subsets, differ between apheresis and bone marrow harvests.[92] Enhanced in vitro responses to mitogens and recall antigens were also observed after BSCT (2–3 months) compared with bone marrow.[91] Whether this contributes to a lower incidence of infectious complications is not yet known. T-cell depletion has been used in allogeneic transplantation to reduce the incidence of GVHD. However, this may jeopardize graft function and the graft-versus-leukaemia effect. The risks and benefits need careful study.[93,94] Whether earlier immune reconstitution in BSC autografts will result in a graft-versus-tumour effect and enhanced disease-free survival, as suggested by the Nebraska group, is yet to be determined.[95] The potential to manipulate the graft, either in vitro or in vivo, with immunomodulatory agents may also prove beneficial.[96]

CONCLUSIONS

The use of blood stem cells for autologous and allogeneic transplantation following myeloablative therapy leads to earlier haematological and immunological engraftment than the use of bone marrow. This has improved the risk-to-benefit ratio of the procedures, making it possible to offer high-dose treatment for a wider range of indications and to more patients.

Rapid haematopoietic recovery depends on collecting adequate numbers of blood stem cells for reinfusion. The patient's age, diagnosis, marrow involvement and prior exposure to cytotoxics and radiotherapy can affect the harvest, in addition to the choice of mobilizing regimen itself. At transplantation, the choice of high-dose regimen, autologous or allogeneic BSC and the use of haematopoietic growth factors influences engraftment. After this, infection, GVHD, hepatic veno-occlusive disease and tumour relapse can retard engraftment.

Because so many factors interact, recommendations for safe cell numbers for transplantation must have a wide safety margin. Clinicians need to be aware of the importance of reinfusing adequate numbers of early and late repopulating cells. Local guidelines should be developed that take into account the patient population and treatment protocols in use. Once validated, simple methods can be used to guide routine practice.

REFERENCES

1. Moore MA, Metcalf D, Ontogeny of the haemopoietic system: yolk sac origin of in vivo and in vitro colony forming cells in the developing mouse embryo. *Br J Haematol* 1970; **18:** 279–96.
2. Wong PM, Chung SW, Chui DH, Eaves CJ, Properties of the earliest clonogenic hemopoietic precursors to appear in the developing murine yolk sac. *Proc Natl Acad Sci USA* 1986; **83:** 3851–4.
3. Tavassoli M, Embryonic and fetal hemopoiesis: an overview. *Blood Cells* 1991; **17:** 269–81.
4. Broxmeyer HE, Self-renewal and migration of stem cells during embryonic and fetal hematopoiesis: important, but poorly understood events. *Blood Cells* 1991; **17:** 282–6.
5. Fliedner TM, Steinbach KH, Repopulating potential of hematopoietic precursor cells. *Blood Cells* 1988; **14:** 393–410.
6. Lajtha LG, Stem cell concepts. *Differentiation* 1979; **14:** 23–34.
7. Jordan CT, Lemischka IR, Clonal and systemic analysis of long-term hematopoiesis in the mouse. *Genes Develop* 1990; **4:** 220–32.
8. Van Zant G, Chen JJ, Scott-Micus K, Developmental potential of hematopoietic stem cells determined using retrovirally marked allophenic marrow. *Blood* 1991; **77:** 756–63.
9. Cairns J, Mutation selection and the natural history of cancer. *Nature* 1975; **255:** 197–200.

10. Brenner MK, Rill DR, Holladay MS et al, Gene marking to determine whether autologous marrow infusion restores long-term haemopoiesis in cancer patients. *Lancet* 1993; **342:** 1134–7.

11. Baumann I, Swindell R, Van Hoeff MEHM et al, Mobilisation kinetics of primitive haemopoietic cells following G-CSF with or without chemotherapy for advanced breast cancer. *Ann Oncol* 1996; **7:** 1051–7.

12. Weaver A, Ryder D, Crowther D et al, Increased numbers of long-term culture-initiating cells in the apheresis product of patients randomized to receive increasing doses of stem-cell factor administered in combination with chemotherapy and a standard-dose of granulocyte-colony-stimulating factor. *Blood* 1996; **88:** 3323–8.

13. Shapiro F, Yao TJ, Moskowitz C et al, Effects of prior therapy on the in-vitro proliferative potential of stem cell factor plus filgrastim mobilized CD34-positive progenitor cells. *Clin Cancer Res* 1997; **3:** 1571–8.

14. Jones RJ, Wagner JE, Celano P et al, Separation of pluripotent haematopoietic stem cells from spleen colony-forming cells. *Nature* 1990; **347:** 188–9.

15. Uchida N, Aguila HL, Fleming WH et al, Rapid and sustained hematopoietic recovery in lethally irradiated mice transplanted with purified Thy-1.1lo Lin-Sca-1+ hematopoietic stem cells. *Blood* 1994; **83:** 3758–79.

16. Winton EF, Colenda KW, Use of long-term human marrow cultures to demonstrate progenitor cell precursors in marrow treated with 4-hydroperoxycyclophosphamide. *Exp Hematol* 1987; **15:** 710–14.

17. Yeager AM, Kaizer H, Santos GW et al, Autologous bone marrow transplantation in patients with acute nonlymphocytic leukemia, using ex vivo marrow treatment with 4-hydroperoxycyclophosphamide. *N Engl J Med* 1986; **315:** 141–7.

18. Sutherland HJ, Hogge DE, Lansdorp PM et al, Quantitation, mobilization, and clinical use of long-term culture-initiating cells in blood cell autografts. *J Hematother* 1995; **4:** 3–10.

19. Sutherland HJ, Eaves CJ, Lansdorp PM et al, Kinetics of committed and primitive blood progenitor mobilization after chemotherapy and growth factor treatment and their use in autotransplants. *Blood* 1994; **83:** 3808–14.

20. Hirao A, Kawano Y, Takaue Y et al, Engraftment potential of peripheral and cord blood stem cells evaluated by a long-term culture system. *Exp Hematol* 1994; **22:** 521–6.

21. Gordon MY, Blackett NM, Lewis JL, Goldman JM, Evidence for a mechanism that can provide both short-term and long-term haemopoietic repopulation by a seemingly uniform population of primitive human haemopoietic precursor cells. *Leukemia* 1995; **9:** 1252–6.

22. Pawliuk R, Eaves C, Humphries RK, Evidence of both ontogeny and transplant dose-regulated expansion of hematopoietic stem-cells in-vivo. *Blood* 1996; **88:** 2852–8.

23. Hayflick L, Moorehead PS, The serial cultivation of human diploid cell strains. *Exp Cell Res* 1961; **25:** 585–621.

24. Vaziri H, Dragowska W, Allsopp RC et al, Evidence for a mitotic clock in human hematopoietic stem cells: loss of telomeric DNA with age. *Proc Natl Acad Sci USA* 1994; **91:** 9857–60.

25. Vaziri H, Schachter F, Uchida et al, Loss of telomeric DNA during aging of normal and trisomy 21 human lymphocytes. *Am J Human Genet* 1993; **52:** 661–7.

26. Holt SE, Wright WE, Shay JW, Regulation of telomerase activity in immortal cell-lines. *Molec Cell Biol* 1996; **16:** 2932–9.

27. Zhu X, Kumar R, Mandal M et al, Cell cycle-dependent modulation of telomerase activity in tumor cells. *Proc Natl Acad Sci USA* 1996; **93:** 6091–5.

28. Engelhardt M, Kumar R, Albanell J et al, Telomerase regulation, cell cycle and telomere stability in primitive hematopoietic cells. *Blood* 1997; **90:** 182–93.

29. Hirao A, Kawano Y, Takaue Y et al, Engraftment potential of peripheral and cord blood stem cells evaluated by a long-term culture system. *Exp Hematol* 1994; **22:** 521–6.

30. Deryugina EI, Muller-Sieburg CE, Stromal cells in long-term cultures: keys to the elucidation of hematopoietic development? *Crit Rev Immunol* 1993; **13:** 115–50.

31. Wineman J, Moore K, Lemischka I, Muller-Sieburg C, Functional heterogeneity of the hematopoietic microenvironment: rare stromal elements maintain long-term repopulating stem cells. *Blood* 1996; **87:** 4082–90.

32. Zhou YQ, Levesque JP, Hatzfeld A et al, Fibrinogen potentiates the effect of interleukin-3 on early human hematopoietic progenitors. *Blood* 1993; **82:** 800–6.

33. Verfaillie CM, Direct contact between human primitive hematopoietic progenitors and bone marrow stroma is not required for long-term in vitro hematopoiesis. *Blood* 1992; **79:** 2821–6.

34. Verfaillie CM, Soluble factor(s) produced by human bone marrow stroma increase cytokine-induced proliferation and maturation of primitive hematopoietic progenitors while preventing their terminal differentiation. *Blood* 1993; **82:** 2045–53.

35. Laver J, Jhanwar SC, O'Reilly RJ, Castro-Malaspina H, Host origin of the human hematopoietic microenvironment following allogeneic bone marrow transplantation. *Blood* 1987; **70:** 1966–8.

36. Simmons PJ, Przepiorka D, Thomas ED, Torok-Storb B, Host origin of marrow stromal cells following allogeneic bone marrow transplantation. *Nature* 1987; **328:** 429–32.

37. Molineux G, Testa NG, Massa G, Schofield R, An analysis of haemopoietic and microenvironmental populations of mouse bone marrow after treatment with busulphan. *Biomed Pharmacother* 1986; **40:** 215–20.

38. Neben S, Marcus K, Mauch P, Mobilization of hematopoietic stem and progenitor cell subpopulations from the marrow to the blood of mice following cyclophosphamide and/or granulocyte colony-stimulating factor. *Blood* 1993; **81:** 1960–7.

39. Schick F, Einsele H, Weiss B et al, Assessment of the composition of bone marrow prior to and following autologous BMT and PBSCT by magnetic resonance. *Ann Hematol* 1996; **72:** 361–70.

40. Gisselbrecht C, Prentice HG, Bacigalupo A et al, Placebo-controlled phase III trial of lenograstim in bone-marrow transplantation. *Lancet* 1994; **343:** 696–700.

41. Stewart FM, Crittenden RB, Lowry PA et al, Long-term engraftment of normal and post-5-fluorouracil murine marrow into normal non-myeloablated mice. *Blood* 1993; **81:** 2566–71.

42. Naparstek E, Hardan Y, Ben-Shahar M et al, Enhanced marrow recovery by short preincubation of marrow allografts with human recombinant interleukin-3 and granulocyte–macrophage colony-stimulating factor. *Blood* 1992; **80:** 1673–8.

43. Ratajczak MZ, Ratajczak J, Kregenow DA, Gewirtz AM, Growth factor stimulation of cryopreserved CD34$^+$ bone marrow cells intended for transplant: an in vitro study to determine optimal timing of exposure to early acting cytokines. *Stem Cells* 1994; **12:** 599–603.

44. Johnsen HE, Hansen PB, Plesner T et al, Increased yield of myeloid progenitor cells in bone marrow harvested for autologous transplantation by pretreatment with recombinant

45. human granulocyte-colony stimulating factor. *Bone Marrow Transplant* 1992; **10:** 229–34.

45. Beyer J, Schwella N, Zingsem J et al, Hematopoietic rescue after high-dose chemotherapy using autologous peripheral-blood progenitor cells or bone marrow: a randomized comparison. *J Clin Oncol* 1995; **13:** 1328–35.

46. Schmitz N, Linch DC, Dreger P et al, Randomised trial of filgrastim-mobilised peripheral blood progenitor cell transplantation versus autologous bone-marrow transplantation in lymphoma patients. *Lancet* 1996; **347:** 353–7.

47. Smith TJ, Hillner BE, Schmitz N et al, Economic analysis of a randomized clinical trial to compare filgrastim-mobilized peripheral-blood progenitor-cell transplantation and autologous bone marrow transplantation in patients with Hodgkin's and non-Hodgkin's lymphoma. *J Clin Oncol* 1997; **15:** 5–10.

48. Watts MJ, Sullivan AM, Jamieson E, Progenitor-cell mobilization after low-dose cyclophosphamide and granulocyte colony-stimulating factor: an analysis of progenitor-cell quantity and quality and factors predicting for these parameters in 101 pretreated patients with malignant lymphoma. *J Clin Oncol* 1997; **15:** 535–46.

49. Zimmerman TM, Mick R, Myers S et al, Source of stem cells impacts on hematopoietic recovery after high-dose chemotherapy. *Bone Marrow Transplant* 1995; **15:** 923–7.

50. Shpall EJ, Jones RB, Bearman SI et al, Transplantation of enriched CD34-positive autologous marrow into breast cancer patients following high-dose chemotherapy: influence of CD34-positive peripheral-blood progenitors and growth factors on engraftment. *J Clin Oncol* 1994; **12:** 28–36.

51. Civin CI, Trischmann T, Kadan NS et al, Highly purified CD34-positive cells reconstitute hematopoiesis. *J Clin Oncol* 1996; **14:** 2224–33.

52. Mahe B, Milpied N, Hermouet S et al, G-CSF alone mobilizes sufficient peripheral blood CD34$^+$ cells for positive selection in newly diagnosed patients with myeloma. *Br J Haematol* 1996; **92:** 263–8.

53. Lemoli RM, Fortuna A, Motta MR et al, Concomitant mobilization of plasma cells and hematopoietic progenitors into peripheral blood of multiple myeloma patients: positive selection and transplantation of enriched CD34$^+$ cells to remove circulating tumor cells. *Blood* 1996; **87:** 1625–34.

54. Gordon B, Haire W, Ruby E et al, Factors pre-

dicting morbidity following hematopoietic stem cell transplantation. *Bone Marrow Transplant* 1997; **19:** 497–501.

55. Sheridan WP, Begley CG, Juttner CA et al, Effect of peripheral-blood progenitor cells mobilised by filgrastim (G-CSF) on platelet recovery after high-dose chemotherapy. *Lancet* 1992; **339:** 640–4.

56. Pettengell R, Woll PJ, Thatcher N et al, Multicyclic, dose-intensive chemotherapy supported by sequential reinfusion of hematopoietic progenitors in whole blood. *J Clin Oncol* 1995; **13:** 148–56.

57. Pettengell R, Testa NG, Swindell R et al, Transplantation potential of hematopoietic cells released into the circulation during routine chemotherapy for non-Hodgkin's lymphoma. *Blood* 1993; **82:** 2239–48.

58. Ossenkoppele GJ, Schuurhuis GJ, Jonkhoff AR et al, G-CSF (filgrastim)-stimulated whole blood kept unprocessed at 4°C does support a BEAM-like regimen in bad-risk lymphoma. *Bone Marrow Transplant* 1996; **18:** 427–31.

59. Pettengell R, Woll PJ, O'Connor DA et al, Viability of haemopoietic progenitors from whole blood, bone marrow and leukapheresis product: effects of storage media, temperature and time. *Bone Marrow Transplant* 1994; **14:** 703–9.

60. Bensinger WI, Weaver CH, Appelbaum FR et al, Transplantation of allogeneic peripheral blood stem cells mobilized by recombinant human granulocyte colony-stimulating factor. *Blood* 1995; **85:** 1655–8.

61. Kurtzberg J, Laughlin M, Graham ML et al, Placental blood as a source of hematopoietic stem cells for transplantation into unrelated recipients. *N Engl J Med* 1996; **335:** 157–66.

62. Rubinstein P, Carrier C, Adamson J et al, New York Blood Centers program for unrelated placental umbilical-cord blood (PBC) transplantation – 243 transplants in the first 3 years. *Blood* 1996; **88**(Suppl 1): 557.

63. Wagner JE, Kernan NA, Steinbuch M et al, Allogeneic sibling umbilical-cord-blood transplantation in children with malignant and non-malignant disease. *Lancet* 1995; **346:** 214–19.

64. Bensinger WI, Buckner CD, Shannon-Dorcy K et al, Transplantation of allogeneic CD34$^+$ peripheral blood stem cells in patients with advanced hematologic malignancy. *Blood* 1996; **88:** 4132–8.

65. Pettengell R, Morgenstern GR, Woll PJ et al, Peripheral blood progenitor cell transplantation in lymphoma and leukemia using a single apheresis. *Blood* 1993; **82:** 3770–7.

66. Takamatsu Y, Harada M, Teshima T et al, Relationship of infused CFU-GM and CFU-Mk mobilized by chemotherapy with or without G-CSF to platelet recovery after autologous blood stem cell transplantation. *Exp Hematol* 1995; **23:** 8–13.

67. Gianni AM, Where do we stand with respect to the use of peripheral blood progenitor cells? *Ann Oncol* 1994; **5:** 781–4.

68. Dreger P, Kloss M, Petersen B et al, Autologous progenitor cell transplantation: prior exposure to stem cell-toxic drugs determines yield and engraftment of peripheral blood progenitor cell but not of bone marrow grafts. *Blood* 1995; **86:** 3970–8.

69. Mavroudis D, Read E, Cottlerfox M et al, CD34(+) cell dose predicts survival, posttransplant morbidity, and rate of hematologic recovery after allogeneic marrow transplants for hematologic malignancies. *Blood* 1996; **88:** 3223–9.

70. Weaver CH, Hazelton B, Birch R et al, An analysis of engraftment kinetics as a function of the CD34 content of peripheral blood progenitor cell collections in 692 patients after the administration of myeloablative chemotherapy. *Blood* 1995; **86:** 3961–9.

71. Korbling M, Huh YO, Durett A et al, Allogeneic blood stem cell transplantation: peripheralization and yield of donor-derived primitive hematopoietic progenitor cells (CD34$^+$ Thy-1dim) and lymphoid subsets, and possible predictors of engraftment and graft-versus-host disease. *Blood* 1995; **86:** 2842–8.

72. Miflin G, Russell NH, Hutchinson RM et al, Allogeneic peripheral blood stem cell transplantation for haematological malignancies – an analysis of kinetics of engraftment and gvhd risk. *Bone Marrow Transplant* 1997; **19:** 9–13.

73. Bensinger WI, Clift R, Martin P et al, Allogeneic peripheral blood stem cell transplantation in patients with advanced hematologic malignancies: a retrospective comparison with marrow transplantation. *Blood* 1996; **88:** 2794–800.

74. Pettengell R, Luft T, Henschler R et al, Direct comparison by limiting dilution analysis of long-term culture-initiating cells in human bone marrow, umbilical cord blood, and blood stem cells. *Blood* 1994; **84:** 3653–9.

75. Sutherland HJ, Lansdorp PM, Henkelman DH et al, Functional characterization of individual human hematopoietic stem cells cultured at limiting dilution on supportive marrow stromal layers. *Proc Natl Acad Sci USA* 1990; **87:** 3584–8.

76. Breems DA, van Hennik PB, Kusadasi N et al, Individual stem cell quality in leukapheresis products is related to the number of mobilized stem cells. *Blood* 1996; **87:** 5370–8.

77. Bensinger W, Appelbaum F, Rowley S et al, Factors that influence collection and engraftment of autologous peripheral-blood stem cells. *J Clin Oncol* 1995; **13:** 2547–55.

78. Schwartzberg L, Birch R, Blanco R et al, Rapid and sustained hematopoietic reconstitution by peripheral blood stem cell infusion alone following high-dose chemotherapy. *Bone Marrow Transplant* 1993; **11:** 369–74.

79. Zimmerman TM, Lee WJ, Bender JG et al, Quantitative CD34 analysis may be used to guide peripheral blood stem cell harvests. *Bone Marrow Transplant* 1995; **15:** 439–44.

80. Haas R, Mohle R, Fruhauf S et al, Patient characteristics associated with successful mobilizing and autografting of peripheral blood progenitor cells in malignant lymphoma. *Blood* 1994; **83:** 3787–94.

81. Maraninchi D, The clinical consequences of haematological and non-haematological toxicity following bone marrow transplantation and the possible impact of haematopoietic growth factors. *Bone Marrow Transplant* 1993; **11**(Suppl 2): 12–22.

82. Tricot G, Jagannath S, Vesole D et al, Peripheral blood stem cell transplants for multiple myeloma: identification of favorable variables for rapid engraftment in 225 patients. *Blood* 1995; **85:** 588–96.

83. Bentley SA, Brecher ME, Powell E et al, Long-term engraftment failure after marrow ablation and autologous hematopoietic reconstitution: differences between peripheral blood stem cell and bone marrow recipients. *Bone Marrow Transplant* 1997; **19:** 557–63.

84. Mauch P, Hellman S, Loss of hematopoietic stem cell self-renewal after bone marrow transplantation. *Blood* 1989; **74:** 872–5.

85. Voso MT, Murea S, Goldschmidt H et al, High-dose therapy with peripheral blood stem cell transplantation results in a significant reduction of the haemopoietic progenitor cell compartment. *Br J Haematol* 1996; **94:** 759–66.

86. Anasetti C, Rybka W, Sullivan KM et al, Graft-v-host disease is associated with autoimmune-like thrombocytopenia. *Blood* 1989; **73:** 1054–8.

87. Bodey GP, Buckley M, Sathe YS, Freireich EJ, Quantitative relationships between circulating leucocytes and infection in patients with acute leukaemia. *Ann Intern Med* 1966; **64:** 328–40.

88. Nash RA, Gooley T, Davis C, Appelbaum FR, The problem of thrombocytopenia after hematopoietic stem-cell transplantation. *Stem Cells* 1996; **14:** 743.

89. Bernstein SH, Barnett M, Cairo M et al, A multi-center observation study of platelet utilization among recipients of myeloablative therapy and stem cell transplantation (SCT). *Proc Am Soc Clin Oncol* 1996; **15:** 84.

90. Witherspoon RP, Armitage JO, Antman KH, Immunologic reconstitution after high-dose chemoradiotherapy and allogeneic or autologous bone marrow or peripheral blood hematopoietic stem cell transplantation. In: *High-Dose Cancer Therapy. Pharmacology, Hematopoietins, Stem cells.* Baltimore: Williams & Wilkins, 1992: 211–23.

91. Ottinger HD, Beelen DW, Scheulen B, Schaefer UW, Grossewilde H, Improved immune reconstitution after allotransplantation of peripheral-blood stem-cells instead of bone-marrow. *Blood* 1996; **88:** 2775–9.

92. Galy AH, Webb S, Cen D et al, Generation of T cells from cytokine-mobilized peripheral blood and adult bone marrow CD34$^+$ cells. *Blood* 1994; **84:** 104–10.

93. Roberts MM, To LB, Gillis D et al, Immune reconstitution following peripheral blood stem cell transplantation, autologous bone marrow transplantation and allogeneic bone marrow transplantation. *Bone Marrow Transplant* 1993; **12:** 469–75.

94. Scheid C, Pettengell R, Ghielmini M et al, Time-course of the recovery of cellular immune function after high-dose chemotherapy and peripheral blood progenitor cell transplantation for high-grade non-Hodgkin's lymphoma. *Bone Marrow Transplant* 1995; **15:** 901–6.

95. Vose JM, Anderson JR, Kessinger A et al, High-dose chemotherapy and autologous hematopoietic stem-cell transplantation for aggressive non-Hodgkin's lymphoma. *J Clin Oncol* 1993; **11:** 1846–51.

96. Lopez-Jimenez J, Perez-Oteyza J, Munoz A et al, Subcutaneous versus intravenous low-dose IL-2 therapy after autologous transplantation: results of a prospective, non-randomized study. *Bone Marrow Transplant* 1997; **19:** 429–34.

7

The impact of growth factors on hematopoietic recovery after high-dose chemotherapy and autologous stem cell transplantation

Gary Spitzer and Douglas Adkins

ABSOLUTE NEUTROPENIA FOLLOWING HIGH-DOSE THERAPY

The major cause of morbidity and mortality following high-dose chemotherapy is infection secondary to severe prolonged myelosuppression. By shortening the duration of myelosuppression, infusion of stem cells obtained from bone marrow or peripheral blood has permitted the administration of single or repetitive cycles of intensive chemotherapy. However, absolute neutropenia, defined as an absolute neutrophil count (ANC) $\leq 100/\mu l$, is not abolished by infusion of bone marrow or peripheral blood stem cells (PBSC).[1-3] It is during this period that most patients acquire infections or experience febrile neutropenia. We and others have pointed out that resolution of fever with antibiotic therapy occurs in the majority of cases upon the first appearance of circulating neutrophils and is not dependent upon recovery to higher neutrophil levels. Methods to reduce the neutropenic complications of high-dose therapy will have to dramatically reduce the interval to the first evidence of neutrophil recovery.

THEORETICAL CONSIDERATIONS OF GROWTH FACTOR MODIFICATION OF HEMATOPOIETIC TOXICITY

The ability of growth factors to modify the hematopoietic toxicity of chemotherapeutic regimens has been evaluated in a number of studies. Granulocyte colony-stimulating factor (G-CSF) has shown marked effects on the modification of hematopoietic toxicity when the chemotherapy is modestly myelotoxic, resulting in the nadir ANC $< 500/\mu l$ for a short duration (approximately 3 days) and brief absolute neutropenia.[4,5] Higher-dose therapy regimens vary in their marrow-ablative potential, with different spontaneous potentials for trilineage recovery when given without infusion of marrow or peripheral blood stem cells. A common feature of these high-dose regimens, however, is that the CFU-GM (colony-forming unit granulocyte–macrophage) and more mature proliferative myeloid cells are almost totally depleted for several days following the administration of such therapy. The severe neutropenic trough of more myelosuppressive therapy is not necessarily abbreviated by G-CSF alone, suggesting that the primary action of G-CSF in vivo is on recognizable early myeloid cells and possibly on myeloid progenitor cells.[6,7]

Recent studies suggest that G-CSF produces little in vivo expansion of progenitor cells or even blast cells. The action of G-CSF begins at the promyelocyte level, and is most marked on expanding myelocytes and in shortening neutrophil transit time through the marrow.[8] If we deplete the pool of cells upon which G-CSF acts then there is a requisite regeneration time for these cells and an absolute period of neutropenia that growth factors would not be able to modify. The same would apply if PBSC were infused after intensive therapy; an obligate time is necessary to generate promyelocytes and later forms that are expanded by G-CSF to generate neutrophils. There is increasing evidence that G-CSF is important for endogenous regulation of granulopoiesis.[9–11] During neutropenia, elevated levels of endogenous G-CSF occur due to the reverse relation between G-CSF and neutrophil levels. Thus the clinical impact of exogenous G-CSF administration after dose-intense therapy may be minimal.[12–15] In fact, given the falling levels of endogenous G-CSF with higher neutrophil recovery, one could extrapolate that the maximum effect of pharmacological levels of G-CSF achieved by exogenous administration would be after significant spontaneous neutrophil recovery has already occurred, when endogenous G-CSF levels could be consumed by the elevated neutrophil mass.

Bone marrow contains both early and late progenitor cells. Engraftment following autologous bone marrow infusion can be divided into several phases. The initial phase of engraftment is the duration to the appearance of the first neutrophil – the durations to the higher ANC of $100/\mu l$, $500/\mu l$ and $1000/\mu l$ and the period of early platelet recovery usually occurring during the first 2–5 weeks after transplantation. The rate of recovery of the initial phase of engraftment is related, in part, to the numbers and quality of late (mature) progenitor cells infused. The subsequent phases, which are associated with more stable and complete hematopoietic recovery, are secondary to the transplantation of intermediate and early progenitor and stem cells or to the persistence of similar endogenous cells. This latter phase occurs beyond 5 weeks post transplant.[16]

The incidence of infectious complications and fever due to intensive therapy correlates with the duration of absolute neutropenia.[17] The durations of antibiotics and of hospitalization depend not only on the time to the appearance of the first neutrophil but also on variable criteria used by different groups for cessation of antibiotics and discharge (see later). Following autologous bone marrow transplantation (ABMT), the time to the appearance of the first neutrophil is approximately 8–12 days, and the time to recovery to ANC $\geq 500/\mu l$ is frequently a week longer.

G-CSF AND GM-CSF POST STEM CELL INFUSION

Administration of G-CSF or of granulocyte–macrophage colony-stimulating factor (GM-CSF) after high-dose chemotherapy given with ABMT has been evaluated as a potential means to decrease the neutropenic interval and the incidence of infectious complications. The majority of these studies have administered colony-stimulating factors following ABMT alone. Several randomized and non-randomized studies have clearly shown that growth factors accelerate neutrophil recovery by a week or more following ABMT, but have no effect on platelet recovery. Post-transplant administration of growth factors minimally effects the time to the appearance of the first neutrophil, but does result in a more rapid rise in the terminal component of neutrophil recovery. Thus administration of growth factors following ABMT has not been consistently associated with a reduction of febrile days. Some studies have demonstrated a minor reduction in the frequency of documented culture-positive infections and duration of hospitalization.[18–27] Unfortunately, these studies do not provide much data on comparisons of recovery to neutrophils of 100/μl or less (Table 7.1). One wonders about the clinical significance of reduced positive cultures or abnormal chest roentgenograms: better endpoints would be febrile episodes with unstable circulatory or respiratory parameters, which are episodes that definitely require hospitalization and are asso-

ciated with significant morbidity or potential mortality.

It has been reported that PBSC, harvested during the rapid upswing of white blood cells following chemotherapy or following several days of G-CSF and/or GM-CSF, result in equivalently rapid neutrophil recovery as ABMT given with recombinant growth factors; however, platelet recovery appears to be enhanced with PBSC over the latter.[28–42] This is assumed to be related to the capture and subsequent infusion of a greater number of progenitor cells.

Infusion of greater numbers of progenitor cells with PBSC may obviate the requirements for post-transplant administration of growth factors, to ensure rapid hematopoietic recovery. Conceptually, why would one expect the effect

Table 7.1 Impact of G-CSF or GM-CSF on recovery following ABMT

Reference	Drug and dose	Diagnosis	Days to ANC > 500/μl	Days to ANC > 1000/μl	Febrile days (% patients or days)	Documented infections
Link et al[25]	GM-CSF CI 250 μg/m²	NHL and ALL with TBI	15 vs 28	18 vs 33	79.5% vs 77.5%	36% vs 62.5%
Gorin et al[23]	GM-CSF CI 250 μg/m²	NHL and non-TBI	14 vs 21	17 vs 30	4 vs 2	36% vs 46%
Nemunaitis et al[26]	GM-CSF 2-h infusion 250 μg/m²	NHL, Hodgkin's and ALL, mainly TBI	19 vs 26	26 vs 33	97% vs 97%	17% vs 30%
Khwaja et al[24]	GM-CSF 250 μg/m² s.c.	Lymphoma, BEAC	14 vs 20		8 vs 6	14[a] vs 13
Gisselbrecht et al[22]	G-CSF 5 μg/kg 30-min infusion	Lymphoma, ALL, myeloma, solid tumor	14 vs 20	16 vs 27	3 vs 5	6 vs 8
Stahel et al[27]	G-CSF 10-20 μg/kg s.c. infusion	Lymphoma		10 vs 18	1 vs 4	24% vs 29%
Advani et al[19]	GM-CSF 10 μg/kg		12 vs 16	15 vs 24		6/16 vs 6/33

[a] Number of patients. Key: CI = continuous infusion; NHL = non-Hodgkin's lymphoma; ALL = acute lymphoblastic leukaemia; TBI = total body irradiation; BEAC = carmustine, etoposide, cytarabine, cyclophosphamide.

of growth factors post transplant to be less noticeable on early recovery with higher numbers of progenitor cells infused? As will be seen later, this is certainly the case clinically. One explanation could be that regulatory mechanisms sense higher numbers of progenitor cells and drive differentiation, whereas lesser numbers may home to marrow, undergo limited self-renewal, and require high levels of growth factors to shift them from the self-renewal mode to the differentiation mode that is so important in protecting the host early after high-dose therapy. Indeed, the difference in neutrophil recovery with the use of growth factors post PBSCT is less marked than that following ABMT (see below); therefore, the value of growth factors post PBSCT is more questionable than in ABMT.

ROLES OF NEUTROPHIL GROWTH FACTORS POST PBSCT

We have explored the mobilization of peripheral blood and bone marrow progenitor cells with G-CSF and GM-CSF to increase the progenitor cell pool available for stem cell infusion after intensive therapy, in the hope of shortening the interval of neutropenia and thereby decreasing hematopoietic toxicity.[43] Given the unclear role of growth factors administered after ABMT and/or PBSCT in reducing the frequency of infectious complications and the duration of absolute neutropenia, additional studies were needed to determine whether these expensive biological agents are of clinical benefit in this setting or could be used more selectively. Although hematopoietic recovery after high-dose therapy given with and without growth factors post infusion has been reported in phase II studies of mobilized PBSC,[28–42] it is unclear from these reports if granulocyte recovery is indeed significantly slower when growth factors are not administered post transplantation. We therefore evaluated this question in a randomized trial. Because of the potential variability in harvest quality between successive cohorts of patients, we initiated this phase III study to evaluate early engraftment kinetics,

morbidity and duration of hospitalization in patients who were randomly assigned in a non-blinded fashion to receive or to not receive G-CSF and GM-CSF after high-dose chemotherapy given with growth-factor-mobilized PBSC and ABMT.[43]

Patients randomized to arm 1 did not receive any G-CSF or GM-CSF after ABMT and PBSCT. However, if the ANC remained less than 500/μl at 18 days post transplant, patients in arm 1 were allowed to receive growth factors. Patients randomized to arm 2 received G-CSF 7.5 μg/kg as a 2-hour i.v. infusion given every 12 hours and GM-CSF 2.5 μg/kg as a 2-hour i.v. infusion given every 12 hours. Growth factors were discontinued when the ANC recovered to more than 1500/μl for two successive days. Upon recovery of the platelet count to 100 000/μl and of the ANC to 1500/μl, a second cycle of high-dose chemotherapy was given if indicated, and growth factors were administered only if the patient was previously randomized to arm 2.

The supportive-care aspects of this study are important. Patients received prophylactic antimicrobial agents, including vancomycin, ciprofloxacin, fluconazole and acyclovir. Infection was presumed in patients who developed a temperature of 38°C or more when their ANC was less than 1000/μl. Patients with neutropenic fever had appropriate cultures and chest X-ray performed, and were empirically placed on a therapeutic dose of vancomycin and ceftazidime, along with discontinuation of ciprofloxacin. Patients with clinically or microbiologically documented infections who had responded to initial antimicrobial therapy were treated for a total of 10–14 days. In patients with documented infections who had defervesced but remained neutropenic after 14 days of antibiotics, antibiotics were cautiously discontinued, but were re-instituted if fever recurred. If the initial fever was of undetermined origin (the majority) and the patient defervesced with empiric therapy, antibiotics were usually discontinued with the return of the ANC to 500/μl or more on two consecutive days. However, if patients were afebrile and clinically stable with no systemic signs of infection then antibiotics were frequently discontinued before reaching this level. Patients received irradiated leucocyte filtered prophylactic single donor platelet concentrate transfusions if the platelet count was less than 20 000/µl and 2 units of packed red blood cells if the hemoglobin was less than 8.0 g/dl.

In this study, we observed that growth factors administered post stem cell infusion did significantly accelerate neutrophil recovery and shorten the duration of hospitalization (Figure 7.1; Tables 7.2 and 7.3). Despite the more rapid neutrophil recovery and a modest shortened duration of hospitalization observed with the administration of growth factors following PBSC and ABMT infusion, the clinical significance of this observation needs to be examined further. It has been suggested that patients could either be discharged earlier in their hospitalization with equal confidence at lower absolute neutrophil counts than the value of 500 or 1000/µl that is so frequently utilized as a guideline for hospital discharge, or alternatively managed with febrile neutropenia as

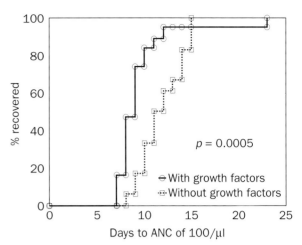

Figure 7.1 Time to neutrophil recovery to 100 neutrophils/µl with (○) and without (□) growth factors after PBSCT.

outpatients if their clinical condition is stable.[44–48] In this study, the small difference (2 days) in duration of hospitalization favoring the use of growth factors was not associated with a significantly lower incidence of days

Table 7.2 Hematopoietic recovery (cycle 1) after high-dose therapy and PBSCT with or without growth factors post transplant

Recovery to	Positive factors	Negative factors	p value[a]
Neutrophils of			
100/µl	9 (8–9)[b]	11.5 (10–14)	0.0005
	9.5 ± 3.5[c]	11.8 ± 2.3	
500/µl	10 (10–12)	16 (14–20)	0.0004
	11.5 ± 3.3	17.8 ± 8.9	
1000/µl	12 (11–13)	21 (16–26)	0.0008
	12.4 ± 3.8	22.4 ± 11.9	
Platelets of			
20 × 10³/µl	13 (11–22)	12 (8–37)	0.4918
	17 ± 8.6	14.8 ± 7.7	
50 × 10³/µl	16 (13–25)	14 (8–37)	0.3446
	23 ± 15.6	17 ± 7.1	

[a] Mann–Whitney. [b] Median (range). [c] Mean ± SD.
Reproduced with permission from *J Clin Oncol* 1994; **12**: 661–70[43].

Table 7.3 Number of febrile episodes, transfusions and duration of hospitalization in cycle 1 after high-dose therapy and PBSCT with or without growth factors post-transplant

Parameter	Positive factors	Negative factors	p value[a]
Days febrile	2 (0.5)[b]	3 (0–13)	
	2.7 (±2.8)[c]	3.7 (±3.1)	0.2060
Hospital days	19 (15–35)	21 (17–35)	
	19.3 (±4.4)	21.7 (±7.2)	0.0112
Erythrocyte transfusions	4 (0–13)	4 (0–16)	
	3.7 (±2.89)	4.1 (±3.5)	0.4866
Platelet transfusions	4.5 (3–12)	4.0 (3–21)	
	5.7 (±2.8)	5.2 (±4.3)	0.3850
Documented infections	2	1	

[a] Mann–Whitney. [b] Median (range). [c] Mean ± SD.
Reproduced with permission from *J Clin Oncol* 1994; **12**: 661–70.

febrile, of documented septic episodes, or of decreased transfusion requirements. The earlier discharge observed in the arm receiving growth factors was not due to earlier resolution of fever or infection, but may be due to a tendency by physicians to relate hospital discharge to both a rapid upward and a sustained recovery to an ANC of 500–1000/μl, both of which would occur earlier with those patients receiving growth factors. With experience, our clinical group is gaining confidence that the withdrawal of systemic antibiotics and hospital discharge in these patients should be guided by absence of fever for 48 hours or more, increasing neutrophil counts, stable vital signs and good performance status. The treatment duration of a clinical event, such as febrile neutropenia, in this patient population should be monitored and determined by clinical parameters and not by the ANC alone.

The impact of growth factors given after infusion of PBSC may vary depending on the method of mobilization of the PBSC. One argument against the general validity of these phase III trial results could be that the quality of the apheresis product mobilized by the combined use of G-CSF and GM-CSF is inferior to that of alternative methods of PBSC mobilization, such as high-dose cytoxan given with or without growth factors or G-CSF alone. The combination of growth factors used in this study to facilitate the collection of PBSC is at least equivalent to other mobilization methods, as demonstrated by the relatively rapid platelet recovery (a median of 12–13 days to a platelet count of 20 000/μl and 14–16 days to a count of 50 000/μl), which is certainly equivalent to other reports utilizing PBSC support. In addition, neutrophil recovery to 500/μl in arm 1 is also similar to a number of studies that have not used growth factors post PBSC infusion.

A review of reported randomized and non-randomized studies evaluating G-CSF post PBSC infusion (Table 7.4)[43,49,50] repeatedly shows a variable enhancement of neutrophil recovery, no statistical impact on platelet recovery and no evidence of any decrease in morbidity or mortality. Not one study shows a

Table 7.4 Impact of G-CSF or GM-CSF on recovery following PBSCT

Author	Drug	Diagnosis	Days to ANC > 100/μl	Days to ANC > 500/μl	Febrile days
Spitzer et al[43]	G-CSF and GM-CSF	Breast and lymphoma	9 vs 11.5	10 vs 16	2 vs 3
Klumpp et al[49]	G-CSF	Breast		10.5 vs 16	5 vs 3
Cortelazzo et al[50]	G-CSF	Lymphoma		10 vs 12	4 vs 3.5
To et al[42]	Historical–nothing		10	11	

decrease in febrile days post PBSCT. Discharge from hospital is in our view a non-objective endpoint, and is clouded by many subjective components in the decision analysis as discussed above. These observations suggest that at least those patients who mobilize adequate PBSC products may safely have growth factors excluded after PBSCT without negative clinical consequences. Growth factors given after stem cell infusion are expensive and cloud the information gathered from studies designed to address the difference in hematopoietic recovery after high-dose therapy utilizing different strategies to mobilize PBSC. If growth factors were not given after PBSC infusion, it would be easier to evaluate the clinical significance of different approaches to mobilizing PBSC. As a logical extension of our work, we have investigated in a randomized method if there is any advantage in terms of hematopoietic recovery after high-dose therapy to adding GM-CSF to G-CSF to mobilize PBSC. To increase the ability to evaluate this endpoint, we do not administer growth factors post PBSC infusion.

DELAYED PLATELET RECOVERY OBSERVED WITH SUCCESSIVE CYCLES OF HIGH-DOSE THERAPY

There are potential negative aspects of the routine use of growth factors post PBSCT, other than cost and side-effects. We evaluated further the pattern of platelet recovery following PBSC infusion in the randomized studies of growth factors post PBSC.[51] The study apheresed PBSC over four successive days following 4–5 days of combination growth factors including G-CSF and GM-CSF. Apheresis products from days 1 and 3 or from days 2 and 4 were alternately used to support either the first or the second cycle of high-dose therapy in consecutive patients. The intent of this specific design was to ensure that the composition of the infused PBSC product that contributed to platelet recovery would be distributed equally between the two cycles. Patients received ABMT in addition to PBSCT, unless there was evidence of bone or bone marrow involvement or in patients with lymphoma who only received PBSC (not bone marrow) after each cycle of high-dose therapy. Examining platelet recovery after successive cycles in individual patients by a paired *t*-test revealed a significant delay in early platelet recovery with cycle 2 compared with cycle 1 (Table 7.5 and Figure 7.2).[51] Growth factors were stopped at a median of 14 days – suggesting that platelet recovery is rapid upon cessation of these factors, and that recovery may be diverted toward neutrophil maturation with their use and can be rapidly reversed upon their cessation. Given that essentially equivalent quantities of stem cells were infused after each cycle of high-dose therapy for any given patient,

Table 7.5 Delayed early platelet recovery with use of growth factors with serial high-dose therapy and PBSCT

Platelet count	Cycle 1: + growth factors	Cycle 1: no growth factors	p value[a]	Cycle 2: + growth factors	Cycle 2: no growth factors	p value
>20	11[b] (9–22)	12 (9–14)	0.53	15 (9–42)	11 (9–16)	0.04
>50	14 (10–25)	14 (12–18)	0.25	16 (10–135)	16 (11–106)	0.85

[a] Log rank. [b] Median (range).
The median number of platelet transfusions in arm 1 was 5 and that in arm 2 was 3; $p = 0.059$.

this suggests that there is an endogenous component to platelet recovery. It is possible that the first cycle of high-dose therapy depletes this important component, which becomes more obvious after administration of the second cycle of high-dose therapy. This endogenous component must be a factor separate from the apheresis product, because the apheresis collections were infused via random distribution between the two cycles of high-dose therapy. This design should distribute an equal quality and quantity of apheresis product between the two cycles of therapy, supporting the hypothesis that the delay in platelet recovery observed with the second cycle of high-dose therapy is unrelated to any difference in the quality of the

PBSC. The delayed platelet recovery to 20 000/µl in the arm receiving growth factors post transplant, which become statistically evident only after two cycles of high-dose therapy, may be more apparent in the larger number of patients receiving only one cycle of therapy, especially if these patients were heavily pretreated. A recent large multivariate analysis of the factors predicting platelet recovery following either ABMT or PBSCT showed that G-CSF slowed platelet recovery and that its use may contribute to costs and the morbidity from platelet transfusions.[52]

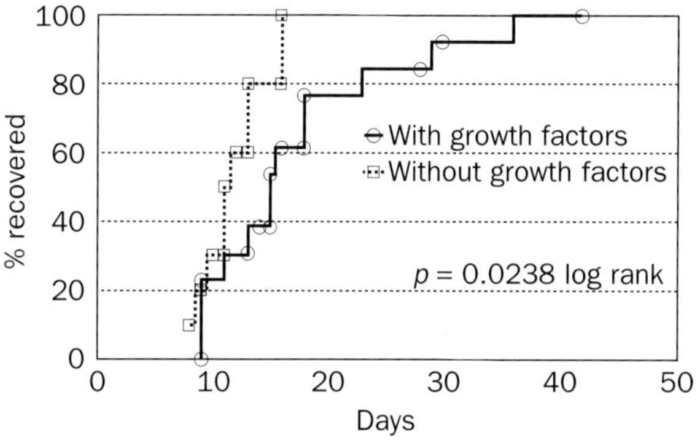

A ROLE FOR NEW THROMBOPOIETINS FOLLOWING ABMT OR PBSCT?

Recently, there has been much excitement due to the cloning of the ligand thrombopoietin (TPO) for the c-mpl receptor present on megakaryocytes, on platelets and on primitive hematopoietic cells. This is truly the equivalent of thrombopoietin, generating impressive thrombocytosis in mice and man, and modifying thrombocytopenia after chemotherapy and sublethal irradiation in primate models.[53–65] The question is whether TPO will be able to either modify the potential obligate period of approximately 12 days to platelet independence of 20 000 platelets/µl or the delayed platelet recovery following infusion of suboptimal stem cell products. The unknown impact of this cytokine is confounded by questions of possible

Figure 7.2 Platelet recovery following a second cycle of high-dose therapy with (○) and without (□) use of G-CSF after PBSCT.

diversion of maturation from neutrophil recovery (lineage steel) and other unknown interactions with neutrophil growth factors. In vivo studies suggest that the mpl ligand does take several (6–8) days to show an increment in platelet counts above baseline – kinetics slower than those of G-CSF or GM-CSF. This may hint at an inadequate immediate effect: for clinical impact, it is the very early part of recovery that will reduce platelet transfusions most – the recovery to above 10 000/μl. Recently published murine transplant experiments suggest that a pegylated truncated form of the mpl ligand called megakarocytic growth and differentiation factor (MGDF) enhances platelet recovery of G-CSF-mobilized PBSC without impacting on the enhanced neutrophil recovery, and is effective when used with G-CSF post-transplant.[66] Clinical trials in humans are awaited with interest.

NEWER INTERLEUKINS POST ABMT

A number of studies have evaluated, in phase II design, newer growth factors such as interleukin (IL)-6, IL-3 and IL-11, either as single agents or in combinations with G-CSF or GM-CSF. Trials of IL-3 alone have not been impressive compared with historical controls in improving neutrophil or platelet recovery.[67] A sequential trial of IL-3 followed by GM-CSF suggested that platelet recovery was enhanced compared with GM-CSF alone,[68] but subsequent randomized studies have not borne this out (unpublished). The toxicity profile of IL-3 post ABMT is complicated by a number of non-life-threatening dose-limiting systemic side-effects, including fever.

IL-6 alone, or in combination with GM-CSF, has been evaluated following ABMT. In a phase I study, recovery of neutrophils and platelets was slower than that expected of G-CSF or GM-CSF post transplant.[69] A small study using GM-CSF at doses of 3 or 5 μg/kg with IL-6 at doses of 0.5 or 1 μg/kg reported an impressive recovery of neutrophils to 500/μl at 11 days and platelet transfusion independence at 12 days.[70] However, a subsequent study of G-CSF at a dose of 5 μg/kg with or without IL-6 at doses of 0.5 or 2.5 μg/kg/day failed to show any differences in neutrophil or platelet recovery: a range of 11–12 days to an ANC of 500/μl in all groups, and 20 days to a platelet count of 20 000/μl in all groups. A number of patients developed moderate veno-occlusive disease; however, the relationship of the latter complication to IL-6 is unclear.[71]

IL-11 has also been given with G-CSF post ABMT. IL-11 was given post transplant in escalating doses, with G-CSF at 5 μg/kg/day. Neutrophil recovery is as expected with G-CSF (12 days to an ANC of 500/μl), but platelet recovery to more than 20 000/μl was not impressive at 21 days.[72]

PIXY321, a genetically engineered molecule combining yeast-derived GM-CSF with IL-3 through an amino acid linker protein with promising synergistic in vitro activity, has been evaluated in phase II studies post ABMT. Neutrophil recovery has been similar to that with GM-CSF alone, but platelet recovery has been reported to be enhanced (17 days to platelet independence compared with 26 days historical experience with GM-CSF alone).[73] Unfortunately, like IL-3 trials, recent multi-institutional phase III trials have not confirmed this advantage and are a constant reminder of the danger of using historical data to reach conclusions.[74]

POSSIBLE RECOMMENDATIONS TO REDUCE POST-TRANSPLANT USE OF GROWTH FACTORS

It is clear that CFU-GM predicts the rapidity of hematopoietic recovery, particularly of neutrophils, after both ABMT and PBSCT.[16,75] A rough approximation of these correlations is summarized in Tables 7.6 and 7.7. However, these assays are cumbersome, time-consuming and non-reproducible between different laboratories, and results are delayed. Correlations of variable degrees between peripheral CD34+ cell concentration and CFU-GM have been established between different laboratories.[76–78] Correlations between CD34+ cell numbers

Table 7.6 Components of hematopoietic recovery

Days 7–14	Days 14–28	>Day 28
Lots of progenitor cells cause rapid recovery >20 × 10⁴/kg	Modest numbers of progenitors (1–20) × 10⁴/kg. Recovery will occur in this period: faster if growth factors given	Permanent recovery depends on stem cells rather than progenitor cells. However, it is uncommon for more stem cells to exist in the face of absent CFU-GM except following chemical purging

Table 7.7 Relationship of CFU-GM and CD34⁺ numbers infused and hematopoietic recovery

CFU-GM	Neutrophil recovery	Platelet recovery	Trough week 5 or 6[a]
>20 × 10⁴/kg or CD34 >5 × 10⁶/kg	<14 days	<21 days	Occasional
(5–20) × 10⁴/kg or CD34 (2–5) × 10⁶/kg	<14 days	<28 days	Frequent if ablative therapy is used
(1–5) × 10⁴/kg or CD34 (1–2) × 10⁶/kg	14–28 days	Median 4–7 weeks; may not occur	NR
<1 × 10⁴/kg or CD34 <1 × 10⁶/kg	>28 days	Frequently may not occur	NR

[a] More frequently if heavily pretreated or acute myelogenous leukaemia.
NR, not reported.

infused and hematopoietic recovery, particularly platelet recovery, has been reported by several groups.[79–84] Recovery is strongly related to CD34⁺ cell numbers infused and less so to other factors such as prior therapy, preparative therapy and second transplant when patients are minimally pretreated or have been less intensively treated (e.g. breast cancer patients), but other factors are more appreciated in more heavily pretreated patients such as those with leukemia, lymphoma and myeloma.[85,86] This would suggest that CD34⁺ cells are really surrogate markers whose relationship to hematopoietic recovery is more unpredictable when patients are more heavily pretreated, or alternatively that significant endogenous intermediate or primitive stem cells are not retained following treatment and the stem cell infusion is called upon to modify more than just very early recovery. It has been reported in patients with significant prior therapy that, despite generous CD34⁺ cell collection of (2–5) × 10⁶/kg, recovery of platelets can be significantly delayed.[86] Furthermore, CD34⁺ cell enumeration is not always reproducible between different centers; therefore one has to be cautious in being overconfident with recommendations based on CD34⁺ cell numbers alone.

From an overview of the literature, one can generalize, despite all the considerations above, that hematopoietic recovery is rapid when CFU-GM are above $(5–20) \times 10^4$/kg or CD34$^+$ cells above 2×10^6/kg.[41,75,80,84] However, many of the studies correlating CD34$^+$ cell numbers infused and recovery used post-PBSCT growth factors. Nevertheless, the impact of lower number of CD34$^+$ cells ($<(2–2.5) \times 10^6$/kg) shows a modest slowing of neutrophil recovery, and growth factors may be advantageous in this subset following PBSCT. It would appear that a CD34$^+$ cell number above this threshold does not effectively distinguish clinically significant recovery patterns, and we would consider that growth factors may show no clinical benefit from this group. However, because CD34$^+$ cell numbers do not predict all the factors responsible for hematopoietic recovery – particularly in more heavily pretreated patients, and with more intensive regimens of conditioning, primary marrow disorders or repetitive high-dose therapy – allowance should be made to introduce growth factors at some point where there may be a significant proportion of delayed-recovery patients. We have chosen day 12 post infusion without an ANC of 100/μl, which is a few days after the median recovery time to this

level, to introduce growth factors if they are not routinely used, regardless of CD34$^+$ cell numbers infused. Using these guidelines, 75% of all patients, regardless of CD34 numbers collected (but probably even more with adequate collections), would not require the use and cost of recombinant growth factors post PBSCT (Figure 7.1 and Table 7.8). This would also eliminate a number of the side-effects related to growth factors, which, even if not life-threatening, may be quite uncomfortable.

CONCLUSIONS

Growth factors administered post PBSCT and ABMT are associated with modestly faster neutrophil recovery and fewer hospital days. However, these endpoints are influenced extensively by clinical individuality related to discharge policies and confidence in managing modestly neutropenic patients ($<500/\mu$l) in an outpatient setting. Other clinical variables, febrile days and septic episodes have never been reported in randomized studies to be reduced with the use of post PBSCT growth factors. The use of growth factors post PBSCT has not been associated with any clinical benefit in terms of the prevention of infectious complications in the majority of patients. This may be related to the minimal effect on the early part of neutrophil recovery, to an ANC of 100/μl. The difference with use of PBSC is even less than that following ABMT.

Growth factors post PBSCT could be of value in patients with poor stem cell collections or slow neutrophil recovery; however, growth factors post PBSC cell infusions can be associated with slower platelet recovery and more platelet transfusion with repeated cycles of high-dose therapy. The questionable value (in some instances a potentially negative impact) and the costs of these drugs ($2000–3000 for a 14-day course) should make us examine their use more critically and selectively in patients undergoing PBSCT.

Table 7.8 Recommendations for growth factors post PBSCT

- Stem cell collection low, $<2 \times 10^6$/kg CD34$^+$ cells: administer growth factors

- Standard collection, $>2 \times 10^6$/kg CD34$^+$ cells: no growth factors
- ANC still $<100/\mu$l by day 12 post transplant: administer growth factors (this would eliminate need in approximately $\geqslant$75% of patients)

REFERENCES

1. Spitzer G, Deisseroth A, Ventura G et al, Use of recombinant human hematopoietic growth factors and autologous bone marrow transplantation to attenuate the neutropenic trough of high-dose therapy. *Int J Cell Cloning* 1990; 8(Suppl 1): 249–59.

2. Spitzer G, Adkins DR, Persistent problems of neutropenia and thrombocytopenia with peripheral blood stem cell transplantation. *J Hematother* 1994; **3**: 193–8.

3. Spitzer G, Spencer V, Dyson P et al, Does peripheral blood further enhance hematopoietic recovery after autologous bone marrow transplantation and post transplantation recombinant growth factor? *Int J Cell Cloning* 1992; **10**: 146–8.

4. Crawford J, Ozer H, Stoller R et al, Reduction by granulocyte colony-stimulating-factor of fever and neutropenia induced by chemotherapy in patients with small-cell lung cancer. *N Engl J Med* 1991; **325**: 164–70.

5. Gabrilove J, Jakubowski A, Scher H et al, Effect of granulocyte colony-stimulating factor on neutropenia and associated morbidity due to chemotherapy for transitional carcinoma of the urothelium. *N Engl J Med* 1988; **318**: 1414–22.

6. Neidhart J, Mangalik A, Kohler W et al, Granulocyte colony-stimulating factor stimulates recovery of granulocytes in patients receiving dose-intensive chemotherapy without bone marrow transplantation. *J Clin Oncol* 1989; **7**: 1685–92.

7. Neidhart J, Kohker W, Stidley C et al, Phase 1 study of repeated cycles of high-dose cyclophosphamide, etoposide and cisplatin administered without bone marrow transplantation. *J Clin Oncol* 1990; **8**: 1728–38.

8. Price TH, Chatta GS, Dale DC, Effect of recombinant granulocyte colony-stimulating factor on neutrophil kinetics in normal young and elderly human. *Blood* 1996; **88**: 335–40.

9. Lieschke G, Grail D, Hodgson G et al, Mice lacking granulocyte colony-stimulating factor have chronic neutropenia, granulocyte and macrophage progenitor deficiency, and impaired neutrophil mobilization. *Blood* 1994; **84**: 1737–46.

10. Hammond W, Csiba E, Canin A et al, Chronic neutropenia. A new canine model induced by human granulocyte-stimulating factor. *J Clin Invest* 1991; **87**: 704–10.

11. Layton JE, Hockman H, Sheridan WP, Morstyn G, Evidence for a novel in vivo control mechanism of granulopoiesis: Mature cell related control of a regulatory growth factor. *Blood* 1989; **74**: 1303–7.

12. Cairo MS, Suen Y, Sender L et al, Circulating granulocyte colony-stimulating factor (G-CSF) levels after allogeneic and autologous bone marrow transplantation: Endogenous G-CSF production correlates with myeloid engraftment. *Blood* 1992; **79**: 1869–73.

13. Geissler D, Niederwieser D, Aulitzky WE et al, Serum colony stimulating factors in patients undergoing bone marrow transplantation: enhancing effect of recombinant human GM-CSF. *Behring Institut Mitteilungen* 1988; **83**: 289–300.

14. Sallerfors B, Olofsson T, Lenhoff S, Granulocyte–macrophage colony-stimulating factor (GM-CSF) and granulocyte colony-stimulating factor (G-CSF) in serum in bone marrow transplanted patients. *Bone Marrow Transplant* 1991; **8**: 191–5.

15. Watari K, Asano S, Shirafuji N, Serum granulocyte colony-stimulating factor levels in healthy volunteers and patients with various disorders as estimated by enzyme immunoassay. *Blood* 1989; **73**: 117–22.

16. Spitzer G, Verma DS, Fisher R et al, The myeloid progenitor cell – its value in predicting hematopoietic recovery after autologous bone marrow transplantation. *Blood* 1980; **55**: 317–23.

17. Bodey G, Buckley M, Sathe Y et al, Quantitative relationship between circulating leukocytes and infection in patients with acute leukemia. *Ann Intern Med* 1966; **64**: 328–40.

18. Taylor K, Jagannath S, Spitzer G et al, Recombinant human granulocyte colony-stimulating factor hastens granulocyte recovery after high-dose chemotherapy and autologous bone marrow transplantation in Hodgkin's disease. *J Clin Oncol* 1989; **7**: 1791–9.

19. Advani R, Chao NJ, Horning SJ et al, Granulocyte–macrophage colony-stimulating factor (GM-CSF) as an adjunct to autologous hematopoietic stem cell transplant for lymphoma. *Ann Intern Med* 1992; **116**: 183–9.

20. Brandt S, Peters W, Atwater S et al, Effect of recombinant human granulocyte–macrophage colony-stimulating factor on chemotherapy-induced myelosuppression. *N Engl J Med* 1988; **318**; 869–76.

21. Devereux S, Linch D, Gribben J et al, GM-CSF accelerates neutrophil recovery after autologous

bone marrow transplantation for Hodgkin's disease. *Bone Marrow Transplant* 1989; **4**: 49–54.

22. Gisselbrecht C, Prentice HG, Bacigalupo A et al, Placebo-controlled phase III trial of lenograstim in bone-marrow transplantation. *Lancet* 1996; **343**: 696–700.

23. Gorin N, Coiffer B, Pico J et al, Granulocyte–macrophage colony-stimulating factor (GM-CSF) shortens aplasia duration after autologous bone marrow transplantation (ABMT) in non-Hodgkin's lymphoma. A randomized placebo-controlled double blind study [abstract]. *Blood* 1996; **76**: 542a.

24. Khwaja A, Linch DC, Goldstone AH et al, Recombinant human granulocyte–macrophage colony-stimulating factor after autologous bone marrow transplantation for malignant lymphoma: a British National Lymphoma Investigation double-blind, placebo-controlled trial. *Br J Hematol* 1992; **82**: 317–23.

25. Link H, Boogaerts MA, Carella A et al, A controlled trial of recombinant human granulocyte–macrophage colony-stimulating actor after total body irradition, high-dose chemotherapy, and autologous bone marrow transplantation for acute lymphoblastic leukemia and malignant lymphoma. *Blood* 1992; **80**: 2188–95.

26. Nemunaitis J, Rabinowe S, Singer J et al, Recombinant granulocyte–macrophage colony-stimulating factor after autologous bone marrow transplantation for lymphoid malignancy: Pooled results from three randomized double-blind, placebo controlled trials. *N Engl J Med* 1991; **324**: 1773–8.

27. Stahel RA, Jost LM, Cerny T et al, Randomized study of recombinant human granulocyte colony-stimulating factor after high-dose chemotherapy and autologous bone marrow transplantation for high-risk lymphoid malignancies. *J Clin Oncol* 1994; **12**: 1931–8.

28. Bensinger W, Singer J, Appelbaum F et al, Autologous transplantation with peripheral blood mononuclear cells collected after administration of recombinant granulocyte stimulating factor. *Blood* 1993; **81**: 3158–63.

29. Blanco R, Birck R, Schwartzberg L, Rapid and sustained hematopoietic reconstitution by peripheral blood stem cell infusion alone following high-dose chemotherapy. *Bone Marrow Transplant* 1993; **11**: 369–74.

30. Boiron J, Marit G, Faberes C et al, Collection of peripheral blood stem cells in multiple myeloma following single high-dose cyclophosphamide

with and without recombinant human granulocyte–macrophage colony-stimulating factor (rhGM-CSF). *Bone Marrow Transplant* 1993; **12**: 49–55.

31. Bolwell BJ, Lichtin A, Anderesen S et al, G-CSF and peripheral primed progenitor cells (PPPC) enhances engraftment in autologous bone marrow transplantation (ABMT) for non-Hodgkin's disease (NHD) [abstract]. *Blood* 1991; **78**: 242a.

32. Bregni M, Siena S, Bonadonna G et al, Clinical utilization of human haematopoietic progenitors elicited in peripheral blood by recombinant human granulocyte colony-stimulating factor (rHuG-CSF). *Eur J Cancer* 1994; **30**: 235–8.

33. Brice P, Marolleau J, Dombret H et al, Autologous peripheral blood stem cell transplantation after high dose therapy in patients with advanced lymphomas. *Bone Marrow Transplant* 1992; **9**: 337–42.

34. Brugger W, Birken R, Bertz H et al, Peripheral blood progenitor cell mobilized by chemotherapy plus granulocyte-colony stimulating factor accelerate both neutrophil and platelet recovery after high-dose VP16, ifosamide and cisplatin. *Br J Haematol* 1993; **84**: 402–7.

35. Chao NJ, Schriber JR, Grimes K et al, Granulocyte colony-stimulating factor 'mobilized' peripheral blood progenitor cells accelerate granulocyte and platelet recovery after high dose chemotherapy. *Blood* 1993; **81**: 2031–5.

36. Gianni AM, Siena S, Bregni M, Granulocyte–macrophage colony-stimulating factor to harvest circulating haemopoietic stem cells for autotransplantation. *Lancet* 1989; **ii**: 580–4.

37. Grigg A, Begley CG, Juttner CA et al, Effect of peripheral blood progenitor cells mobilized by filgrastim (G-CSF) on platelet recovery after high-dose chemotherapy. *Bone Marrow Transplant* 1993; **11**: 23–8.

38. Huan SD, Hester J, Spitzer G et al, Influence of mobilized peripheral blood cells on the hematopoietic recovery by autologous marrow and recombinant human granulocyte–macrophage colony stimulating factor after high-dose cyclophosphamide, etoposide, and cisplatin. *Blood* 1992; **79**: 3388–93.

39. Peters W, Kurtzberg J, Atwater S et al, Comparative effects of rhuG-CSF and rhuGM-CSF on hematopoietic reconstitution and granulocyte function following high-dose chemotherapy and autologous bone marrow transplantation (ABMT) [abstract]. *Proc Am Soc Clin Oncol* 1989; **8**: 181.

40. Roberts MM, To LB, Haylock DN et al, Comparison of hematological recovery times and supportive care requirements of autologous recovery phase peripheral blood stem cell transplants, autologous bone marrow transplants and allogenic bone marrow transplants. *Bone Marrow Transplant* 1992; **9**: 277–84.

41. Sheridan WP, Begley CG, Juttner CA et al, Effect of peripheral-blood progenitor cells mobilized by filgrastim (G-CSF) on platelet recovery after high-dose chemotherapy. *Lancet* 1992; **399**: 640–4.

42. To LB, Dyson PG, Branford AL, Peripheral blood stem cells collected in very early remission produce rapid and sustained autologous hemopoietic reconstitution in acute nonlymphoblastic leukemia. *Bone Marrow Transplant* 1989; **2**: 103–8.

43. Spitzer G, Adkins D, Spencer V et al, Randomized study of growth factors post-peripheral-blood stem-cell transplant: Neutrophil recovery is improved with modest clinical benefit. *J Clin Oncol* 1994; **12**: 661–70.

44. Pizzo PA, Robichaud KJ, Wesley R et al, Fever in the pediatric and young adult patient with cancer: A prospective study of 1001 episodes. *Medicine* 1982; **61**: 153–65.

45. Bash R, Katz J, Cash J, Buchanan G, Safety and cost effectiveness of early hospital discharge of lower risk children with cancer admitted with fever and neutropenia. *Cancer* 1994; **74**: 189–96.

46. Rubenstein EB, Rolston K, Benjamin RS, Outpatient treatment of febrile episodes in low-risk neutropenic patients with cancer. *Cancer* 1993; **71**: 3640–6.

47. Mullen CA, Buchanan GR, Early hospital discharge of children with cancer treated for fever and neutropenia: Identification and management of the low-risk patient. *J Clin Oncol* 1990; **8**: 1998–2004.

48. Gilbert C, Meisenberg B, Vrendenburgh J et al, Sequential prophylactic oral and empiric once-daily parenteral antibiotics for neutropenia and fever after high-dose chemotherapy and autologous bone marrow support. *J Clin Oncol* 1994; **12**: 1005–11.

49. Klumpp TR, Mangan KM, Goldberg SL Granulocyte colony-stimulating factor accelerates neutrophil engraftment following peripheral-blood stem cell transplantation: a prospective, randomized trial. *J Clin Oncol* 1995; **13**: 1323–7.

50. Cortelazzo S, Viero P, Bellavita P et al, Granulocyte colony-stimulating factor following peripheral-blood progenitor-cell transplant in

non-Hodgkin's lymphoma. *J Clin Oncol* 1995; **18**: 935–41.

51. Spitzer G, Adkins D, McIntyre W, A randomized study showing delayed early platelet recovery after tandem peripheral blood stem cell (PBSC) transplant with use of growth factors post transplant [abstract]. *Blood* 1995; **86**: 103a.

52. Bernstein S, Barnett M, Cairo R et al, A multicenter observational study of platelet utilization among recipients of myeloablative therapy and stem cell transplantation [abstract]. *Proc Am Soc Clin Oncol* 1996; **15**: 84.

53. Bartley TD, Bogenberger J, Hunt P et al, Identification and cloning of a megakaryocyte growth and development factor that is a ligand for the cytokine receptor Mpl. *Cell* 1994; **77**: 1117–24.

54. de Sauvage FJ, Hass PE, Spencer SD et al, Stimulation of megakaryocytopoiesis and thrombopoiesis by the c-Mpl ligand. *Nature* 1994; **369**: 533–8.

55. Farese AM, Hunt P, Boone T, MacVittie TJ, Recombinant human megakaryocyte growth and development factor stimulates thrombocytopoiesis in normal nonhuman primates. *Blood* 1995; **86**: 54–9.

56. Fielder P, Gurney A, Stefanich E et al, Regulation of thrombopoietin levels by c-mpl-mediated binding to platelets. *Blood* 1996; **87**: 2154–61.

57. Gurney AL, Carver-Moore K, de Sauvage F, Moore MW, Thrombocytopenia in c-mpl-deficient mice. *Science* 1994; **265**: 1445–7.

58. Kaushansky K, Lok S, Holly RD et al, Promotion of megakaryocyte progenitor expansion and differentiation by the c-Mpl ligand thrombopoietin. *Nature* 1994; **369**: 568–71.

59. Kaushansky K, Broudy VC, Grossmann, A et al, Thrombopoietin expands erythroid progenitors, increases red cell production and enhances erythroid recovery after myelosuppressive therapy. *J Clin Invest* 1995; **96**: 1683–7.

60. Kaushansky K, Broudy VC, Lin N et al, Thrombopoietin, the Mpl ligand, is essential for full megakaryocyte development. *Proc Natl Acad Sci USA* 1995; **92**: 3234–8.

61. Kuter DJ, Beeler DL, Rosenberg RD, The purification of megapoietin: A physiological regulator of megakaryocyte growth and platelet production. *Proc Natl Acad Sci USA* 1994; **91**: 11 104–8.

62. Kutter DJ, Rosenberg RD, The reciprocal relationship of thrombopoietin (c-Mpl ligand) to changes in the platelet mass during busulfan-induced thrombocytopenia in the rabbit. *Blood* 1995; **85**: 2720–30.

63. Lok S, Kaushansky K, Holly RD et al, Cloning and expression of murine thrombopoietin cDNA and stimulation of platelet production in vivo. *Nature* 1994; **369:** 565–8.

64. Ulich TR, del Castillo J, Yin S et al, Megakaryocyte growth and development factor ameliorates carboplatin-induced thrombocytopenia in mice. *Blood* 1995; **86:** 971–6.

65. Wendling F, Maraskovsky E, Debili N et al, cMpl ligand is a humoral regulator of megakaryocytopoiesis. *Nature* 1994; **369:** 571–4.

66. Molineux G, Harley C, McElroy P et al, Megakaryocyte growth and development factor accelerates platelet recovery in peripheral blood progenitor cell transplant recipients. *Blood* 1996; **88:** 366–76.

67. Nemunaitis J, Appelbaum F, Singer J et al, Phase I trial with recombinant human interleukin-3 in patients with lymphoma undergoing autologous bone marrow transplantation. *Blood* 1993; **82:** 3272–8.

68. Fay J, Lazarus H, Herzig R et al, Sequential administration of interleukin-3 (rhIL-3) and granulocyte–macrophage colony stimulating factor after autologous bone marrow transplantation. *Blood* 1994; **84:** 2151–7.

69. Lazarus H, Winton E, Williams S et al, Phase I study of recombinant human interleukin-6 (IL-6) after autologous bone marrow transplant (ABMT) in patients with poor-prognosis breast cancer [abstract]. *Blood* 1993; **82**(Suppl 1): 677a.

70. Fay J, Collins R, Pineiro L et al, Concomitant administration of interleukin-6 (rhIL-6) and leukomax (rhGM-CSF) following autologous bone marrow transplantation – a phase I trial [abstract]. *Blood* 1993; **82**(Suppl 1): 1707a.

71. Devine S, Winton E, Holland H et al, Simultaneous administration of interleukin-6 (rhIL-6) and Neupogen (rhG-CSF) following autologous bone marrow transplantation (ABMT) for breast cancer [abstract]. *Blood* 1994; **84**(Suppl 1): 343a.

72. Champlin R, Mehra R, Kaye J et al, Phase I study of recombinant interleukin-11 following autologous BMT in patients with breast cancer [abstract]. *Proc Am Soc Oncol* 1994; **13:** 201a.

73. Vose JM, Anderson J, Bierman P et al, Initial trial of PIXY321 (GM-CSF/IL-3 fusion protein) following high-dose chemotherapy and autologous bone marrow transplantation (ABMT) for lymphoid malignancy [abstract]. *Proc Am Soc Oncol* 1993; **12:** 1237a.

74. Vose JM, Pandite L, Beveridge RA et al, The PIXY321 ABMT study group. Phase III study comparing PIXY321 and GM-CSF following autologous bone marrow transplantation (ABMT) in patients with non-Hodgkin's lymphoma (NHL) [abstract]. *Blood* 1994; **84:** 3876.

75. Reiffers J, Faberes C, Boiron JM et al, Peripheral blood progenitor cell transplantation in 118 patients with hematological malignancies: Analysis of factors affecting the rate of engraftment. *J Hematother* 1994; **3:** 185–92.

76. Siena S, Bregni M, Brando L, Flow cytometry for clinical estimation of circulating progenitors for autologous transplantation in cancer patients. *Blood* 1991; **77:** 400–9.

77. Siena S, Bregni M, Brando B, Circulation of CD34⁺ hematopoietic stem cells in the peripheral blood of high dose cyclophosphamide-treated patients: enhancement by recombinant human granulocyte–macrophage colony stimulating factor. *Blood* 1989; **74:** 1905–14.

78. Bender JG, Lum L, Unverszager KL et al, Correlation of colony-forming cells, long-term-initiating cells and CD34⁺ cells in apheresis products with different regimens. *Bone Marrow Transplant* 1994; **13:** 479–85.

79. Bensinger W, Longin K, Appelbaum FR et al, Peripheral blood stem cells (PBSCs) collected after recombinant granulocyte colony stimulating factor (rhG-CSF): An analysis of factors correlated with the tempo of engraftment after transplantation. *Br J Haematol* 1994; **87:** 825–31.

80. Bensinger W, Appelbaum F, Rowley S et al, Factors that influence collection and engraftment of autologous peripheral-blood stem cells. *J Clin Oncol* 1994; **13:** 2547–55.

81. Bolwell J, Fishleder A, Andersen W et al, G-CSF primed peripheral blood progenitor cells in autologous bone marrow transplantation. Parameters affecting bone marrow engraftment. *Bone Marrow Transplant* 1993; **12:** 609–14.

82. Schiller G, Rosen L, Vescio R et al, Threshold dose of autologous CD34⁺ positive peripheral blood progenitor cells required for engraftment after myeloablative treatment for multiple myeloma [abstract]. *Blood* 1994; **84**(Suppl):207a.

83. Smith D, Bregni M, Brando B et al, Flow cytometry for clinical estimation of circulating hematopoietic progenitors for autologous transplantation in cancer patients. *Blood* 1991; **2:** 400–9.

84. Weaver CH, Hazelton B, Birch R et al, An analysis of engraftment kinetics as a function of the CD34 content of peripheral blood progenitors

cell collections in 692 patients after the administration of myeloablative chemotherapy. *Blood* 1995; **10:** 3961–9.

85. Dreger P, Kloss M, Petersen B et al, Autologous progenitor cell transplantation: prior exposure to stem cell toxic drugs determines yield and engraftment of peripheral blood progenitor cell but not of bone marrow grafts. *Blood* 1995; **86:** 3970–8.

86. Tricot G, Jagannath S, Vesole D et al, Peripheral blood stem cell transplants for multiple myeloma – identification of favorable variables for rapid engraftment in 225 patients [abstract]. *Blood* 1994; **84**(Suppl): 180a.

8

CD34$^+$ blood stem cell transplantation

Yago Nieto and Elizabeth J Shpall

INTRODUCTION

Tumor cell contamination of stem cell grafts

Peripheral blood progenitor cells (PBPC) have replaced bone marrow as the primary source for autologous stem cell transplantation. Although tumor burden appears to be lower in PBPC fractions than in bone marrow,[1] modern immunocytochemistry with an antibody panel can detect breast cancer tumor cells in PBPC fractions of 20% of stage IV patients and 11% of patients with stage II disease.[2] Sharp et al[3] reported higher relapse rates for breast cancer or non-Hodgkin's lymphoma patients who received autologous peripheral blood grafts contaminated with malignant cells identified in a long-term culture assay, compared with those with no identifiable tumor cells in their graft. Another study suggests that the presence of occult micrometastases is a poor prognostic factor in patients with high-risk breast cancer treated with high-dose chemotherapy and autologous bone marrow and PBPC support.[4] The majority of stage IV breast cancer patients relapse in sites of previous bulky disease, which may suggest an insufficient cytotoxic capacity of the high-dose chemotherapy regimen, rather than a direct effect of the reinfused tumor cells in those patients. Whether breast cancer cells in the graft are a marker of systemic tumor burden or whether they contribute to relapse post transplant remains unclear.

Brenner et al[5] used a neomycin-resistance gene to mark the marrow cells that were reinfused into children with neuroblastoma or acute leukemia following high-dose therapy administration. Gene-marked tumor cells were detected in the majority of patients who relapsed after the transplant, demonstrating that malignant cells contaminating a stem cell graft are associated with disease recurrence.[5] Gene-marked Philadelphia-positive (Ph$^+$) cells have also been identified at relapse after autologous bone marrow transplant for chronic myelogeneous leukemia.[6] Gribben et al[7,8] reported that follicular non-Hodgkin's lymphoma patients whose marrow stem cell product was purged from bcl-2 positive to negative, assessed by polymerase chain reaction, had a lower relapse rate than comparable patients who remained bcl-2 positive after the immunologic purging procedure. Nonrandomized comparisons between patients with acute myeloid leukemia (AML) in first remission, who received pharmacologically purged versus unpurged autologous marrow support, suggest a clinical benefit for the purge in the former group.[9,10]

Negative purging procedures

Purging, or negative-selection procedures – either pharmacologic[11] or immunologic[12] – have been primarily used to purge bone marrow. These procedures can damage or deplete the normal progenitors, delay engraftment, and increase the patient's risk of myelosuppressive complications. Because of the potential tumor cell contamination, purging PBPC could be important. In two clinical studies that used immunologically purged PBPC grafts in non-Hodgkin's lymphoma[13] or breast cancer,[14] tumor cell removal was achieved without prolongation of the engraftment rates compared with historical controls. However, because of its potential toxicity to the normal stem cells, negative purging of PBPC, particularly with chemotherapy, is not commonly performed.

THE CD34 ANTIGEN

CD34 antigen expression on normal progenitors

The CD34 antigen is a 115 kDa surface glycophosphoprotein, expressed on 1–3% of normal bone marrow cells, including both the committed and probably the long-term reconstituting progenitor cells.[15] In vitro data suggest that the human bone marrow CD34+ cell compartment contains primitive multipotential hematopoietic cells, responsible for both short- and long-term repopulation.[16]

The positive selection of normal hematopoietic progenitors takes advantage of the fact that malignant cells in many tumors do not express the CD34 antigen, as opposed to the normal immature progenitor hematopoietic cells. CD34 selection is a strategy that has been employed more commonly than negative-purging strategies in the eradication of cancer cells from PBPC autografts.

Flow cytometric analysis can distinguish two different populations of CD34+ hematopoietic cells that differ in their relative levels of CD34 expression.[17,18] The CD34bright population contains the majority of the immature progenitor cells, whereas the CD34dim population contains more lineage-committed progenitors. The CD34bright compartment is enriched for differentiated progenitors (CFU-GM, BFU-E and CFU-Meg), and even more enriched for the early multipotential CFU-GEMM, CFU-blast and long-term culture-initiating cells (LTC-IC). The LTC-IC and CFU-blast assays are considered to be the most relevant in vitro assays for the hypothetical stem cell, although these cells may be functionally different from the true stem cell.

Very immature lymphoid cells are also CD34+, and this antigen expression decreases from the maturation point where lymphoid cells rearrange the immunoglobulin (B cells) or antigen-receptor (T cells) genes.[19,20] Combined, these data strongly suggest that CD34 is expressed at high levels on the earliest hematopoietic cells, and its surface expression decreases to undetectable levels progressively during maturation.

CD34+ cells are identifiable at very low levels (<1%) in steady-state non-mobilized peripheral blood, but, after mobilization, they may increase to 1–5%.[21] CD34 is also normally expressed in vascular endothelial cells.[22]

CD34 expression on malignant cells (Table 8.1)

Tumor expression of CD34 tends to mirror normal tissue expression, and therefore antibodies targeting the CD34 antigen bind strongly to vascular tumor cells, including angiosarcoma, hepatic hemangioendothelioma and Kaposi's sarcoma, especially around the vascular sprouts where active angiogenesis is taking place.[22] In adults, most other nonhematologic tumors reported are CD34−, other than a report of four cases of CD34+ squamous cell lung carcinoma.[23] Neuroblastoma[24] and peripheral neuroepithelial (PNET)/Ewing's sarcoma[25] are also reportedly CD34−.

Table 8.1 CD34 antigen expression in malignancies	
CD34$^+$ malignancies	**CD34$^-$ malignancies**
Acute myelogenous leukemia	Chronic lymphocytic leukemia
Acute lymphoblastic leukemia	Hodgkin's disease
Chronic myeloid leukemia	Non-Hodgkin's lymphomas
Myelodysplastic syndromes	Multiple myeloma
Tumors of vascular origin	Breast carcinoma
	Most adult solid tumors[a]
	Neuroblastoma
	PNET/Ewing's sarcoma

[a] Four cases of CD34$^+$ squamous cell lung carcinoma have been reported.

About 40% of acute myeloid leukemias[26] and 65% of common (pre-B) acute lymphoblastic leukemias[27] are reactive, whereas only 1–5% of acute T-lymphoid leukemias express the CD34 antigen.[28] Chronic lymphoproliferative disorders[29] and most lymphomas[30] are CD34$^-$. Malignant cells in multiple myeloma do not express CD34 antigen.[31] In chronic myelogenous leukemia, data from the literature appear to be inconsistent, although in the largest series published so far, all patients in accelerated phase and blastic crisis, and 75% of those in chronic phase, had CD34$^+$ tumors, with the percentage of positivity increasing significantly as the disease progressed.[32] In myelodysplastic syndromes, marrow cells from a significant percentage of patients with refractory anemia with excess of blasts (RAEB), RAEB in transformation, and chronic myelomonocytic leukemia express CD34.[33] So do alkylator-associated secondary myelodysplasias and acute myelogenous leukemias.[34] CD34 expression in myelodysplastic syndromes has been shown to be an independent and significant predictor of poor survival.[35] In fact, those data suggest that an increase in the number of CD34$^+$ cells in the marrow or blood of a patient with myelodysplasia may be a harbinger of blast crisis.

METHODS OF CD34 SELECTION

CD34 selection is often preceded by a non-immunologic procedure to remove the mononuclear cell compartment from the remaining fractions by exploiting the physical and functional differences between the two populations. The most widely used method is density gradient centrifugation, which separates the buffy coat containing the mononuclear cells from the erythrocytes and polymorphonuclear cells.[36,37]

The development of monoclonal antibodies that identify different epitopes of the CD34 antigen[38] has generated a number of immunologic technologies for positive selection of cells labeled with an anti-CD34 monoclonal antibody. Most of them use a solid-phase matrix to remove the labeled target cells from the remaining mononuclear cell product.

Immunoadsorption CD34-selection method

This method, based on a biotin–avidin immunoaffinity system, was initially developed by Berenson et al.[39] The Ceprate clinical device (CellPro Inc) uses the anti-CD34 monoclonal antibody 12.8 identified by Andrews et al.[40] The hematopoietic cell product is incubated with biotinylated 12.8 antibody. After a wash to remove the unbound antibodies, the sample is passed through a column of avidin-coated poly-acrylamide beads. CD34$^+$ cells are retained in the column by the beads and are subsequently eluted at the end of the procedure, following gentle mechanical agitation.

Animal studies have shown that CD34$^+$ cells isolated with the Ceprate device can success-fully engraft myeloablated dogs[41] and baboons.[42] Subsequent clinical trials have confirmed the feasibility of CD34 selection with the immuno-adsorption method in patients.

The CellPro column is currently being evalu-ated in a wide variety of clinical settings, either as a means of depleting autografts of tumor cells for different diseases or for T-cell deple-tion in allo/PBPC transplants, as described below.

Immunomagnetic CD34-selection methods (Table 8.2)

Magnetic microspheres (Dynal Inc) are 45 µm in diameter and contain 20% magnetite by weight dispersed throughout their volume. Initially, these magnetic beads were widely used in negative purging regimens in conjunc-tion with monoclonal antibodies that targeted the tumor cell.[43] More recently, they have been employed in CD34-selection procedures with the Isolex-300 (Baxter Healthcare Corp), a semi-automated device that consists of a stand that holds a disposable chamber and a built-in array of permanent magnets that can be slid into direct contact with the chamber. Target cells were labeled with the monoclonal antibody MY-10, developed by Civin et al,[44] which results in rosetting between the target cells and the immunobeads. Rosseted CD34$^+$ cells are isolated in the magnetic separator as the non-labeled cells are drained from the chamber by gravity. Target cells are subsequently released from the magnetic beads by incubation with chymopapain, specific for a certain epitope on the CD34 antigen.[45]

The Isolex-300 system has been clinically used by Civin et al[46] in marrow grafts from pediatric patients with advanced refractory solid tumors. Three of the 13 patients had a final CD34$^+$ product of poor purity and received their unprocessed back-up marrow. The median purity of the 13 selected products was 80%, and the median CD34$^+$ cell recovery was 33%.

More recently, a direct immunomagnetic separation method that uses microspheres pre-coated with anti-CD34 monoclonal antibody (Dynabeads CD34) has been developed. At the end of the selection procedure, the beads are detached from the CD34$^+$ cells with an anti-mouse Fab polyclonal antibody, commercially available as 'Detachabead', instead of with chy-mopapain.[47] A pilot clinical trial using the Isolex-300i, a fully automated device, reported prompt engraftment in patients transplanted with CD34$^+$ cells selected with this method.[48]

The Magnetic Cell Separator (MACS) (Amcell Corp), originally described by Miltenyi et al,[49] is a preclinical device that employs biodegradable nanoparticles, rather than larger microspheres, as the solid phase for collection of the target CD34$^+$ cells. The hematopoietic cells are incubated with an anti-CD34 mono-clonal antibody, washed, and then mixed with the 60-nm iron–dextran paramagnetic colloid nanoparticles, which are coated with an anti-immunoglobulin that reacts with the anti-CD34 monoclonal antibody. The nanobead–cell com-plexes are passed over a column containing a metallic matrix with a high-gradient magnetic field induced by external permanent magnets. Bead-coated cells are retained in the matrix; nonrosetted cells are washed through. Target cells are very simply eluted by removing the column from the magnetic field and flushing. The eluted product can be passed over a second column to increase the purity. When the proce-dure is over, the selected cells are still attached to the nanobeads, although this does not inter-fere with further analysis of the product (flow cytometry or culture). The small size and low nonspecific binding of the particles confer important advantages, including rapid inter-action with the cells, resulting in a shorter pro-

Table 8.2 Enrichment and recovery of CD34+ bone marrow and peripheral blood progenitor cells with different clinically tested devices

Devices	Bone marrow			
	Purity (% CD34+)	Recovery of CD34+ cells	Fold enrichment	Ref
Ceprate	72%	42%	54×	56
Isolex-300	80%	33%	25×	30
Isolex-300i	No data			
ACS	No data			
	PBPC			
	Purity (% CD34+)	Recovery of CD34+ cells	Fold enrichment	Ref
Ceprate	42%	52%	51×	56
Isolex-300	86%	41%	NR	32
Isolex-300i	97%	50%	NR	32
ACS	95%	65%	NR	34

NR = not reported.

cessing time of about one hour, compared with the other immunomagnetic method, as well as an excellent yield and purity of the CD34-selected product.

A recently developed clinical-scale device, the Amgen Cell Selector (ACS), uses this magnetic cell sorting (MACS) technology. Richel et al[50] showed the safety of this device in a pilot clinical study. Reinfused bead-coated CD34+ cells produced successful engraftment in 12 breast cancer patients treated with high-dose

therapy. The biodegradable beads have not interfered with the CD34+ cell engraftment to date.

Flow cytometry

Flow cytometry can successfully isolate highly purified CD34+ subpopulations on the basis of multiple surface antigens from small hematopoietic samples.[51] However, sorting of CD34+

cells from large volumes for clinical use presents important problems, which unlikely to be overcome, since the cell yield is insufficient and the procedure is time-consuming.

A system has been developed by Systemix Inc in which a series of previous depletion steps eliminate the committed (lineage-positive) progenitors prior to high-speed cell sorting for CD34+ cell enrichment. Clinically, the pre-depletion steps make cell sorting easier. Furthermore, malignant cells have been shown to be eradicated when highly purified noncommitted CD34+/lineage-negative subpopulations are isolated. However, this pre-enrichment is labor-intensive, and at present, flow cytometry is not widely employed outside highly specialized laboratories. The advantage of using flow cytometry is that it produces a CD34+ cell product of higher purity than methods currently employed. A preliminary preclinical study with this high-speed method showed substantial (up to >7 logs) depletion of myeloma cells.[52] Clinical trials using the technology developed by Systemix are currently in progress.

CLINICAL DATA ON CD34-SELECTED AUTOGRAFTS

Breast cancer

A pilot clinical trial with a small number of breast cancer and neuroblastoma patients first suggested that human marrow cells that were CD34-selected with the CellPro immuno-adsorption column were capable of multi-lineage hematopoietic reconstitution in vivo.[53] Reinfusion of nonselected buffy coats often causes nausea or vomiting, hypertension, bradycardia, abdominal cramps, dysgeusia and arrhythmias. Life-threatening complications, such as acute renal failure acute respiratory failure, anaphylactoid reactions, and severe cardiovascular events, although rare, have been reported. A prospective randomized trial using the CellPro column was performed in 98 breast cancer patients who received high-dose chemotherapy followed by either CD34-selected or buffy coat fraction of marrow.[54] No

acute toxicities were observed during infusion of the CD34+ cell fractions, a much smaller volume than the nonselected marrow, buffy coat or peripheral stem cell fractions. A statistically significant reduction in minor adverse cardiovascular and life-threatening events was noted for patients who received CD34+ marrow when compared with nonselected marrow products.

The University of Colorado Bone Marrow Transplant Program has reported the largest series of breast cancer patients who received a CD34-selected graft after high-dose chemotherapy.[55] Updated results confirmed that CD34-selected stem cells effectively reconstituted immediate and long-term hematopoiesis in 120 breast cancer patients.[56] Immunohistochemical staining was performed on all grafts before and after CD34 selection. An average 2-log tumor depletion (ranging from 1 to >4 logs) was achieved following the procedure.[55] An interim data analysis showed a statistically significant difference in disease-free survival (DFS) between patients whose graft was purged to immunohistochemical negativity versus those who remained immunohistochemically positive after CD34 selection (45% vs 13%, $p = 0.002$).[56] However, in the most recent data update, the DFS difference is no longer statistically significant.[57] Since the majority of patients with breast cancer still had detectable cancer cells present in their stem cell grafts following CD34 selection, maximally effective purging may require a combination of positive- and negative-selection procedures.

A controlled trial randomized breast cancer patients to receive unmanipulated or CD34-selected autologous marrow.[58] There were no differences between the two arms in short- and long-term multilineage hematopoietic reconstitution, relating to granulocyte recovery and reconstitution of cellular and humoral immunity. However, patients who received a CD34-selected autograft, with a final product less than 1.2×10^6 CD34+/kg, had a significant 11-day delay in platelet recovery, compared to patients who received more than 1.2×10^6 CD34+/kg.

Recent use of retroviral gene marking technology has confirmed that CD34+ cells from both peripheral blood and bone marrow contribute to sustained engraftment of both hematopoietic and immune systems in breast cancer and multiple myeloma patients.[59]

Multiple myeloma

Although multiple myeloma is characterized by the growth of a clonal population of plasma cells in the bone marrow, circulating myeloma cells can be detected in the peripheral blood at a concentration as high as 10%.[60] Furthermore, stem cell mobilization with granulocyte colony-stimulating factor (G-CSF) or granulocyte–macrophage colony-stimulating factor (GM-CSF), with or without chemotherapy, results in a 10- to 50-fold increase of circulating myeloma cells.[61,62]

Normal plasma cells do not express CD34, since this antigen expression is gradually lost during normal hematopoietic cell maturation. A study that used the genetic sequence of the immunoglobulin heavy chain variable region as a marker of clonality showed that the malignant monoclonal plasma cells do not express CD34 antigen either.[35]

A phase II trial has been conducted in 37 patients who received PBPC, CD34-selected with the Ceprate column, after high-dose busulfan and cyclophosphamide.[63] A 2.7–4.5 log myeloma cell depletion was demonstrated following the selection process. A randomized trial of autologous unselected versus CD34-selected PBPC using the Ceprate column is presently ongoing in multiple myeloma patients.

Non-Hodgkin's lymphoma

Non-Hodgkin's lymphoma cells do not express CD34.[64] Gorin et al[65] transplanted 15 non-Hodgkin's lymphoma patients with marrow cells, harvested while in clinical complete remission, and CD34-selected with the CellPro column. Lymphoma cells expressing the *bcl-2* t(14; 18) translocation were identified by PCR in the buffy coat of nine patients before CD34 selection. Eight of these *bcl-2*-positive marrows

became *bcl-2*-negative after the CD34-selection procedure. With a short follow-up, 73% of all 15 patients remain free of relapse.[65] Other investigators have reported that only 20% of those non-Hodgkin's lymphoma patients, in complete remission or very good partial response at the time of PBPC pheresis, who expressed t(14; 18) by PCR in the leukapheresis products, became PCR-negative after CD34 selection using the CellPro column.[66]

Neuroblastoma

Civin et al treated 13 pediatric neuroblastoma patients with myeloablative chemotherapy and autologous CD34-selected bone marrow stem cells in a pilot clinical trial using the Isolex-300 device.[23] The calculated median tumor-cell depletion following the CD34-selection procedure was 2.6 logs. Normal long-term engraftment was observed in all transplanted patients, compared with historical controls of similarly treated patients who received unmanipulated marrow.

T-CELL DEPLETION FOR MOBILIZED BLOOD ALLOGRAFTS

PBPC are used increasingly in the allogeneic stem cell transplant setting. Compared with historical data with marrow support, the advantages of using PBPC include ease of collection, rapid hematopoietic reconstitution, and possibly less morbidity to the donor. Data from the Fred Hutchinson Cancer Center show that G-CSF-mobilized PBPC contain approximately 1 log more T lymphocytes than bone marrow.[67] Since T lymphocytes are responsible for graft-versus-host disease (GVHD), a potential major disadvantage of allogeneic PBPC is the possibility of an increased rate of GVHD compared with allogeneic marrow transplant. Acute GVHD does not seem to be increased in two pilot studies with small numbers of patients receiving allogeneic non-T-cell-depleted PBPC transplants from an HLA-identical sibling.[68,69] However, a retrospective review of 47 allo/

PBPC recipients treated at the MD Anderson Cancer Center revealed a statistically greater rate of extensive chronic GVHD in that group of patients than in 35 bone-marrow recipients treated at the same institution during the same time period (48% vs 35%, $p = 0.015$). Furthermore, the clinical picture of GVHD varied between both groups: a higher proportion of thrombocytopenia at onset (a marker of high-risk disease); more frequent hepatic, esophageal and gastrointestinal disease; and less mouth and lung involvement in the allo/PBPC group.[70]

Ceprate and Isolex-300, the two most commonly used CD34-selection devices to date, have demonstrated a T-cell depletion capacity equivalent to counterflow centrifugation elutriation or anti-T-cell monoclonal antibody purging, which are the most frequently employed T-cell depletion procedures. Overall, CD34 selection with immunobeads, using the Isolex-300 device, can remove an average 4 logs of T lymphocytes,[71,72] whereas immunoadsorption with the Ceprate column achieves a T-cell depletion of 2–3 logs.[43,73,74] Several pilot clinical trials are in progress using the CellPro[44,75] and Isolex-300[46,76–78] devices to T-deplete allogeneic grafts.

PROMISING FUTURE CLINICAL APPLICATIONS

Ex vivo expansion of the CD34$^+$-enriched peripheral blood product

Preclinical studies have shown the feasibility of growing human progenitors ex vivo in a static liquid culture system containing growth factor support.[79–81] Single growth factors give minimal growth, whereas combinations have been capable of expanding the committed progenitors. Different investigators[82–85] have reported synergistic activity of a number of combinations including stem cell factor (SCF), interleukin (IL)-3, IL-6, G-CSF, IL-1, erythropoietin (EPO) and Flt-3 ligand. In preliminary studies of breast cancer stem cells, these methods of culturing the CD34$^+$-enriched product do not appear to expand the breast cancer cells it contains,[86] although additional studies are needed to confirm these data.

Potential theoretical benefits of ex vivo CD34$^+$ expansion include faster hematopoietic reconstitution following myeloablative therapy, hematopoietic support for multiple repeated cycles of high-dose therapy, a reduced pheresis requirement for mobilized PBPC, the generation of sufficient cells from cord blood to produce hematopoietic support in an adult, and enhanced tumor purging.

There has been concern that the ex vivo culture conditions could promote the differentiation of primitive to committed progenitors, thereby diminishing the number of stem cells capable of long-term hematopoietic repopulation. Selected preclinical data suggest that sufficient pluripotent stem cells for short-term engraftment are present in cultured grafts.[81,87] In a pilot clinical trial,[88] autologous PBPC mobilized with both chemotherapy and G-CSF, collected in a single pheresis procedure, CD34-selected with the CellPro column, and subsequently expanded ex vivo, successfully engrafted patients treated with high-dose, but not truly myeloablative, chemotherapy with ifosfamide, carboplatin, etoposide and epirubicin. Engraftment times were identical to historical controls with nonexpanded peripheral blood CD34$^+$ cells. Clinical studies with myeloablative chemotherapy regimens will be required to definitely determine the short- and long-term reconstitution potential of cultured progenitors.

Ex vivo expansion of cord blood-derived progenitor cells

Preliminary data suggest that umbilical cord blood contains eightfold higher numbers of early hematopoietic progenitors than adult marrow.[89] Cord blood transplantation has been performed over the past five years, predominantly in the pediatric population. Its use in adults is presently under investigation. Currently, many cord blood banks are actively collecting units for use in the unrelated allogeneic transplant setting. A major concern for adult recipients is that the relatively small number of hematopoietic progenitors in cord blood samples may be inadequate for prompt and durable engraftment. Ex vivo expansion of cord blood progenitors has shown an enhanced proliferative potential of the cord-derived cells when compared with marrow-derived progenitors.[90]

In pediatric cord blood transplant recipients, preliminary studies suggest that the incidence of GVHD is less than that seen in bone marrow transplant patients. Whether this low incidence of GVHD is caused by cord-derived lymphocytes being immunologically naive or is just an effect of the patients' young age is not clear yet. However, in vitro data show that umbilical cord blood T lymphocytes are as alloreactive as those of adult peripheral blood, with a similar capacity to cause a GVHD reaction.[91]

T-cell depletion of the cord blood product can be effectively achieved with CD34+ selection. The Ceprate column yields approximately 2 logs of T-lymphocyte depletion, with a corresponding 1-log reduction in CFU-GM.[92] Expansion of the CD34+-enriched, T-cell-depleted product could potentially compensate for the loss of CFU-GM committed progenitors. In vitro[93] and animal studies[66] suggest the capacity of expanded cord-derived progenitors to engraft. Ongoing clinical studies are testing its feasibility in patients.

Immunotherapy with dendritic cells developed in vitro from CD34+ progenitors

Dendritic cells are professional antigen-presenting cells, considered to be among the most effective stimulators of T-cell immunity. They are found in many non-lymphoid tissues, including skin (Langerhans cells) and gastrointestinal mucosa. They migrate after antigen capture through the afferent lymph or bloodstream to lymphoid organs, where they present the antigen to the T cells.

Reid et al[94] and Caux et al[95] demonstrated in 1992 that dendritic cells are contained in the CD34+ population, from which they can be isolated. Since then, different groups have cultured dendritic cells from bone marrow, cord

blood and peripheral blood-derived CD34+-enriched cells by in vitro culture with different growth factor combinations. The specific growth factors vary according to the source of the progenitors and the type of dendritic cell desired. GM-CSF + tumor necrosis factor-α (TNF-α) are effective for bone marrow,[55] cord blood[56] and G-CSF-mobilized peripheral blood.[96] IL-4 + GM-CSF are used with steady-state peripheral blood.[57] The stem cell-targeted growth factors SCF[97,98] and Flt-3 ligand[99] further augment the effect of those combinations. These dendritic cells, cultured ex vivo, possess normal antigen-presenting capacity.[100]

By retroviral transduction of the human tumor antigen MUC-1 on CD34+ cells, and their subsequent cytokine-induced differentiation into dendritic cells, investigators from the University of Pittsburgh obtained a population of dendritic cells with stable and high-level expression of MUC-1. MUC-1(+)-transduced dendritic cells showed a more potent allostimulation of CD4+ T cells in vitro than MUC-1(−) dendritic cells.[101]

Ongoing clinical studies with dendritic cells, isolated CD34+ cells and cultured ex vivo, will determine their capacity to generate therapeutic T-cell responses to tumor antigens in cancer patients.

Gene therapy with retroviral-mediated gene-transferred CD34+ stem cells

Gaucher's disease is a congenital metabolic storage disease that is characterized by deficient activity of the glucocerebrosidase enzyme, which takes part in lipid metabolism. In 1992, it was first reported[102] that retroviral vectors could efficiently transfer the glucocerebrosidase gene into bone-marrow hematopoietic progenitor cells of patients with this disease, and that normal levels of glucocerebrosidase enzyme activity were subsequently expressed by these cells. CD34+ cell enrichment is performed to increase the retrovirus : cell ratio, since retroviral infection of stem cells has low efficiency, and high titers of the appropriate retrovirus cannot yet be obtained. CD34+ PBPC have produced higher transfection rates than CD34$^+$ marrow cells,[103,104] and are being used with increasing frequency in gene transfer studies.

An ongoing clinical trial at the University of Pittsburgh is testing the capacity of these genetically modified CD34-selected cells for competitive engraftment in Gaucher's disease patients with no prior myelosuppressive therapy. Cytokine-mobilized PBPC are CD34-selected with the Ceprate device. Subsequently, they are retrovirally transduced with the glucocerebrosidase gene, and finally returned to the patient in adequate numbers, and with a normal glucocerebrosidase enzyme activity.[105] Patients with other diseases caused by a bone-marrow-derived gene deficiency, such as Fan-

coni anemia,[106] or X-linked severe combined immunodeficiency syndrome,[107] may benefit from this promising therapy in the future.

CONCLUSIONS

Since first described ten years ago, CD34$^+$ cell selection has gained increasing acceptance in bone marrow and peripheral stem cell transplant settings. Ongoing clinical trials will address the utility of the procedure for both autologous and allogeneic transplant recipients. In the next few years, we hope to see further refinements of this technology and definition of its clinical indications.

REFERENCES

1. Ross AA, Cooper BW, Lazarus HM et al, Detection and viability of tumor cells in peripheral blood stem cell collections from breast cancer patients using immunocytochemical and clonogenic assay techniques. *Blood* 1993; **82:** 2605.

2. Franklin W, Shpall EJ, Archer P et al, Immunocytochemical detection of breast cancer cells in marrow and peripheral blood of patients undergoing high dose chemotherapy with autologous stem cell support. *Breast Cancer Res Treat* 1996; **41:** 1–13.

3. Sharp JC, Kessinger A, Mann S et al, Detection and clinical significance of minimal tumor cell contamination of peripheral blood stem cell harvests. *Int J Cell Clon* 1992; **10**(Suppl 1): 92–4.

4. Vredenburgh J, Silva O, De Sombre K et al, The significance of bone marrow micrometastases for patients with breast cancer and ⩾10+ nodes treated with high-dose chemotherapy and hematopoietic support [Abstract]. *Proc Am Soc Clin Oncol* 1995; **14:** 217.

5. Brenner MK, Rill DR, Moen RC et al, Gene-marking to trace origin of relapse after autologous bone marrow transplantation. *Lancet* 1993; **341:** 85–6.

6. Deisseroth AB, Zu Z, Claxton D et al, Genetic marking shows that Ph$^+$ cells present in autologous transplants of chronic myelogenous leukemia (CML) contribute to relapse after autologous bone marrow transplantation in CML. *Blood* 1994; **83:** 3068–76.

7. Gribben JG, Freedman AS, Neuberg D et al, Immunologic purging of marrow assessed by PCR before autologous bone marrow transplantation for B-cell lymphoma. *N Engl J Med* 1991; **325:** 1525–33.

8. Freedman AS, Gribben JG, Neuberg D et al, High-dose therapy and autologous bone marrow transplantation in patients with follicular lymphoma during first remission. *Blood* 1996; **88:** 2780–6.

9. Gorin NC, Aegerter P, Auvert B et al, Autologous bone marrow transplantation for acute myelocytic leukemia in first remission: A European survey of the role of marrow purging. *Blood* 1990; **75:** 1606–14.

10. Chao NJ, Stein AS, Long GD et al, Busulfan/etoposide – Initial experience with a new preparatory regimen for autologous bone marrow transplantation in patients with acute nonlymphoblastic leukemia. *Blood* 1993; **81:** 319–23.

11. Shpall EJ, Jones RB, Bast RC et al, 4-Hydroperoxycyclophosphamide purging of breast cancer from the mononuclear cell fraction of bone marrow in patients receiving high-dose chemotherapy and autologous marrow support: A phase I trial. *J Clin Oncol* 1991; **9:** 85–93.

12. Shpall EJ, Bast RC, Joines WT et al, Immunomagnetic purging of breast cancer from bone marrow for autologous transplantation. *Bone Marrow Transplant* 1991; **7:** 145–51.

13. Negrin RS, Kusnier-Glaz CR, Still BJ et al,

Transplantation of enriched and purged peripheral blood progenitor cells from a single apheresis product in patients with non-Hodgkin's lymphoma [Abstract]. *Blood* 1994; **84**(Suppl 1): 396a.

14. Vredenburgh JJ, Hussein A, Rubin P et al, High-dose chemotherapy and immunomagnetically purged peripheral blood progenitor cells and bone marrow for metastatic breast carcinoma [Abstract]. *Proc Am Soc Clin Oncol* 1996; **15**: 339.

15. Krause DS, Fackler MJ, Civin CI, Stratford May W, CD34: structure, biology and clinical utility. *Blood* 1996; **87**: 1–13.

16. Srour EF, Brandt JE, Briddell RA et al, Human CD34(+) HLA DR(−) bone marrow cells contain progenitor cells capable of self-renewal, multilineage differentiation, and long-term in vitro hematopoiesis. *Blood Cells* 1991; **17**: 287–95.

17. Civin CI, Banquerigo ML, Strauss LC, Loken MR, Antigenic analysis of hematopoiesis. VI. Flow cytometric characterization of My-10 positive progenitor cells in normal human bone marrow. *Exp Hematol* 1987; **15**: 10.

18. Andrews RG, Singer JW, Bernstein ID, Precursors of colony-forming cells in humans can be distinguished from colony-forming cells by expression of the CD33 and CD34 antigens and light scatter properties. *J Exp Med* 1989; **169**: 1721.

19. Loken MR, Shah VO, Dattilio KL, Civin CI, Flow cytometric analysis of human bone marrow. II. Normal B lymphocyte development. *Blood* 1987; **70**: 1316.

20. Gore SD, Kastan MB, Civin CI, Normal human bone marrow precursors that express terminal deoxynuclotidyl transferase include T-cell precursors and possible lymphoid stem cells. *Blood* 1991; **77**: 1681.

21. Siena S, Bregni M, Gianni M, Estimation of peripheral blood CD34$^+$ cells for autologous transplantation in cancer patients. *Exp Hematol* 1993; **21**: 203.

22. Fina L, Molgaard HV, Robertson D et al, Expression of the CD34 gene in vascular endothelial cells. *Blood* 1990; **75**: 2417–26.

23. Berenson RJ, Andress RG, Bensinger WI et al, Selection of CD34$^+$ marrow cells for autologous marrow transplantation. In: *Autologous Bone Marrow Transplantation. Proceedings of the Fourth International Symposium. The University of Texas, MD Anderson Cancer Center, Houston, TX* (Dicke KA, Spitzer G, Jagannath S, Evinger-Hodges MJ, eds). 1989: 55–60.

24. Bensinger WI, Berenson RJ, Andrews RJ et al, Positive selection of hematopoietic progenitors from marrow and peripheral blood for transplantation. *J Clin Apheresis* 1990; **5**: 74–6.

25. Krauth KA, Dockhom-Dwomiczak B et al, RT-PCR controlled reverse purging of autologous peripheral stem cell grafts. *Proc Annu Meet Soc Clin Oncol* 1995; **14**: A1450.

26. Civin CI, Strauss LC, Brovall C et al, Antigenic analysis of hematopoiesis. III. A hematopoietic progenitor cell surface antigen defined by a monoclonal antibody raised against KG-1a cells. *J Immunol* 1984; **133**: 157.

27. Borowitz MJ, Shuster JJ, Civin CI et al, Prognostic significance of CD34 expression in childhood B-precursor acute lymphocytic leukemia: A Pediatric Oncology Group Study. *J Clin Oncol* 1990; **8**: 1389.

28. Gore SD, Kastan MB, Civin CI, Normal human bone marrow precursors that express terminal deoxynucleotidyl transferase include T-cell precursors and possible lymphoid stem cells. *Blood* 1991; **77**: 1681.

29. Civin CI, Trischman T, Fackler MJ et al, Report of CD34 cluster workshop section. In: *Leucocyte Typing IV. White Cell Differentiation Antigens* (Knapp W, Dorken B, Gilks WR et al, eds). Oxford: Oxford University Press, 1990: 818–25.

30. Berenson RJ, Andrews RG, Bensinger WI et al, Selection of CD34$^+$ marrow cells for autologous marrow transplantation. *Hematol Oncol Ann* 1994; **2**: 78.

31. Vescio RA, Hong CH, Cao J et al, The hematopoietic stem cell antigen, CD34, is not expressed on the malignant cells in multiple myeloma. *Blood* 1994; **84**: 3283–90.

32. Banavali S, Silvestri F, Hulette B et al, Expression of hematopoietic progenitor cell-associated antigen CD34 in chronic myeloid leukemia. *Leuk Res* 1991; **15**: 603–8.

33. Soligo D, Delia D, Oriani A et al, Identification of CD34$^+$ cells in normal and pathological bone marrow biopsies by QBEND10 monoclonal antibody. *Leukemia* 1991; **5**: 1026–39.

34. Borowitz MJ, Gockerman JP, Moore JO et al, Clinicopathologic and cytogenetic features of CD34 (My-10)-positive acute nonlymphocytic leukemia. *Am J Clin Pathol* 1989; **91**: 265.

35. Guyotat D, Campos L, Thomas X et al, Myelodysplastic syndromes: A study of surface markers and in vitro growth patterns. *Am J Hematol* 1990; **34**: 26–31.

36. Schriber JR, Dejbakhsh-Jones S, Kusnierz-Glaz CR et al, Enrichment of bone marrow and blood progenitor (CD34$^+$) cells by density gradients

with sufficient yields for transplantation. *Exp Hematol* 1995; **23:** 1024–9.

37. Ficoll-Paque: For In Vitro Isolation of Lymphocytes (booklet). 1983. Uppsala, Sweden: Pharmacia.

38. Civin CI, Strauss LC, Brovall C et al, A hematopoietic progenitor cell surface antigen defined by a monoclonal antibody raised against KG-1a cells. *J Immunol* 1984; **133:** 157–65.

39. Berenson RJ, Bensinger WI, Kalamasz D, Positive selection of viable cell populations using avidin–biotin immunoadsorption. *J Immunol Meth* 1986; **91:** 11–16.

40. Andrews RG, Singer JW, Bernstein ID, Monoclonal antibody 12-8 recognizes a 115-kD molecule present on both unipotent hematopoietic colony-forming cells and their precursors. *Blood* 1986; **67:** 842–5.

41. Berenson RJ, Bensinger WI, Kalamasz WI, Kalamasz D et al, Engraftment of dogs with Ia-positive marrow cells isolated by avidin–biotin immunoadsorption. *Blood* 1987; **69:** 1363–7.

42. Berenson RJ, Andrews RG, Bensinger WI et al, Antigen CD34$^+$ marrow cells engraft lethally irradiated baboons. *J Clin Invest* 1988; **81:** 951–5.

43. Shpall EJ, Bast RC, Joines W et al, Immuno-pharmacologic purging of breast cancer for autologous bone marrow transplantation: preclinical and clinical results. *Prog Clin Biol Res* 1990; **333:** 321–35.

44. Civin C, Strauss LC, Brovall C et al, Antigenic analysis of hematopoiesis. III. A hematopoietic progenitor cell surface antigen defined by a monoclonal antibody raised against KG1a cells. *J Immunol* 1984; **133:** 157.

45. Hardwick A, Law P, Mansour V et al, Development of a large-scale immunomagnetic separation systems for harvesting CD34-positive cells from bone marrow. In: *Advances in Bone Marrow Purging and Processing* (Gross S, Gee AP, Worthington-White D, eds). New York: Wiley-Liss, 1992: 583–9.

46. Civin CI, Trischmann T, Kadan NS et al, Highly purified CD34-positive cells reconstitute hematopoiesis. *J Clin Oncol* 1996; **14:** 2224–33.

47. Herikstad BV, Lien E, Hematopoietic stem cells. In: *The Mulhouse Manual* (Wunder E, Sovalat H, Henon P et al, eds). Dayton, OH: AlphaMed, 1994: 149–60.

48. Marolleau JP, Brice P, Dal Cortivo L et al, CD34$^+$ selection by immunomagnetic selection (Isolex 300) for patients with malignancies. *Blood* 1996; **88:** 110a.

49. Miltenyi S, Muller W, Weichel W, Radbruch A, High gradient magnetic cell separation with MACS. *Cytometry* 1990; **11:** 231–8.

50. Richel D, Johnsen H, Canon J et al, Highly purified CD34$^+$ cells isolated with the Amgen Cell Selector provide rapid engraftment following high dose chemotherapy in breast cancer patients. *Blood* 1996; **88:** 110a.

51. Uchida N, Combs A, Conti S, et al, The in vivo hematopoietic population of a rhodamine-123 low population of human marrow. *Exp Hematol* 1994; **22:** 755.

52. Redding C, Sasaki D, Leemhuis T et al, Clinical scale purification of CD34$^+$Thy$^+$Lin$^-$ stem cells from mobilized peripheral blood by high speed fluorescence-activated cell sorting for use as an autograft for multiple myeloma patients. *Blood* 1994; **84:** 399a.

53. Berenson RJ, Bensinger WI, Hill RS et al, Engraftment after infusion of CD34$^+$ marrow cells in patients with breast cancer or neuroblastoma. *Blood* 1991; **77:** 1717–22.

54. Jacobs CA, Shpall EJ, Ball ED et al, A prospective randomized phase III study using the Ceprate SC Stem Cell Concentrator to isolate CD34$^+$ hematopoietic progenitors for autologous marrow transplantation after high-dose chemotherapy. In: *Proceedings of the Seventh International Symposium on Autologous Marrow and Blood Transplantation* 1994: 669–78.

55. Shpall EJ, Jones RB, Bearman SI et al, Transplantation of enriched CD34-positive autologous marrow into breast cancer patients following high-dose chemotherapy: influence of CD34-positive peripheral-blood progenitors and growth factors on engraftment. *J Clin Oncol* 1994; **12:** 28–36.

56. Cagnoni PJ, Jones RB, Franklin W et al, Use of CD34-positive autologous hematopoietic progenitors to support patients with breast cancer after high-dose chemotherapy [Abstract]. *Blood* 1995; **86:** 386a.

57. Shpall EJ, Bearman SI, Cagnoni PJ et al, Long-term follow-up of CD34-positive hematopoietic progenitor cell support for breast cancer patients receiving high-dose chemotherapy. Submitted to *J Clin Oncol*.

58. Champlin R, Ball E, Holland K et al, Importance of cell dose with CD34-selected autologous marrow transplants: Results of a controlled trial. *Blood* 1995; **86:** 293a.

59. Dunbar CE, Cottler-Fox M, O'Shaughnessy JA et al, Retrovirally marked CD34-enriched

peripheral blood and bone marrow cells contribute to long-term engraftment after autologous transplantation. *Blood* 1995; **85**: 3048–57.

60. Billadeau D, Quam L, Thomas W et al, Detection and quantitation of malignant cells in the peripheral blood of multiple myeloma patients. *Blood* 1992; **80**: 1818–24.

61. Lemoli RM, Fortuna A, Motta MR et al, Concomitant mobilization of plasma cells and hematopoietic progenitors into peripheral blood of multiple myeloma patients: positive selection and transplantation of enriched CD34$^+$ cells to remove circulating tumor cells. *Blood* 1996; **87**: 1625–34.

62. Corradini P, Voena C, Astolfi M et al, High-dose sequential chemotherapy in multiple myeloma: residual tumor cells are detectable in bone marrow and peripheral blood harvests and after autografting. *Blood* 1995; **85**: 1596–1602.

63. Schiller G, Vescio R, Freytes C et al, Transplantation of CD34$^+$ peripheral blood progenitor cells after high-dose chemotherapy for patients with advanced multiple myeloma. *Blood* 1995; **86**: 390–7.

64. Berenson RJ, Andrews RG, Bensinger WI et al, Selection of CD34$^+$ marrow cells for autologous marrow transplantation. *Hematol Oncol Ann* 1994; **2**: 78.

65. Gorin NC, Lopez M, Laporte JP et al, Preparation and successful engraftment of purified CD34$^+$ bone marrow progenitor cells in patients with non-Hodgkin's lymphoma. *Blood* 1995; **85**: 1647–54.

66. Mahe B, Milpied N, Hermouet S et al, G-CSF alone mobilizes sufficient peripheral blood CD34$^+$ cells for positive selection in newly diagnosed patients with myeloma and lymphoma. *Br J Haematol* 1996; **92**: 263–8.

67. Weaver CH, Longin K, Buckner CD, Bensinger W, Lymphocyte content in peripheral blood mononuclear cells collected after the administration of recombinant human granulocyte colony-stimulating factor. *Bone Marrow Transplant* 1994; **13**: 411–15.

68. Bensinger WI, Weaver CH, Appelbaum FR et al, Transplantation of allogeneic peripheral blood stem cells mobilized by recombinant human granulocyte colony-stimulating factor. *Blood* 1995; **85**: 1655–8.

69. Korbling M, Przepiorka D, Huh YO et al, Allogeneic blood stem cell transplantation for refractory leukemia and lymphoma: potential advantage of blood over marrow allografts. *Blood* 1995; **85**: 1659–65.

70. Anderlini P, Przepiorka D, Khouri I et al, Chornic graft-vs-host disease after allogeneic marrow or blood stem cell transplantation. *Blood* 1995; **86**: 109a.

71. Dreger P, Viehmann K, Steinmann J et al, G-CSF-mobilized peripheral blood progenitor cells for allogeneic transplantation: comparison of T cell depletion strategies using different CD34$^+$ selection systems or CAMPATH-1. *Exp Hematol* 1995; **23**: 147–54.

72. Bensinger WI, Rowley S, Appelbaum FR et al, CD34 selected allogeneic peripheral blood stem cell transplantation in older patients with advanced hematologic malignancies [Abstract]. *Blood* 1995; **86**: 97a.

73. Cottler-Fox M, Cipolone K, Yu M et al, Positive selection of CD34$^+$ hematopoietic cells using an immunoaffinity column results in T cell-depletion to elutriation. *Exp Hematol* 1995; **23**: 320–2.

74. Schiller G, Rowley S, Buckner CD et al, Transplantation of allogeneic CD34$^+$ peripheral blood stem cells in older patients with advanced hematologic malignancy [Abstract]. *Blood* 1995; **86**: 389a.

75. Cornetta K, Gharpure V, Abonour R et al, Sibling-matched allogeneic bone marrow transplantation using CD34 cells obtained by immunomagnetic bead separation. *Blood* 1995; **86**: 389a.

76. Link H, Arseniev L, Bahre O et al, Combined transplantation of allogeneic bone marrow and CD34 blood cells. *Blood* 1995; **86**: 2500–8.

77. Holland HK, Bray AM, Geller RB et al, Transplantation of HLA-identical positively selected CD$^+$ cells of peripheral blood and marrow from related donors results in prompt engraftment and low incidence of GVHD in recipients undergoing allogeneic transplantation [Abstract]. *Blood* 1995; **86**: 389a.

78. Finke J, Brugger W, Bertz H et al, Allogeneic transplantation of peripheral blood derived CD34$^+$ selected progenitor cells from matched related donors: Results of a clinical phase I/II study [Abstract]. *Blood* 1995; **86**: 290a.

79. Haylock DN, To LB, Dowse TL et al, Ex vivo expansion and maturation of peripheral blood CD34$^+$ cells into the myeloid lineage. *Blood* 1992; **80**: 1405–12.

80. Shapiro F, Yao TJ, Raptis G et al, Optimization of conditions for ex vivo expansion of CD34$^+$ cells from patients with stage IV breast cancer. *Blood* 1994; **84**: 3567–74.

81. Henschler R, Brugger W, Luft T et al, Maintenance of transplantation potential in ex vivo expanded CD34(+)-selected human peripheral blood progenitor cells. *Blood* 1994; **84:** 2898–2903.

82. Lill MC, Lynch M, Fraser JK et al, Production of functional myeloid cells from CD34-selected hematopoietic progenitor cells using a clinically relevant ex vivo expansion system. *Stem Cells* 1994; **12:** 626–37.

83. Purdy MH, Hogan CJ, Hami L et al, Large volume ex vivo expansion of CD34-positive hematopoietic progenitor cells for transplantation. *J Hematother* 1995; **4:** 515–25.

84. Brugger W, Mocklin W, Heimfeld S et al, Ex vivo expansion of enriched peripheral blood CD34$^+$ progenitor cells by stem cell factor, interleukin-1β (IL-1β), IL-6, IL-3, interferon-γ, and erythropoietin. *Blood* 1993; **81:** 2579–84.

85. McKenna HJ, De VriesP, Brasel K et al, Effect of flt3 ligand on the ex vivo expansion of human CD34$^+$ hematopoietic progenitor cells. *Blood* 1995; **86:** 3413–20.

86. Vogel W, Behringer D, Scheding S et al, Ex vivo expansion of CD34$^+$ peripheral blood progenitor cells: implications for the expansion of contaminating epithelial tumor cells. *Blood* 1996; **88:** 2707–13.

87. Muench MO, Firpo MY, Moore MA, Bone marrow transplantation with interleukin-1 plus kit-ligand ex vivo expanded bone marrow accelerates hematopoietic reconstitution in mice without the loss of stem cell lineage and proliferative potential. *Blood* 1993; **81:** 3463–73.

88. Brugger W, Heimfeld S, Berenson RJ et al, Reconstitution of hematopoiesis after high-dose chemotherapy by autologous progenitor cells generated ex vivo. *N Engl J Med* 1995; **333:** 283–7.

89. Traycoff C, Abboud M, Laver J et al, Evaluation of the in vitro behavior of phenotypically defined populations of umbilical cord blood hematopoietic progenitor cells. *Exp Hematol* 1994; **22:** 215–22.

90. Traycoff C, Abboud MR, Laver J et al, Human umbilical cord blood hematopoietic progenitor cells: Are they the same as their adult bone marrow counterparts? *Blood Cells* 1994; **20:** 382–90.

91. Deacock SJ, Schwarer AP, Bridge J et al, Evidence that umbilical cord blood contains a higher frequency of HLA class II-specific alloreactive T cells than adult peripheral blood. *Transplantation* 1992; **53:** 1128–34.

92. Laver J, Traycoff CM, Abdel-Mageed A et al, Effects of CD34$^+$ selection and T cell immunodepletion on cord blood hematopoietic progenitors: relevance to stem cell transplantation. *Exp Hematol* 1995; **23:** 1492–6.

93. Moore MA, Hoskins T, Ex vivo expansion of cord blood-derived stem cells and progenitors. *Blood Cells* 1994; **20:** 468–79.

94. Reid CD, Stackpoole A, Meager A, Tikerpae J, Interactions of tumor necrosis factor with granulocyte–macrophage colony-stimulating factor and other cytokines in the regulation of dendritic cell growth in vitro from early bipotent CD34$^+$ progenitors in human bone marrow. *J Immunol* 1992; **149:** 2681–8.

95. Caux C, Dezutter-Dambuyant C, Schmitt D, Banchereau J, GM-CSF and TNF-α cooperate in the generation of dendritic Langerhans cells. *Nature* 1992; **360:** 258–61.

96. Romani N, Gruner S, Brang D et al, Proliferating dendritic cell progenitors in human blood. *J Exp Med* 1994; **180:** 83–93.

97. Santiago-Schwarz F, Rappa DA, Laky K, Carsons SE, Stem cell factor augments TNF/GM-CSF-mediated dendritic cell hematopoiesis. *Stem Cells* 1995; **13:** 186–97.

98. Young JW, Skabolcs P, Moore MA, Identification of dendritic cell colony-forming units among normal human CD34$^+$ progenitors that are expanded by c-kit-ligand and yield pure dendritic cell colonies in the presence of GM-CSF and TNF-α. *J Exp Med* 1995; **182:** 1111–19.

99. Siena S, Di Nicola M, Bregni M et al, Massive ex vivo generation of functional dendritic cells from mobilized CD34$^+$ blood progenitors from anticancer therapy. *Exp Hemat* 1995; **23:** 1463–71.

100. Bernhard H, Disis ML, Heimfeld S et al, Generation of immunostimulatory dendritic cells from human CD34$^+$ hematopoietic progenitor cells of the bone marrow and peripheral blood. *Cancer Res* 1995; **55:** 1099–104.

101. Henderson RA, Nimgaonkar MT, Watkins SC et al, Human dendritic cells genetically engineered to express high levels of the human epithelial tumor antigen (MUC-1). *Cancer Res* 1996; **56:** 3763–70.

102. Nolta JA, Yu XJ, Bahner I, Kohn DB, Retroviral-mediated transfer of the human glucocerebrosidase gene into cultured Gaucher bone marrow. *J Clin Invest* 1992; **90:** 342–8.

103. Bregni M, Magni M, Siena S et al, Human peripheral blood hematopoietic progenitors are

optimal targets of retroviral-mediated gene transfer. *Blood* 1992; **80:** 1418–22.

104. Dunbar CE, Cottler-Fox M, O'Shaughnessy JA et al, Retrovirally marked CD34-enriched peripheral blood and bone marrow cells contribute to long-term engraftment after autologous transplantation. *Blood* 1995; **85:** 3048–57.

105. Nimgaokar M, Mierski J, Beeler M et al, Cytokine mobilization of peripheral blood stem cells in patients with Gaucher disease with a view to gene therapy. *Exp Hematol* 1995; **23:** 1633–41.

106. Walsh CE, Grompe M, Vanin E et al, A functionally active retrovirus vector for gene therapy in Fanconi anemia group C. *Blood* 1994; **84:** 453–9.

107. Qazilbash MH, Walsh CE, Russell SM et al, Retroviral vector for gene therapy of X-linked severe combined immunodeficiency syndrome. *J Hematother* 1995; **4:** 91–8.

9

Therapeutic use of cells expanded ex vivo from blood stem cells

James G Bender

INTRODUCTION

The ability to separate cell populations from blood or marrow, combined with the availability of a vast array of cytokines, has focussed significant attention and resources on the concept of producing therapeutic cell products from in vitro cultures of cells stimulated with combinations of cytokines. The studies that initially explored this concept began in the mid-1980s and were aimed at the production of therapeutic lymphocyte populations for use in the treatment of cancer. Interleukin (IL)-2 was available and peripheral blood lymphocytes were easy to obtain. Since then, a variety of interleukins, chemokines, cytokines, colony-stimulating factors and other growth-promoting and controlling factors have been identified and characterized.[1] In a parallel path, the understanding of compartments of hematopoietic differentiation has been refined using improved assays for early and intermediate stages, and the ever-growing number of surface antigens have been used to classify the cell populations and their differentiation stages.[2] In addition, technologies have emerged using antibodies directed against differentiation antigens to fractionate cell mixtures and prepare enriched populations of cells. This interface between the understanding of cellular differentiation and the array of regulatory molecules controlling this process presents an opportunity to produce a variety of therapeutic cell products ex vivo. Significant effort has been directed at using many of these cytokines as in vivo therapeutics. However, because of the pleiotropic action of many cytokines, their widespread use as pharmaceuticals has been limited by toxicities. Ex vivo expansion therefore provides an opportunity to eliminate these toxicities by using recombinant cytokines to produce cell populations that can then be washed free of cytokines and media before reinfusion.

Exploring the combinations of cytokines and cell populations that are possible requires a focus on defining approaches that bring value to patient treatment. These approaches can enhance or replace current cell therapies or identify new cell products with therapeutic value. Table 9.1 is a list of potential applications for ex vivo cell expansion either through producing therapeutic cell products or by impacting transplantation by purging cell populations or eliminating the need for apheresis or bone marrow harvest. Cell therapies currently being tested in the clinic include those for treating

Table 9.1   Applications for expansion of blood stem cells

Therapeutic cell products
  Neutropenia
  Thrombocytopenia
  Antigen-specific lymphocytes
  Genetically modified cells for:
    hereditary diseases – chronic
      granulomatous disease (CGD)
    anti-tumor cells – thymidine kinase
      (TK)-transfected lymphocytes
    stem cell protection – mdr transfection

Purging
  Lymphocytes (allogeneic)
  Tumor cells (autologous)

Reduce harvesting requirements
  Eliminate bone marrow harvest or apheresis
  Use cord blood for adult transplants

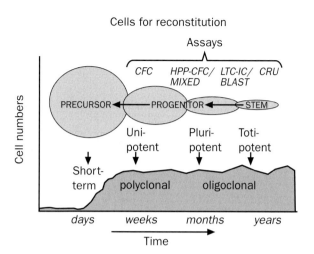

Figure 9.1 Cells for reconstitution.

cytopenias associated with cancer therapies, immune therapies to eradicate residual tumor cells or to treat relapse, and genetically modified cells for the treatment of immunodeficiency and hereditary diseases. Concepts for new therapeutic cell preparations that are in preclinical testing include in vitro expansion to produce antigen-specific lymphocytes for the treatment of cancer or viral infections,[3,4] the expansion of natural killer (NK) cells,[5] as well as new variations of the lymphokine-activated killer (LAK) cell therapies.[6] The discussion here will focus on cells expanded from blood stem cells for hematopoietic reconstitution.

POTENTIAL VALUE OF EXPANDED BLOOD STEM CELL PRODUCTS

Blood stem cells expanded ex vivo could be used as a supplement to augment current transplant protocols, as the sole support of hematopoietic reconstitution, or for purging unwanted cell populations. Currently, blood

stem cells are the primary treatment used for hastening hematopoietic recovery after high-dose therapy. The use of blood stem cells rather than marrow has been driven by the more rapid platelet and granulocyte recoveries observed with mobilized blood compared with marrow.[7] The cells responsible for this effect are not well understood. A model that depicts the cell types involved in hematopoietic recovery during transplantation is shown diagrammatically in Figure 9.1. In this model, various compartments of stem cells, progenitors and precursors provide differentiation stages that contribute at different stages of hematopoietic recovery. In vitro and in vivo assays described to characterize these populations are also included to give possible points of reference for considering how these compartments may be defined. A small population of primitive stem cells is most likely responsible for later long-term hematopoiesis, and data from allogeneic transplants support the concept that only a few stem cell clones are responsible for the long-term oligoclonal hematopoiesis.[8] Early recovery has been considered to be due to the committed progenitors in the colony-forming cell (CFC) or pre-CFC compartments. Studies in mice have suggested that clonogenic cells are responsible for the early phase of engraftment,[9] as have human transplants, where delayed engraftment was observed when clonogenic cells were removed from the graft by treatment with 4-hydroperoxy-cyclophosphamide (4HC).[10] More recently, this concept has been challenged in mouse studies using fractionated cell preparations.[11] In these studies, clonogenic cells were not found to affect early engraftment, suggesting that this engraftment comes from a more primitive pre-CFU cell population.

Although it is not yet clear which cell populations in blood stem cell products cause the early hematopoietic recovery, studies with CD34[+]-enriched cells indicate that the reconstituting cells are within this population of immature cells.[12] However, regardless of the dose of CD34[+] cells, an obligate period of neutropenia of about 10 days is required for the immature CD34[+] cells to differentiate into mature neutrophils and platelets. One strategy then for treating this cytopenic period is to provide partially differentiated neutrophilic and/or megakaryocytic precursor cells that would rapidly mature upon reinfusion.[13–15] This use of expanded blood stem cells as a supplement to current blood stem cell therapies would provide further reduction or elimination of these cytopenias.

An alternative strategy of using expanded cells as the sole support for reconstitution would reduce the harvesting of stem cells. In this approach, expansion of more primitive stem cells as well as committed progenitors would reduce or potentially eliminate the need for apheresis or bone marrow harvest.[16] This concept also applies to the transplantation of umbilical cord blood cells, where the dose of progenitors obtainable from a single cord blood has limited the scope of this stem cell source to transplantion in children and delayed engraftment is often observed.[17] Expansion of progenitors to provide an adequate dose would permit transplantation in adults and greatly extend the use of this stem cell source. Although this approach is conceptually attractive, it is often difficult to authenticate the in vitro maintenance of expansion of these most primitive stem cell populations.

In addition to reducing the starting stem cell dose requirements and providing supplements for transplantation, ex vivo culturing also provides a mechanism for eliminating unwanted cells in the product as an alternative or adjunct to cell fractionation techniques. This can be used with either of the preceding strategies. Previously this has been explored in the treatment of chronic myeloid leukemia, in which culturing was used to eliminate malignant cells while retaining normal progenitors.[18] Although still not an established therapy, this concept may also apply to other tumor types, since there is substantial evidence that cells from solid tumors do not proliferate well in ex vivo culture systems.[19] With allogeneic transplantation or with the use of cord blood, there is also the potential for reducing graft-versus-host disease by using culturing to decrease numbers of lymphocytes in grafts, since these cells rapidly decline in ex vivo cultures lacking IL-2.[20]

ANIMAL MODEL DATA

Experimental approaches to studying biological effects of ex vivo treated cell products in animal models have ranged from short-term ex vivo exposure to cytokines (hours to days) to longer-term cultures (days to weeks). The mouse has been a primary model for studying hematopoietic stem cell engraftment. The short-term exposure to cytokines that results in little in vitro proliferation may affect an activation or priming of the cells that upon reinfusion may accelerate in vivo proliferation or enhance homing to the appropriate microenvironment. Data supporting this concept have come from mouse studies showing enhanced recovery of mice given marrow cells cultured in cytokines.[21–24] Short-term incubation with growth factors for 2–4 hours has been shown to enhance the initial hematopoietic recovery of neutrophils and platelets.[22,23] Peters et al,[25] using cultured bone marrow cells that were not obtained after 5-fluorouracil (5-FU) treatment, observed a long-term engraftment defect in cells cultured for 48 hours in cytokines. These data suggest that inducing quiescent stem cells into the cell cycle may interfere with their homing and subsequent long-term engraftment.

Longer-term culture for either three,[24] six[26] or seven days [21,27] of bone marrow harvested after 5-FU administration in combinations of kit ligand, IL-1, IL-3 and IL-6 have also been shown to enhance recovery. In these studies, transplantation of the cultured cells resulted in long-term engraftment of donor cells at 120–280 days. The cells responsible for this recovery were not characterized. Some characterization of Thy1[+] Lin[−] cells in cultures of bone marrow cells indicate that the engraftment potential of this phenotype declines during culture.[28] Recently, a study has shown that 6 days of culture in stem cell factor (SCF) and IL-11 results in cells that can rescue lethally irradiated mice and be serially transplanted through four transfers.[29] Overall, mouse studies have demonstrated that cultured cells can hasten short-term engraftment, and in some reports can provide for long-term engraftment. Further studies that characterize the populations responsible for each phase of engraftment will be useful in defining desirable cell compositions.

HUMAN DATA

Short-term culturing

Recent studies using human cells[13,30] have shown that significant expansions of colony-forming cells are possible in ex vivo cultures of mononuclear cells or purified CD34[+] cells. A clinical trial of bone marrow transplantation using allogeneic marrow that was incubated for 4 days in IL-3 and granulocyte–macrophage colony-stimulating factor (GM-CSF) showed a reduction in the period of neutropenia.[31] In contrast, another study in which allogeneic bone marrow was incubated for 1 hour showed no effect on engraftment.[32] Other studies using mobilized mononuclear cells cultured for 3 days showed no side-effects of the reinfusion, but also no clinical benefit in the reduction of neutropenia.[33] Together, these limited studies are inconclusive, and indicate that short-term ex vivo exposure to cytokines may not be adequate for providing a useful cell product. Alternatively, the appropriate cytokine or combination of cytokines

may not have been applied to this strategy of short-term exposure.

Longer-term culturing

Investigators have also used longer culture periods of 7 days to 3 weeks to stimulate proliferation and differentiation and provide a supplemental cell preparation to impact cytopenia. One study[34] reported transient recovery of neutrophil counts by the reinfusion of culture-derived mature neutrophils from three-week cultures of peripheral blood. No adverse reactions were observed in these studies after the administration of 1.5×10^9 cultured cells. These data are consistent with other studies[35] of the reinfusion of granulocytes harvested after mobilization of allogeneic donors with granulocyte colony-stimulating factor (G-CSF). In these studies, no toxicities were observed after an average of 4×10^{10} neutrophils were reinfused and a transient recovery of granulocyte counts occurred. These studies indicate that high doses of mature cells may be required to impact neutropenia, but that this can be done safely. More recently, CD34[+] cells expanded in PIXY321 (IL-3/GM-CSF) to produce neutrophil precursors also showed no toxicities at cell doses over 10^{10}, and a reduction in the neutropenia in patients given higher doses of cultured cells was observed.[14]

Other investigators have expanded cells to reduce harvesting requirements, and have used the cultured cells as the sole support for hematopoietic reconstitution. In one study,[16] 11×10^6 CD34[+] cells (approximately one-tenth of a therapeutic dose) were expanded 62-fold in a cocktail of factors to provide a dose of 11×10^6 cultured cells/kg containing 12×10^4 colony-forming cells/kg. As above, no toxicities of the cultured cells were observed. In addition, these patients had neutrophil and platelet recovery within the same time as patients receiving a conventional dose of CD34[+] cells. In another study of 10 patients using a different culture system and a myeloablative conditioning regimen that included radiotherapy,[36] a 20-fold expansion of cells was achieved and no toxicities were observed when cultured cells were reinfused as a supplement. In two additional patients,[37] the cultured cells were used as the sole support for recovery. One patient who received a high dose of expanded CFU-GM (1033×10^4/kg) had prompt engraftment while a second patient whose cells did not expand required infusion of backup products. These data support the safety of expanded cells and the concept of expanding cells to reduce the need for harvesting bone marrow or apheresis. The data also suggest that a threshold of in vitro expansion will be required. Definitive evidence supporting this approach may be obtained using gene-marking strategies, and will require randomized trials.

DIMENSIONS OF THE EXPANDED CELL PRODUCT

Product that is sole transplantation support

The hematopoietic system in humans contains a total of $(5–10) \times 10^{11}$ cells, with the production of 4×10^{11} cells/day, including 7×10^{10} neutrophils per day for a 70 kg adult.[38] From numbers obtained from blood stem cell transplants, the number of CFU-GM required for engraftment is approximately 2×10^5/kg, or 1.4×10^7 total for a 70 kg patient.[39] Although a correlation with engraftment using this measurement is observed, as discussed earlier, it is still not clear what population is the major contributor to early recovery. A major dilemma in this approach is measuring the primitive population for engraftment and establishing maintenance or expansion of these cells during culture. Clearly, the most primitive cells are required, and an assay currently used to quantitate these early cells in humans is the long-term culture-initiating cell (LTCIC) assay, which measures the cells that produce colony-forming cells after five weeks of culture on stroma.[40] Alternative assays using repopulation of mice with human cells provide data that support the definition of the primitive cell population, but are often not quantitative.[41] Extrapolations made from mouse competitive repopulation experiments[42] have sug-

gested that 10 000–30 000 LTCIC may be sufficient for long-term repopulation. This provides a target number to either maintain or expand in culture.

Many groups have explored the appropriate conditions for maintaining or expanding primitive cells in vitro. Studies in mice have demonstrated that long-term repopulation cells will indeed divide and can be maintained in vitro.[43] Some studies of human cells using the LTCIC assay to quantitate primitive cells have indicated that LTCIC can be maintained when CD34$^+$ cells are cultured in liquid cultures with recombinant cytokines.[42] Others have reported that stromal layer formation is required to maintain or expand the more primitive cells that are required for long-term recovery.[44] Alternatively, studies by Verfaillie and Miller[45] have demonstrated that stromal contact may not be required, but soluble cytokines from stroma in combination with IL-3 and macrophage inflammatory protein 1α (MIP-1α) can result in expansion of LTCIC. Issues arising in translating this into the clinic include whether the LTCIC assay is quantitating the primitive population that results in long-term engraftment and whether sufficient numbers of the appropriate primitive cells can be obtained from ex vivo cultures to provide long-term engraftment. There is an indication that the source of the starting cells may be important, with cord blood and fetal CD34$^+$ cells providing more sustained expansion in culture.[46] This possibility suggests that cord blood transplants may benefit most from this strategy of ex vivo expansion.

Product to augment neutrophil/platelet recovery

A critical issue in producing cells to augment recovery is whether the numbers of appropriate cells can be produced to provide clinical benefit. In normal adults, circulating granulocytes are produced at a rate of 1.5×10^9/kg body weight/day,[38] with approximately 0.7×10^9 granulocytes/kg body weight in the blood and a 10-fold higher reserve of granulocytes in the marrow.[47] To restore a circulating granulocyte count to 0.5×10^9/liter in a neutropenic patient, it has been estimated that 2×10^{11} neutrophils would be needed over a 10-day period.[13] This number is significantly higher than that obtainable in granulocyte products from allogeneic donors mobilized with G-CSF.[35] In addition, an optimal maintenance of the counts would require the production of a steady supply of mature cells rather than a bolus infusion of mature cells. Assuming that 10^8 CD34$^+$ cells containing approximately 10^7 CFU-GM can be recovered from a single apheresis product from a patient mobilized with cyclophosphamide and G-CSF, adequate numbers of appropriate cells may be generated if a 50-fold expansion of cells can be obtained using an optimal combination of factors. This culture would theoretically give rise to 5×10^9 cells containing 50% neutrophil precursors (promyelocytes and myelocytes) that would proliferate in vivo another 10-fold in 1–3 days, giving rise to 2.5×10^{10} neutrophils. In addition, the numbers of CFU-GM might increase 20-fold from 10^7 to 2×10^8, ultimately giving rise in vivo to an additional 10^{11} neutrophils. Clearly these calculations are only hypothetical, but suggest the requirements for a starting cell preparation and the performance of a culture system. Mathematical modeling may provide a more sophisticated strategy for estimating the cell types and mixture that would be required for developing this therapeutic approach. Some models are predictive of the recoveries seen with radiation-induced aplasia and after bone marrow transplantation.[48] More recently, this modeling approach has been applied to the application of cultured cells for the treatment of neutropenia.[49] In vitro studies of proliferation and differentiation kinetics, in combination with modeling provide a strategy to define the dosages and compositions that will be needed clinically.

CULTURE SYSTEM APPROACHES

Mononuclear cell products from leukapheresis are complex mixtures of lymphocytes, monocytes and a few granulocytes with a low content of proliferating progenitors. Efforts to culture mononuclear cells in static cultures without perfusion or regular feeding have had limited success, because the predominant (>96%) population of non-proliferating cells dies out early in the culture, releasing their cytoplasmic contents. The most effective approach to optimizing the expansion of progenitors in a static culture has been to enrich the CD34$^+$ cell population and seed the cells at densities of 10^4–10^5/ml.[13,30] Alternatively, the use of perfusion or regular feeding has shown that equivalent cell compositions can be obtained using mononuclear cells as the starting population, with a better overall performance.[20] Possibly, perfusion, by providing a more homogeneous environment, may dampen some of the variability seen with hematopoietic cell cultures.

Static systems – gas permeable bags

The need for large-scale cultures of cells to be used clinically began with the LAK cell trials in the early 1980s and continued with the tumor infiltrating lymphocytes (TIL) trials in the mid-1980s. As the dose of cells tested increased, the cell culture volumes ranged into many liters, creating logistical problems when using conventional polystyrene tissue culture flasks and roller bottles.[50] The need for a closed cell culture system that would minimize microbial contamination and simplify the handling of these cultures led to the development of the Lifecell technology, that utilized gas-permeable cell culture bags that can be sterilely connected by means of a 'sterile connect device'.[51] The cell culture bags, used in conjunction with the Lifecell solution transfer pump, provide an easy way to handle large cultures with a reduced risk of contamination to the cells as well as reduced exposure of biohazards to the clinician. More recently, gas-permeable bags with polystyrene coatings, which are more compatible with culturing of CD34$^+$ cells, have been developed and scaled-up for clinical use.[14,52]

Perfusion systems

Perfusion systems for cell culture are widely used to produce soluble proteins and other biologics. Only recently have there been efforts to develop perfusion systems to produce therapeutic cell products. There are a variety of issues involved in designing a system in which the cells are the product, but the main ones include (1) providing a homogeneous environment such that cell viability is maintained; (2) identifying a design that allows easy inoculation and retrieval of the cells. Approaches that address these issues include flat plate chambers with radial or rectangular geometries[20,53] and stirred suspension chambers.[54,55] Flat plate chambers have used membranes[53] or smooth surfaces[56] to provide for stromal development and thereby retain the cells. Alternatively, parallel grooves perpendicular to the fluid flow have been used successfully to retain and perfuse non-adherent cells.[20] More traditional designs such as hollow fiber cartridges have been used successfully to culture lymphocytes,[57] but have not been widely used for progenitor cultures – probably because of biocompatibility issues associated with the materials used as well as problems in maintaining a homogeneous environment.

Besides the fundamental issues of environment and cell retrieval, other issues also come into play when using perfusion for this type of application. One question is whether the same cell population can be derived with a perfused method as with a static method or with a method using a fractionated population such as the CD34-selected preparation. Studies comparing mononuclear cells cultured with perfusion have been shown to result in cell preparations similar to those obtained using CD34+ cells in static culture.[20]

GROWTH FACTORS

Many studies have demonstrated the in vitro proliferation of CD34+ cells stimulated with recombinant cytokines. It is beyond the scope of this chapter to discuss all of these data. There are several reviews of this area.[58–60] Clearly, however, cytokines are fundamental to the success of producing ex vivo expanded cell products. Earlier attempts at culturing cells in

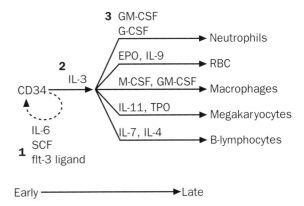

Figure 9.2 Factors for CD34+ cell culture.

Dexter-type long-term cultures in the absence of cytokines resulted in delayed engraftment.[61] The exact combination of cytokines that will prove to be the most useful is not known and will depend upon the type of cell product desired. This will be discussed below, where it is clear that the combination of factors defines the types of cells produced in vitro. Figure 9.2 summarizes diagrammatically how different combinations of factors can be used to expand different lineages. One principle that has emerged from the extensive amount of work done in this area is that combinations of growth-promoting factors work together synergistically to proliferate and differentiate progenitor cells.[13] With limited combinations, early-acting and late-acting (i.e. more lineage-specific) give best results in stimulating differentiation. IL-3 appears to be an important intermediate-stage (multilineage) factor.[13,62,63]

MEDIA

With growing regulatory concern regarding disease transmission and immunization to foreign proteins, the use of animal serum in cell culture media for clinical use is coming under greater scrutiny. These concerns have led to the development of serum-free and defined media for hematopoietic cell culturing. A variety of formulations have been described,[64] and several are commercially available from BioWhittaker and Life Technologies. Usually these media have complex base formulations such as McCoy's or Iscove's Modified Dulbecco's Medium (IMDM), and require the addition of albumin as a protein source. Although these media support the expansion of progenitors,[64] there have been few reports of serum-free growth of stromal cells. However, growth of megakaryocytes is enhanced in serum-free media.[15] An alternative to the use of serum-free media or the addition of animal serum has been to add autologous plasma or pooled AB serum.[16,63,65] The logistics of preparing and utilizing pooled serum components as culture supplements makes these reagents a difficult choice for wide-scale implementation of a therapy. Autologous plasma, however, is readily available from the apheresis process, and therefore may be considered. It would not likely have the inhibitory effects on megakaryocyte growth ascribed to transforming growth factor-β (TGF-β).[66] However, because of the variation in mobilization regimens and patient variability, significant variation has been observed in the effects of adding autologous plasma to cultures of CD34+ cells.[67] Because little is known about the metabolic requirements of progenitors and stem cells or the complete spectrum of cytokines that regulate their growth, an opportunity exists for the development of media formulations for these applications.

CHARACTERIZATION OF CULTURED CELLS

An assumption in exploring the approach of using cultured cells is that cells produced by in vitro techniques will be equivalent or similar to those normally generated in vivo. Although there are data showing normal in vitro function of culture-derived populations,[13,68] little is known of their fate when returned to the in vivo environment. Will they home to the bone marrow, or is that necessary? Will the neutrophils function normally in chemotaxis and bactericidal killing? Will mature megakaryocytes that

normally do not circulate survive the shear forces encountered in the circulation? Preclinical studies will be required to characterize the composition of cells produced ex vivo. Clinical trials will ultimately answer questions of homing and function.

In considering the characterization of the neutrophil lineage, a variety of myeloid antigens have been used with flow cytometry to provide rapid information on the cell composition of cells in culture. Initial studies of normal bone marrow indicated that CD15 was one of the first antigens expressed as cells differentiate from CD34+ cells into the neutrophil lineage.[69] Other antigens such as CD64 and CD67 are also expressed at this time, with CD64 being present on an earlier CD34+ CFU-GM phenotype.[70] As promyelocytes then differentiate further into myelocytes, they express CD11b, and when fully mature bands and segmented neutrophils they express CD16.[69] Several investigators have studied the sequence of antigen expression on cells from cultures of mononuclear cells or selected CD34+ cells with various combinations of factors.[30,71-73] Differences within in vitro derived cells were observed. CD16, normally expressed on mature granulocytes, was only expressed at low levels in a small proportion of the neutrophils produced in vitro.[30,72] Likewise, differences have been observed in phenotypes when different growth factor combinations are used,[74] as well as when different media formulations are used. Significant differences are seen when G-CSF is compared with GM-CSF – with G-CSF stimulating more terminal differentiation of function as well as antigen expression.[68,71] Serum-free media typically do not sustain neutrophil differentiation to mature granulocytes,[63] and the level of some antigens may be reduced.[52] Together, these data suggest that additional cytokines or other nutrients in serum are likely required to result in terminal differentiation of granulocytes in vitro. One example of a cytokine that may be involved is interferon γ. It has been reported to act on the progenitor stage to affect the differentiation and function of the mature cells.[75]

Besides surface antigen expression, morphology, enzyme expression and function have been used to characterize cultured granulocytic cells. In general, the morphology is similar to normal cells, but not identical – causing confusion in performing differentials. Granule size and number may be different, and nuclear-to-cytoplasm ratios are often higher in cultured cells. Studies of chemotaxis and phagocytic and oxidative killing have demonstrated that cells derived from serum-containing cultures are functional.[63,68]

Megakaryocyte differentiation follows similar patterns of differentiation, with sequential changes in antigen expression and morphology. There is much less proliferation; however, endoreplication continues, resulting in large polyploid mature cells that are normally at low frequencies of 0.1–0.5% in bone marrow. Early clonogenic progenitors are found within the CD34 population, and also express CD41.[76] They subsequently express CD4 transiently during an immature megakaryocyte stage.[77] As they mature, other platelet antigens are expressed, including CD61, CD36, CD49 and CD9.[78,79] In vitro cultures of mononuclear cells or CD34$^+$ cells have shown expansion of megakaryocyte CFC, with differentiation to mature megakaryocytes.[15,80] A number of factors including IL-3, IL-6, IL-11 and SCF, have been shown to stimulate earlier stages of megakaryocyte development, with thrombopoietin (c-mpl ligand) stimulating terminal maturation.[80] Generally, CD41a has been the most widely used to characterize immature and maturing megakaryocytes produced in vitro.

Overall, the characterization of culture-derived cells indicates that these precursors have the potential to differentiate into normal functional cells upon reinfusion. In moving these studies to the clinic, it will be important to have a thorough understanding of the composition of cell products tested. This will require a variety of assays to validate the cell composition produced in a culture system.

ISSUES AND CHALLENGES

Reliability

The strategy of using cultured cells as a supplement to augment engraftment does not endanger the patient to graft failure in the advent of culture failure or contamination. If, however, the cultured product is the sole support for transplantation, failure in the culturing process can be catastrophic and life-threatening to the patient. This requires systems used for this application to be very robust, and emphasizes designs that are reliable and that do not have catastrophic failure modes. The ability to cryopreserve the cultured cell product would diminish some of the absolute requirement for reliability, in that cells could be prepared in advance of the conditioning regimen to insure a safe and effective cell product. Cultured cells that have been aliquoted and cryopreserved would be useful for multiple cycles of therapy.

Reproducibility

Significant patient variability in expansion of progenitors has been observed, the source of which is not well understood. A complex process is required to produce cells ex vivo suggesting multiple sources of variability, including the following:

1. There may be inherent variability between cells from individual patients.
2. There may be adverse effects from the ex vivo processing prior to culture, such as fractionation from hydrodynamic damage, hypoxic conditions, and physical damage from enzymatic or physical release.
3. There may be variability in the culturing process related to differential consumption of factors or nutrients, as well as density or environmental effects from non-homogeneous distribution of cells within the culture. The biocompatibility of materials and surfaces can also affect the outcome, with the most primitive progenitors preferring stromal contact. When non-fractionated cells such as mononuclear cells are used, there can be effects of the non-proliferating contaminating cells, depending on their composition.

What are the strategies to diminish this variability? This becomes a critical area in developing therapies that are widely used. The key lies in controlling the process. Simplifying it through automation will provide more consistency and also control labor costs. Defining biocompatible materials and configurations will improve performance, as will better definition of nutrient and factor requirements, leading to better media. Control of feeding (or perfusion rates) will optimize the cell microenvironment and reduce variability in results. As this technology advances, the clinical application of cell culture will evolve from a highly technical art form requiring intensive knowledge and mastery to a routine non-labor-intensive activity. Although patient variability will always be an issue, advances in mobilization regimens as well as treatment of patients earlier in the course of their disease will likely help to dampen some of the interindividual variability.

CONCLUSIONS

The notion of using ex vivo expansion to produce therapeutic cell products is attractive for many reasons, and is part of a larger field of ex vivo cell and tissue engineering. Although there is great potential for the use of cultured hematopoietic cells, few clinical trials have established the value of this approach. In this rapidly moving field, where new cytokines are discovered almost monthly and effector cells within cell mixtures are more precisely defined every year, the balance shifts back and forth between cellular and cytokine therapies. A combined strategy will be based upon benefit as well as cost. Better methods for expanding cells in vivo, using the next generation of growth factors, may obviate some need for ex vivo expansion to provide primitive stem cells. For example, expansion of granulocytes in vivo in allogeneic donors or in autologous patients prior to transplant with improved cryopreservation techniques may provide one alternative to treating the period of absolute neutropenia. In addition, new factors, such as thrombopoietin, may influence the need for platelet transfusions and the requirements for the use of blood stem cells. In contrast, when the source of starting cells is limited, such as with cord blood or in patients who have had extensive prior chemotherapy and do not mobilize adequately, ex vivo expansion might be the only alternative. The development of technology to implement these processes will provide the tools to optimize the use of ex vivo expansion in the clinic.

REFERENCES

1. Vose JM, Armitage JO, Clinical applications of hematopoietic growth factors. *J Clin Oncol* 1995; **13**: 1023–35.
2. Pinto A, Gattei V, Soligo D et al, New molecules burst at the leukocyte surface. A comprehensive review based on the 15th International Workshop on Leukocyte Differentiation Antigens, Boston, USA, 3–7 November, 1993. *Leukemia* 1994; **8**: 347–58.
3. Stevens EJ, Jacknin L, Robbins PF et al, Generation of tumor-specific CTLs from melanoma patients by using peripheral blood stimulated with allogeneic melanoma tumor cell lines: Fine specificity and MART-1 melanoma antigen recognition. *J Immunol* 1995; **154**: 762–71.
4. Chang AE, Yoshizawa H, Sakai K et al, Clinical observations on adoptive immunotherapy with vaccine-primed T-lymphocytes secondarily sensitized to tumor in vitro. *Cancer Res* 1993; **53**: 1043–50.
5. Miller JS, Alley KA, McGlave P, Differentiation of natural killer (NK) cells from human primitive marrow progenitors in a stroma-based long-term culture system: identification of a CD34$^+$7$^+$ NK progenitor. *Blood* 1994; **83**: 2594–601.
6. Fefer A, Benyunes M, Higuchi C et al, Interleukin-2 ± lymphocytes as consolidative immunotherapy after autologous bone marrow transplantation for hematologic malignancies. *Acta Haematol* 1993; **89**(Suppl 1): 2–7.
7. To LB, Roberts MM, Haylock DN et al, Comparison of hematological recovery times and supportive care requirements of autologous recovery phase peripheral blood stem cell trans-

plants, autologous bone marrow transplants and allogeneic bone marrow transplants. *Bone Marrow Transplant* 1992; **9:** 277–84.

8. Turhan AG, Humphries RK, Phillips GL et al, Clonal hematopoiesis demonstrated by X-linked DNA polymorphisms after allogeneic bone marrow transplantation. *N Engl J Med* 1989; **320:** 1655–61.

9. Jones RJ, Celano P, Sharkis SJ, Sensenbrenner LL, Two phases of engraftment established by serial bone marrow transplantation in mice. *Blood* 1989; **73:** 397–401.

10. Rowley SD, Davis JM, Piantadosi S et al, Density-gradient separation of autologous bone marrow grafts before ex vivo purging with 4-hydroperoxycyclophosphamide. *Bone Marrow Transplant* 1990; **6:** 321–7.

11. Zijlmans JM, Kleiverda K, Heemskerk DPM et al, No role for committed progenitor cells in engraftment following transplantation of murine cytokine-mobilized blood cells [abstract]. *Blood* 1995; **86:** 435a.

12. Shpall EJ, Jones RB, Bearman SI et al, Transplantation of enriched CD34-positive autologous marrow into breast cancer patients following high-dose chemotherapy: influence of CD34-positive peripheral-blood progenitors and growth factors on engraftment. *J Clin Oncol* 1994; **12:** 28–36.

13. Haylock DN, To LB, Dowse TL et al, Ex vivo expansion and maturation of peripheral blood CD34$^+$ cells into the myeloid lineage. *Blood* 1992; **80:** 1405–12.

14. Williams SF, Lee WJ, Bender JG et al, Selection and expansion of peripheral blood CD34$^+$ cells in autologous stem cell transplantation for breast cancer. *Blood* 1996; **87:** 1687–91.

15. Qiao X, Loudovaris M, Unverzagt K et al, Immunochemistry and flow cytometry evaluation of human megakaryocytes in fresh samples and cultures of CD34$^+$ cells. *Cytometry* 1996; **23:** 250–9.

16. Brugger W, Heimfeld S, Berenson RJ et al, Reconstitution of hematopoiesis after high-dose chemotherapy by autologous progenitor cells generated ex vivo. *N Engl J Med* 1995; **333:** 283–7.

17. Wagner JEJ, Umbilical cord and placental blood transplantation: analysis of the clinical results. *J Hematother* 1993; **2:** 265–8.

18. Barnett MJ, Eaves CJ, Phillips GL et al, Successful autografting in chronic myeloid leukaemia after maintenance of marrow in culture *Bone Marrow Transplant* 1989; **4:** 345–51.

19. Brugger W, Vogel W, Scheding S et al, Epithelial tumor cells are not expanded concomitantly during cytokine-mediated ex vivo expansion of peripheral blood CD34$^+$ progenitor cells. *Blood* 1995; **86:** 1165A(Abst).

20. Sandstrom CE, Bender JG, Papoutsakis ET, Miller WM, Effects of CD34$^+$ cell selection and perfusion on ex vivo expansion of peripheral blood mononuclear cells. *Blood* 1995; **86:** 958–70.

21. Muench MO, Moore MAS, Accelerated recovery of peripheral blood cell counts in mice transplanted with in vitro cytokine-expanded hematopoietic progenitors. *Exp Hematol* 1992; **20:** 611–18.

22. Fabian I, Bleiberg I, Riklis I, Kletter Y, Enhanced reconstitution of hematopoietic organs in irradiated mice, following their transplantation with bone marrow cells pretreated with recombinant interleukin 3. *Exp Hematol* 1987; **15:** 1140–44.

23. Tavassoli M, Konno M, Shiota Y et al, Enhancement of the grafting efficency of transplanted marrow cells by preincubation with interleukin-3 and granulocyte macrophage colony-stimulating factor. *Blood* 1991; **77:** 1599–606.

24. Serrano F, Varas F, Bernad A, Bueren JA, Accelerated and long-term hematopoietic engraftment in mice transplanted with ex vivo expanded bone marrow. *Bone Marrow Transplant* 1994; **14:** 855–62.

25. Peters SO, Kittler EL, Ramshaw HS, Queensberry PJ, Ex vivo expansion of murine marrow cells with interleukin-3 (IL-3), IL-6, IL-11, and stem cell factor leads to impaired engraftment in irradiated hosts. *Blood* 1996; **87:** 30–7.

26. Bodine DM, Orlic D, Birkett NC et al, Stem cell factor increases colony-forming unit–spleen number in vitro in synergy with interleukin-6, and in vivo in Sl/Sld mice as a single factor. *Blood* 1992; **79:** 913–19.

27. Muench MO, Firpo MT, Moore MA, Bone marrow transplantation with interleukin-1 plus kit-ligand ex vivo expanded bone marrow accelerates hematopoietic reconstitution in mice without the loss of stem cell lineage and proliferative potential. *Blood* 1993; **81:** 3463–73.

28. Knobel KM, McNally MA, Berson AE et al, Long-term reconstitution of mice after ex vivo expansion of bone marrow cells: Differential activity of cultured bone marrow and enriched stem cell populations. *Exp Hematol* 1994; **22:** 1227–35.

29. Holyoake TL, Freshney MG, McNair L et al, Ex

vivo expansion with stem cell factor and inter-leukin-11 augments both short term recovery posttransplant and the ability to serially transplant marrow. *Blood* 1996; **87:** 4589–95.

30. Smith SL, Bender Jg, Maples PB et al, expansion of neutrophil precursors and progenitors in suspension cultures CD34$^+$ cells enriched from human bone marrow. *Exp Hematol* 1993; **21:** 870–7.

31. Naparstek E, Hardan Y, Ben-Shahar M et al, Enhanced marrow recovery by short term preincubation of marrow allografts with human recombinant interleukin-3 and granulocyte-macrophage colony stimulating factor. *Blood* 1992; **80:** 1673–8.

32. Atkinson K, Bartlett A, Dodds A, Rallings M, Lack of efficacy of a short ex vivo incubation of human allogeneic donor marrow with recombinant human GM-CSF prior to its infusion into the recipient. *Bone Marrow Transplant* 1994; **14:** 573–7.

33. Chang Q, Hanks S, Akard L et al, Maturation of mobilized peripheral blood progenitor cells: preclinical and phase 1 clinical studies. *J Hematother* 1996; **4:** 289–97.

34. Gluck S, Chadderton T, Porter K et al, Characterization and transfusion of in vitro cultivated hematopoietic progenitor cells *Transfus Sci* 1995; **16:** 273–81.

35. Caspar CB, Seger RA, Burger J, Gmur J, Effective stimulation of donors for granulocyte transfusions with recombinant methionyl granulocyte colony-stimulating factor. *Blood* 1993; **81:** 2866–71.

36. Alcorn MJ, Holyoake TL, Richmond L et al, CD34-positive cells isolated from cryopreserved peripheral blood progenitor cells can be expanded ex vivo and used for transplantation with little or no toxicity [abstract]. *J Clin Oncol* 1996; **14:** 1839–47.

37. Holyoake TL, Alcorn MJ, Richmond L et al, A phase 1 study to evaluate the safety of re-infusing CD34 cells expanded ex vivo as part or all of a PBPC transplant procedure [abstract]. *Blood* 1995; **86:** 1161.

38. Dancey JT, Duebelbeiss KA, Harker LA, Finch CA, Neutrophil kinetics in man. *J Clin Invest* 1976; **58:** 705–9.

39. Bender JG, To LB, Williams SF, Schwartzberg L, Defining a therapeutic dose of peripheral blood stem cells. *J Hematother* 1992; **1:** 329–41.

40. Sutherland HJ, Eaves CJ, Eaves AC et al, Characterization and partial purification of human marrow cells capable of initiating long-term hematopoiesis in vitro. *Blood* 1989; **74:** 1563–70.

41. Vormoor J, Lapidot T, Pflumio F et al, Immature human cord blood progenitors engraft and proliferate to high levels in severe combined immunodeficient mice. *Blood* 1994; **83:** 2489–97.

42. Henschler R, Brugger W, Luft T et al, Maintenance of transplantation potential in ex vivo expanded CD34(+)-selected human peripheral blood progenitor cells. *Blood* 1994; **84:** 2898–903.

43. Fraser CC, Eaves CJ, Szilvassy SJ, Humphries RK, Expansion in vitro of retrovirally marked totipotent hematopoietic stem cells. *Blood* 1990; **76:** 1071–6.

44. Koller MR, Emerson SG, Palsson BO, Large scale expansion of human stem and progenitor cells from bone marrow mononuclear cells in continuous perfusion culture. *Blood* 1993; **82:** 378–84.

45. Verfaillie CM, Miller JS, CD34$^+$/CD33$^-$ cells reselected from macrophage inflammatory protein 1alpha + interleukin-3-supplemented 'stromalnoncontact' cultures are highly enriched for long-term bone marrow culture initiating cells. *Blood* 1994; **84:** 1442–9.

46. Lansdorp PM, Dragowska W, Mayani H, Ontogeny-related changes in proliferative potential of human hematopoietic cells. *J Exp Med* 1993; **178:** 787–91.

47. Tavassoli M, Expansion of blood stem cell pool or mobilization of its marrow counterpart? *Exp Hematol* 1993; **21:** 1205–6.

48. Tibken B, Hofer EP, A biomathematical model of granulocytopoiesis for estimation of stem cell numbers. *Stem Cells* 1995; **13**(Suppl 1): 283–9.

49. Scheding S, Franke H, Brugger W et al, How many post-progenitor cells have to be transplanted to completely abrogate neutropenia after high-dose chemotherapy and peripheral blood progenitor cell transplantation? [abstract]. *Blood* 1995; **86:** 884a.

50. Muul LM, Director EP, Hyatt CL, Rosenberg SA, Large scale production of human lymphokine activated killer cells for use in adoptive immunotherapy. *J Immunol Meth* 1986; **88:** 265–75.

51. Carter CS, Leitman SF, Cullis H et al, Technical aspects of lymphokine-activated killer cell production. *J Clin Apheresis* 1988; **4:** 113–17.

52. Zimmerman TM, Bender JG, Lee WJ et al, Large scale selection of CD34$^+$ peripheral blood progenitors and expansion of neutrophil precursors

for clinical applications. *J Hematother* 1996; **5:** 247–54.

53. Koller MR, Manchel I, Newsom BS et al, Bioreactor expansion of human bone marrow: Comparison of unprocessed, density-separated, and CD34 enriched cells. *J Hematother* 1995; **4:** 159–69.

54. Zandstra PW, Eaves CJ, Piret JM, Expansion of hematopoietic progenitor cell populations in stirred suspension bioreactors of normal human bone marrow cells. *Biotechnology* 1994; **12:** 909–14.

55. Sardonini CA, Wu YJ, Expansion and differentiation of human hematopoietic cells from static cultures through small-scale bioreactors. *Biotechnol Prog* 1993; **9:** 131–7.

56. Koller MR, Bender JG, Miller WM, Papoutsakis ET, Expansion of primitive human hematopoietic progenitors in a perfusion bioreactor system with IL-3, IL-6, and stem cell factor. *Biotechnology* 1993; **11:** 358–63.

57. Freedman RS, Edwards CL, Kavanaugh JJ et al, Intraperitoneal adoptive immunotherapy of ovarian carcinoma with tumor-infiltrating lymphocytes and low-dose recombinant interleukin-2: A pilot trial. *J Immunother* 1994; **16:** 198–210.

58. McAdams TA, Sandstrom CE, Miller WM et al, Ex vivo expansion of primitive hematopoietic cells for cellular therapies: An overview. *Cytotechnology* 1996; **18:** 133–46.

59. Moore MA, Expansion of myeloid stem cells in culture. *Semin Hematol* 1995; **32:** 183–200.

60. Emerson SG, Ex vivo expansion of hematopoietic precursors, progenitors and stem cells: The next generation of cellular therapeutics. *Blood* 1996; **87:** 3082–8.

61. Barnett MJ, Eaves CJ, Phillips GL et al, autografting with cultured marrow in chronic myeloid leukemia: results of a pilot study. *Blood* 1994; **84:** 724–32.

62. Sato N, Sawada K, Koizumi K et al, In vitro expansion of human peripheral blood CD34+ cells. *Blood* 1993; **82:** 3600–9.

63. Lill MC, Lynch M, Fraser JK et al, Production of functional myeloid cells from CD34-selected hematopoietic progenitor cells using a clinically relevant ex vivo expansion system. *Stem Cells* 1994; **12:** 626–37.

64. Sandstrom CE, Collins PC, McAdams TA et al, Comparison of serum-deprived media for the ex vivo expansion of hematopoietic progenitor cells from cord blood and peripheral blood mononuclear cells. *J Hematother* 1996 **5:** 461–73.

65. Shapiro F, Yao TJ, Raptis G et al, Optimization of conditions for ex vivo expansion of CD34+ cells from patients with stage IV breast cancer. *Blood* 1994; **84:** 3567–74.

66. Kuter DJ, Gminski DM, Rosenberg RD, Transforming growth factor beta inhibits megakaryocyte growth and endomitosis. *Blood* 1992; **79:** 619–26.

67. Loudovaris M, Smith S, Schilling M et al, Human plasma as a supplement to media for the culture of human CD34+ cells [abstract]. *Blood* 1993; **82:** 650a.

68. Frenck RW, Ventura GJ, Krannig G et al, Studies of the function and structure of in vitro propagated human granulocytes. *Pediatr Res* 1991; **30:** 135–40.

69. Terstappen LW, Safford M, Loken MR, Flow cytometric analysis of human bone marrow. III. Neutrophil maturation. *Leukemia* 1990; **4:** 657–63.

70. Olweus J, Lund Johansen F, Terstappen LW, CD64/Fc gamma RI is a granulo-monocytic lineage marker on CD34+ hematopoietic progenitor cells. *Blood* 1995; **85:** 2402–13.

71. Kerst JM, Slaper-Cortenbach ICM, von dem Borne AEG et al, Combined measurement of growth and differentiation in suspension cultures of purified CD34 positive cells enables a detailed analysis of myelopoiesis. *Exp Hematol* 1992; **20:** 1188–93.

72. Terstappen LW, Buescher S, Nguyen M, Reading C, Differentiation and maturation of growth factor expanded human hematopoietic progenitors assessed by multidimensional flow cytometry. *Leukemia* 1992; **6:** 1001–10.

73. Bender JG, Smith SL, Unverzagt KL, Ex vivo expansion of neutrophil precursors from blood CD34+ cells: Applications for the treatment of neutropenia. In: *Hematopoietic Stem Cells: Biology and Therapeutic Applications* (Levitt D, Mertelsmann R, eds), 1995: 171–84.

74. Scheding S, Buhring HJ, Ziegler B et al, Ex-vivo generation of myeloid post-progenitor cells from mobilized peripheral blood CD34+ cells [abstract]. *Blood* 1995; **86:** 912a.

75. Ezekowitz RAB, Sieff CA, Dinauer MC et al, Restoration of phagocytic function by interferon-gamma in X-linked chronic granulomatous disease occurs at the level of a progenitor cell. *Blood* 1990; **76:** 2443–8.

76. Zucker-Franklin D, Yany J, Grusky G, Characterization of glycoprotein IIb/IIIa-positive cells in human umbilical cord blood: their

potential usefulness as megakaryocyte progenitors. *Blood* 1992; **79:** 347–55.

77. Dolzhanskiy A, Basch RS, Karpatkin S, Development of human megakaryocytes: I. Hematopoietic progenitors (CD34$^+$ bone marrow cells) are enriched with megakaryocytes expressing CD4. *Blood* 1996; **87:** 1353–60.

78. Civin CI, Human monomyeloid cell membrane antigens. *Exp Hematol* 1990; **18:** 461–7.

79. Debili N, Issaad C, Massi JM et al, Expression of CD34 and platelet glycoproteins during human megakaryocytic differentiation. *Blood* 1992; **80:** 3022–35.

80. Kaushansky K, Broudy VC, Lin N et al, Thrombopoietin, the Mp1 ligand, is essential for full megakaryocyte development *Proc Natl Acad Sci USA* 1995; **92:** 3234–8.

10

Allogeneic blood stem cell transplantation

Peter Dreger and Norbert Schmitz

CONTENTS • **Introduction** • **Rationale for allogeneic PBSC transplantation** • **Harvesting PBSC from healthy donors** • **Cellular composition of PBSC grafts** • **Haematopoietic capacity of allogeneic PBSC in vivo** • **GVHR reactions** • **GVL activity** • **Graft engineering** • **Conclusions**

INTRODUCTION

Allogeneic transplantation of haematopoietic stem cells has proven to be an effective treatment for a variety of otherwise incurable diseases, such as chronic myeloid leukaemia, relapsed acute leukaemias and refractory severe aplastic anaemia. For decades, bone marrow (BM) has been the only source of haematopoietic tissue that could be used for allotransplantation. However, harvesting a BM graft provides only a limited number of stem cells and requires a surgical procedure associated with significant risks and discomfort for the donor. Therefore attempts to use blood instead of marrow for allogeneic transplantation were made as early as 30 years ago.[1] Experience from autologous transplantation showed that, in principle, peripheral blood stem cells (PBSC) obtained during steady state could be used for haematopoietic reconstitution of a myeloablated host. Such PBSC did not have striking advantages over autologous BM stem cells in terms of engraftment, but required extensive leukapheresis for collecting sufficient progenitor cell numbers.[2,3] Therefore the use of unmobilized PBSC for allogeneic transplantation was not a reasonable alternative to BM

transplantation (BMT); only a single case of successful allogeneic transplantation of unprimed PBSC has been reported.[4]

With the availability of haematopoietic growth factors, however, harvesting of large numbers of PBSC with few leukapheresis procedures became possible, allowing rapid reconstitution of marrow function after autologous transplantation.[5,6] Given these promising results, trials were initiated to determine whether the main advantages of mobilized PBSC, namely improving the convenience of the donor while providing larger stem numbers and faster haematopoietic recovery, could be transferred to the allogeneic setting.

RATIONALE FOR ALLOGENEIC PBSC TRANSPLANTATION

Allogeneic PBSC transplantation (PBSCT) may have benefits for both the donor and the recipient. The donor avoids the risks and discomfort of the marrow collection procedure, including general anaesthesia, and the cells may be harvested in an outpatient setting. The recipient may experience a more rapid recovery of haematopoiesis and of the immune system, which should reduce treatment-related morbidity, facilitate earlier discharge from hospital and decrease costs. In addition, the large number of lymphocytes conferred with PBSC grafts may enhance graft-versus-leukaemia (GVL) effects. On the other hand, graft-versus-host (GVH) reactions (GVHR) might also be increased after allo-PBSC transplantation. A disadvantage for the donor is the need to undergo leukapheresis. Furthermore, the long-term risks of growth factor administration cannot be precisely evaluated at present.

Thus the most important issues that have to be considered with regard to allo-PBSC transplantation include (1) the safety of the donor, (2) the optimum schedule of PBSC mobilization and harvesting, (3) the haematopoietic capacity of the graft, (4) the immunological characteristics of the graft and their impact on GVH and GVL reactivity, and (5) approaches to manipulate the cellular components of PBSC grafts ex vivo ('graft engineering').

HARVESTING PBSC FROM HEALTHY DONORS

Safety

Since the number of circulating progenitor cells is very small during steady-state conditions ($<5 \times 10^3$ CD34$^+$ cells per ml blood), successful harvesting of PBSC from healthy individuals requires mobilization with haematopoietic growth factors. Granulocyte colony-stimulating factor (G-CSF) is routinely used for this purpose – not only because it appears (as opposed to granulocyte–macrophage colony-stimulating factor (GM-CSF)) to be devoid of T-cell-activating properties,[7,8] but, above all, because it is currently the safest among the agents available for PBSC priming. The predominant side-effect of G-CSF is bone pain, which occurs in the vast majority of donors receiving G-CSF at doses of 7.5 µg/kg/day or more (Table 10.1). The bone pain usually responds well to peripheral analgesics like acetaminophen (paracetamol) and disappears after withdrawal of G-CSF. In addition, 10–30% of healthy individuals treated with G-CSF suffer from symptoms such as headache, fatigue and nausea.[9–11]

Whereas the serum levels of sodium, calcium, urea, creatinine, uric acid and bilirubin remain largely unchanged during G-CSF administration, reversible moderate increases of alkaline phosphatase and lactate dehydrogenase are observed in some donors. Serum potassium tends to decline to subnormal levels with G-CSF administration, necessitating occasional oral potassium substitution. These phenomena are probably due to the increased neutrophil turnover induced by G-CSF.[12] G-CSF results in a rapid and dose-dependent leukocytosis (up to $(50–70) \times 10^9/l$ with 10 µg/kg), but has no immediate influence on haemoglobin levels and platelet counts.[9,12,13] However, some investigators have observed a delayed moderate decrease of platelets, which can occur 6–9 days after start of G-CSF administration in healthy individuals.[9] Since leukapheresis causes additional thrombocyte losses, platelet counts as low as $33 \times 10^9/l$ have occasionally been observed in donors of allogeneic PBSC.[10,12,14] The mechanisms responsible for thrombocytopenia following G-CSF administration are not clear; it has been suggested that platelet production might be downregulated by a direct or indirect effect of higher doses of G-CSF. Another possible explanation could be that the expanding granulopoiesis stimulated by G-CSF suppresses the thrombopoiesis in healthy donors. Although bleeding complications have rarely been observed, some authors recommend re-infusion of apheresed platelets to minimize the risk of critical thrombocytopenia if prolonged G-CSF administration and repeated leukapheresis procedures are necessary, e.g. for harvesting large numbers of PBSC for ex vivo manipulation.[10] After G-CSF is stopped, a transient mild neutropenia may occur, which might be due to the inhibitory activity of other cytokines involved in the regulation of granulopoiesis or to suppression of endogenous G-CSF production.[15]

Although long-term adverse effects cannot be definitely ruled out at this time, G-CSF has been administered safely to large cohorts of patients for treatment of neutropenia or for

Table 10.1 Toxicity of PBSC harvesting: overview of clinical results

Authors	n	G-CSF dose (µg/kg)	Bone pain (%)	Pneumothorax (n/CVA)[a]	Other complications
Dreger et al 1994[12]	9	5–10	78	0/5	0
Azevedo et al 1995[14]	17	10	100	0/0	0
Russell et al 1995[82]	14	6–8	100	1/14	0
Griggs et al 1995[11]	30	3–10	93	0/0	0
Bensinger et al 1996[10]	124	4–16	30	0	Myocardial infarction = 1 Angina pectoris = 1
Dreger et al 1996[36]	42	5–16	90	0/20	Hypocalcaemia = 1 Angina pectoris = 1
Harada et al 1996[33]	9	5–15	100	0/0	0
Rosenfeld et al 1996[83]	19	16	70	0/14	0
Bacigalupo et al 1996[51]	31	10	48	0/1	Hypocalcaemia = 1
Höglund et al 1996[13]	24	3–10	71	0/0	0
Urbano-Ispizua et al 1996[84]	33	4–16	100	1/3	0
Martinez et al 1996[85]	20	10	n.a.	0/0	0
Total	348	4–16	69	2/52	5

[a] Number of patients with pneumothorax/number of patients with central venous access.

PBSC mobilization, and to a considerable number of healthy subjects such as granulocyte donors[10,12,16,18] and volunteers.[19-21] With the longest follow-up being more than four years, no case of late adverse events, in particular neoplastic diseases, have been reported so far.[22,23] Furthermore, BM aspirates of normal donors who received G-CSF five years ago showed no evidence of morphological or cytogenetic abnormalities.[24] Even though G-CSF can stimulate leukaemic blasts under certain conditions in vitro, there is so far no evidence that it exerts leukaemogeneic effects in vivo.[25,26] It is noteworthy that strongly elevated G-CSF levels can also occur due to endogenous release of G-CSF, e.g. during severe infections.[27]

The risks of leukapheresis are low when carried out in an appropriate setting. Among the 348 patients included in the 12 studies reviewed in Table 10.1, one case of myocardial infarction shortly after leukapheresis for PBSC collection has been reported, and two other donors had angina pectoris-like symptoms during leukapheresis. In addition, some donors complained of dysaesthesia during leukapheresis, which was severe in two cases. These symptoms were probably due to a transient hypocalcaemia induced by ACD-A used for anticoagulation during the separation. Approximately 10% of the donors needed a central venous access to assure adequate blood flow. Placement of subclavian or internal jugular catheters was complicated by a pneumothorax on 2 of 52 occasions. Overall, leukapheresis is not a trivial procedure without any risk, but appropriate selection of donors (i.e. exclusion of individuals with cardiovascular risk factors or poor peripheral veins) should help to minimize serious complications.

On the other hand, BM harvesting under general anaesthesia has been reported to be associated with an up to 0.4% incidence of life-threatening complications, which may be reduced to 0.1–0.2% by excluding donors with risk factors such as cardiovascular disease, obesity or greater age.[28,29] In addition, BM collection can result in considerable morbidity due to soft tissue and bone trauma; nausea and associated symptoms occur in a large proportion of donors as a consequence of general anaesthesia. Taken together, the risks of G-CSF priming and leukapheresis in healthy donors appear to be acceptable if compared with those of BM collection.

The only other cytokine that has been used for PBSC mobilization in healthy donors is GM-CSF. Besides its unfavourable toxicity profile, GM-CSF seems to be inferior to G-CSF because of a lower mobilization efficacy.[30,31] The combined use of G-CSF and GM-CSF does not significantly increase the PBSC yield compared with G-CSF alone,[31] while it exposes the donor to the toxicities and potential risks of both cytokines.

Timing of leukapheresis and factors influencing the yield

The peak of CD34[+] cells in the peripheral blood usually occurs on day 5 after the start of G-CSF administration (i.e. after four daily doses of G-CSF), implying that leukapheresis should be commenced after 3–5 days of mobilization. These kinetics were originally described in donors primed with 10 µg/kg,[12] but subsequently confirmed for a variety of doses between 3 and 16 µg/kg,[10,11,32–34] In spite of continued cytokine administration, the levels of circulating progenitor cells significantly decrease after day 7, indicating that appropriate timing of PBSC collection is mandatory to achieve optimum results.[35]

G-CSF at a dose of 10 µg/kg gave significantly higher CD34[+] cell yields than at a dose of 3–5 µg/kg,[11,13] suggesting that the mobilization efficacy depends on the amount of G-CSF used. The use of doses as high as 16 µg/kg may further increase the PBSC yield.[10] Mobilization with 10–16 µg/kg allows harvesting of sufficient numbers of CD34[+] cells with one or two leukapheresis procedures[23,26] in the vast majority of donors. Among 35 donors of allogeneic PBSC primed with 10 µg/kg of filgrastim, we observed only one individual yielding less than 1×10^6/kg CD34[+] cells per 10 l collection volume, while 43% reached the target dose of 4×10^6/kg with a single leukapheresis (Table 10.2). The Houston group reported that 94% of 32 healthy donors stimulated with 12 µg/kg of G-CSF yielded 4×10^6/kg CD34[+] cells or more with a single leukapheresis when PBSC collection was commenced on day 5, whereas only 67% of 45 individuals starting leukapheresis on day 4 reached the target dose on the first day ($p < 0.05$).[34] These data illustrate that an adequate stem cell yield can be achieved with few collections if the harvesting procedure is scheduled properly.

CELLULAR COMPOSITION OF PBSC GRAFTS

Similar to BM, the CD34[+] cells contained in G-CSF-mobilized PBSC allografts comprise a variety of subpopulations, including immature progenitor cells as indicated by negativity for the CD33 or CD38 antigens or co-expression of the CD90 or CD117 antigens (Figure 10.1), and progenitor cells committed to the lymphoid lineages.[20] From animal studies in vitro[37] and in vivo,[38] as well as from humans in vitro,[33] there is an ever-growing body of data indicating that stem cells or cells capable of restoring complete haematopoiesis are contained in G-CSF-

Table 10.2 Harvesting PBSC from healthy donors: CD34⁺ yield (data from 41 individuals treated at Kiel University)

G-CSF dose (μg/kg)	<10	10
n	6	35
CD34⁺ cells ($\times 10^6$/kg/graft)[a]	4.8 (1.5–8.1)	5.5 (1–21.3)
CD34⁺ cells ($\times 10^6$/kg/10 l)[b]	2.4 (0.8–4.1)	3.3 (0.9–10.7)
Donors achieving >4 × 10⁶/kg CD34⁺ cells with a single apheresis	1 (17%)	15 (43%)

[a] Leukaphereses were started on day 5 of G-CSF administration.
[b] Leukapheresis volume.

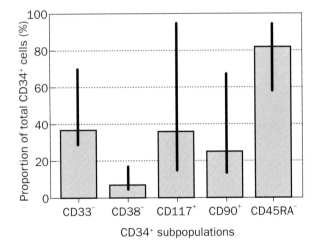

Figure 10.1 Subpopulations of CD34⁺ cells contained in mobilized PBSC products collected from healthy donors.

mobilized CD34⁺ cells. The numbers of long-term culture-initiating cells (LTCIC), which are the most primitive human progenitor cells that can be assayed in vitro, in G-CSF-mobilized blood are comparable to those found in BM.[39]

Compared with values observed in allogeneic marrow grafts, PBSC harvests contain about one log more T cells.[12] This is not only important with regard to potential GVH and GVL activities of the graft, but also has implications for the reconstitution of the immune system post transplant. Recent studies suggest that T-cell regeneration in adult recipients after allogeneic transplantation is mainly determined by the number of mature T cells contained in the allograft.[40] Thus allogeneic PBSC transplantation may be associated with an acceleration of both haematopoietic and immune recovery. Preliminary data indicate that the recovery of T-cell numbers and function after allo-PBSCT is indeed faster than after BMT, resulting in a normalization of the CD4 : CD8 ratio as early as 6 months after transplant, whereas in the BM recipients the CD4 counts remain low for 12 months or longer.[41]

Although all subpopulations contribute to this excess of T cells, detailed subset analyses suggest that the T cells present in PBSC grafts are not only quantitatively but also qualitatively different from those found in BM: Negrin et al[42] reported that a large proportion of CD3[+]CD4[-]CD8[-] T cells is present in PBSC allografts. These cells are believed to play a regulatory role in the development of GVHR. We and two other groups, however, observed much smaller fractions of double negative T cells in allogeneic PBSC products, which were not substantially different from the percentages observed in allogeneic marrow grafts.[18,36,41] Therefore, additional studies have to be performed to clarify the role of this interesting subset in the T-cell repertoire of blood stem cell grafts.

Moreover, murine studies have demonstrated that the T cells contained in G-CSF-mobilized PBSC grafts express predominantly a type 2 cytokine pattern (interleukin (IL)-4 production), whereas the majority of peripheral blood T cells of mice not exposed to G-CSF shows a type 1 pattern (IL-2/interferon-γ production).[8] Interestingly, type 2 T cells can attenuate acute GVHR after allogeneic BMT.[43] In comparison to marrow grafts, PBSC harvests are also characterized by an increased proportion of NK cells,[12] which may be important for GVL activities.[44]

HAEMATOPOIETIC CAPACITY OF ALLOGENEIC PBSC IN VIVO

Primary transplantation of G-CSF-primed PBSC to syngeneic recipients after myeloablative therapy consistently resulted in rapid and sustained haematopoietic recovery. Similar to our experience in five identical twins showing neutrophil and platelet engraftment on day +10 and +9, respectively, the Seattle group observed recovery of neutrophils to more than $0.5 \times 10^9/l$ after 12.5 days and recovery of platelets to more than $20 \times 10^9/l$ after 11 days in five syngeneic recipients.[45,46] These figures compared favourably with a historical Seattle series of 34 transplants using syngeneic BM grafts, where the critical values for both neutrophils and platelets were reached on day +16.[47]

Similarly, the engraftment seen after allogeneic primary transplantation of PBSC is both complete and durable.[23,48,49] The speed of haematopoietic recovery after allo-PBSCT, however, is much more variable than after syngeneic or autologous transplantation. The main reason for this is the genetic difference between donor and recipient, which may delay engraftment per se, causes complications such as GVHR or viral infections, and necessitates the use of cytotoxic drugs like methotrexate. Nevertheless, the reconstitution of haematopoiesis after allogeneic PBSCT seemed to be more rapid than in historical BM controls.[23,49] This impression is supported by the data from larger series reported recently. Table 10.3 summarizes the results of five studies comprising a total of 188 patients. The median time to achieve a neutrophil count of more than $0.5 \times 10^9/l$ and a platelet count of more than $20 \times 10^9/l$ ranged from 14 to 15 days and from 10 to 16 days respectively.[14,50–53] In Seattle, the first 37 patients receiving allogeneic PBSC were compared with 37 historical patients allografted with BM in a matched-pair analysis. A significant difference in favour of the PBSC group was found with regard to neutrophil and platelet engraftment (14 vs 16 and 11 vs 15 days respectively), and the number of red blood cell units transfused (8 vs 17 units). Moreover, the proportion of patients not achieving a durable platelet recovery tended to be lower after PBSCT (14 vs 32%, $p = 0.097$).[54]

An important factor that adversely affects engraftment is the use of methotrexate post transplant,[50,52] while a significant correlation between the speed of engraftment and the number of CD34[+] cells infused cannot be shown yet. Although prompt engraftment was seen with CD34[+] cell numbers below $2 \times 10^6/kg$,[52] above $(4–5) \times 10^6/kg$ are currently regarded as a minimum target dose to ensure engraftment.

The engraftment of allogeneic PBSC is durable, as shown by molecular analysis of chimaerism and blood-group typing.[48,49] The strong haematopoietic capacity of G-CSF-mobilized PBSC is also underlined by trials using PBSC boosts for treatment of engraftment failure of marrow grafts. Similarly to our initial experience, PBSC rescue is successful in a considerable number of patients with non-engraftment after BMT.[22,55,56]

Table 10.3 Haematopoietic recovery and GVHR after allo-PBSCT

Authors	n	ANC >0.5 × 10⁹/l (days)	Platelets >20 × 10⁹/l (days)	Acute GVHR III–IV (%)	Chronic GVHR (%)
Azevedo et al 1995[14]	17	14	14	24	NR[a]
Bensinger et al 1996[50]	40	14	10	13	32
Bacigalupo et al 1996[51]	31	14	14	13	79
Schmitz et al 1997[52]	59	15	16	25	52
Miflin et al 1997[53]	41	14	14	14	43

[a] NR = not reported.

GVHR

Since T cells are the main effector cells of both acute and chronic GVHR, it was a major concern that the large numbers of T cells contained in PBSC grafts might give rise to an increased incidence of severity of GVHR. However, the initial impression was that the incidence of acute GVHR may be even lower than with allogeneic BMT, in particular when severe GVHR are considered.[23,48,49] With increasing patient numbers, it became evident that with standard immunosuppression there is no striking difference between PBSCT and BMT with regard to acute GVHR. In the five larger series mentioned earlier, grade II–IV disease was observed in 38–66% of patients, and grade III–IV in 13–25% (Table 10.3);[14,50–53] this seems similar to what would have been expected after allogeneic BMT. The Seattle matched-pair analysis also suggests that the risk of grade II–IV and grade III-IV GVHR is not higher after PBSCT than after BMT (37% and 14% vs 56% and 33% respectively).[54]

It is not yet understood why the high numbers of T cells infused with the PBSC grafts do not induce an increase of acute GVHR. However, it has been shown earlier that the absolute number of T cells in an allogeneic graft may not be the crucial factor determining the severity of GVHR.[57] Given that a critical number of T cells is already present in the graft, the quality (i.e. specificity) rather than the quantity of donor T cells seems to be the more important determinant influencing GVHR intensity. Another explanation could be that – as already mentioned – the development of GVHR is modulated by regulatory T-cell subsets predominating in PBSC grafts.

Due to the limited number of patients with sufficient follow-up, definite conclusions concerning the impact of allogeneic PBSCT on chronic GVHR cannot be drawn. In the studies previously mentioned, 32–79% of patients at risk developed limited or extensive chronic GVHR (Table 10.3). With one exception, all authors concluded that the incidence of chronic GVHR observed in the respective series seemed comparable to that expected after BMT. It has to be taken into account that the vast majority of these first patients were older or had other risk factors known to be associated with an increase of chronic GVHR. The currently ongoing randomized studies will provide more accurate information on this issue.

GVL ACTIVITY

Since the antileukaemic effects of allogeneic stem cell grafts are mediated predominantly by T cells and NK cells[44,58] the infusion of the large lymphocyte numbers conferred with PBSC allografts could result in increased GVL activity. Although it is far too early for valid conclusions to be drawn, preliminary data observed in patients with CML suggest that complete eradication of disease as revealed by *bcr/abl* PCR may indeed occur more often after PBSCT than after BMT.[59] This is in accordance with our own experience obtained in a mouse model comparing the GVL activity of PBSC and BM allografts: in an MHC-matched setting, transplantation of unmanipulated PBSC into lethally irradiated recipients who had been contaminated with the B-lymphoblastic leukaemia A20 resulted in a reduction of the relapse rate to 29%, which was significantly lower than the relapse rate of 60% observed after transfusion of identical numbers of unmanipulated marrow cells ($p < 0.05$).[60]

Additional evidence for superior in vivo GVL activity of PBSC comes from studies aiming at treatment of leukaemic relapse after BMT using allogeneic PBSC boosts. In comparison with the infusion of unmobilized donor leukocyte infusions (DLI), the potential advantages of PBSC are (1) rapid recovery of donor haematopoiesis without prolonged cytopenias; (2) the possibility to reduce patients' tumour cell load by myelosuppressive chemotherapy prior to PBSC infusion; (3) a possible competition of donor-derived progenitor cells with the malignant clone;[61] (4) a reduction of DLI-associated GVHR due to immune-modulating effects of G-CSF during mobilization. Preliminary data obtained by us and others indicate that indeed durable remissions can be achieved after transfusion of donor-derived mobilized PBSC in patients relapsing with chronic myeloid leukaemia (CML) or acute myeloid leukaemia (AML) after allogeneic BMT. Even in patients who received additional chemotherapy, extensive cytopenias as observed after conventional DLI could be largely avoided, whereas devastating GVHR did not occur.[62,63] Altogether, these observations suggest that mobilized allogeneic PBSC boosts hold promise for immunotherapeutic approaches after allogeneic stem cell transplantation.

GRAFT ENGINEERING

Successful attempts to manipulate allogeneic BM grafts for eliminating GVH-reactive cells were already undertaken in the 1970s.[64] In the clinical situation, however, T-cell depletion (TCD) of marrow grafts has been hampered by two major drawbacks, which were responsible for its overall disappointing results: the reduction of mortality due to GVHR was offset by (1) a dramatic rise in the incidence of engraftment failure and (2) a strongly increased relapse rate[65] due to unspecific stem cell loss and elimination of GVL activity from the graft. To this end, PBSC may help to avoid these problems because of the 'unlimited' amounts of stem cells and immunomodulatory cells that can be harvested from mobilized blood as opposed to BM.

In conjunction with the recent progress in cell separation technology, PBSC appear to be a perfect source for ex vivo graft engineering. We have previously reported that 3–4 logs of T cells can be depleted from PBSC grafts by CD34[+] selection.[66] Meanwhile, others have confirmed these data and used CD34[+]-selected PBPC grafts for clinical allotransplantation[67–71] (Table 10.4). Surprisingly, acute GVHR occurred in a significant proportion of patients in spite of transplanting fewer than 1×10^5/kg T cells. Before the era of CD34[+] selection, it was generally accepted that T-cell numbers higher than 1×10^5/kg are required for the development of GVHR.[72] However, these earlier estimations were based on limiting dilution assays, which are obviously not as precise as immunophenotypic analyses. Therefore more vigorous TCD appears to be necessary for effectively preventing GVHR. Double purging strategies employing CD34[+] selection in combination with T-cell-specific antibodies can achieve TCD of more than 4 log and result in complete elimination of GVHR even in a haplo-identical setting[73–75] (Table 10.5). The incidence of graft failure was very low in these preliminary trials,

Table 10.4 TCD of allo-PBSC using CD34$^+$ selection: clinical experience in HLA-identical siblings

Authors	Device	n	CD34$^+$ ($\times 10^6$/kg)	Neutrophils >0.5 $\times 10^9$/l (days)	Platelets >20 $\times 10^9$/l (days)	Methotrexate[a]	CD3$^+$ ($\times 10^5$/kg)	GVHR II–IV (III–IV)
Link et al 1996[67]	Cellpro	5	6.7	10	13	No	13.5	5/5 (4/5)
	Cellpro	5	8.4	14	16	Yes	6.7	1/5 (1/5)
Finke et al 1996[68]	Cellpro	15	4.3	10	15	No	4.5	3/12 (0/12)
Bensinger et al 1996[69]	Cellpro	5	10.1	13[b]	11	No	9.0	4/5 (3/5)
		5		19[b]	25	Yes		5/5 (2/5)
Bensinger et al 1996[70]	Isolex	20	6.4	13[b]	9	No	0.8	11/5 (2/16)
Corringham and Ho 1995[71]	Isolex	2	>4	10–11	11–12	No	0.3–3	1/2 (0/2)

[a] Short-course methotrexate post transplant.
[b] G-CSF was *not* given post transplant.

Table 10.5 TCD of allo-PBSC using double purging approaches: preliminary clinical experience with haplo-identical recipients

Authors	TCD[a]	n	Age (years)	CD34+ ($\times 10^6$/kg)	CD3+ ($\times 10^5$/kg)	GVHR (III–IV)
Wiesneth et al 1996[73]	Cellpro CD34+ + CD2 beads	7	7 (1–13)	1	0.3	0/7
Handgretinger et al 1996[74]	Cellpro CD34+ + MACS CD34+	6	<18	17	0.6	0/5
Martelli et al 1996[75]	E⁻ + Cellpro CD34+	24	24 (6–48)	13	0.3	0

[a] MACS = Supermacs System (Miltenyi Biotec, Bergisch Gladbach, Germany). E⁻ = sheep erythrocyte rosetting.

indicating that the problem of non-engraftment can indeed be circumvented by the use of PBSC.

In spite of extensive depletion of T cells caused by the double purging strategies mentioned above, immune reconstitution appeared to be sufficient – at least in pediatric recipients.[74] Since in recipients with insufficient thymic function, T-cell regeneration after BMT is largely dependent on the number of mature T cells present in the graft, the restoration of the immune system may be a problem in adult patients receiving heavily T-depleted haplo-identical stem cell grafts.[75]

The increased incidence of leukaemia relapse occurring after TCD will obviously not be overcome with the use of CD34+-selected PBSC alone. However, the large quantities of lymphocytes that can be segregated from PBSC grafts might be used for adding GVL activity to the haematopoietic potential conferred with the isolated CD34+ cells. Supplementing T-cell-depleted allografts with delayed T-cell addbacks, cytokine-activated NK cells, or leukaemia-specific T-cell clones is currently under investigation, and may allow preservation of the GVL effect without inducing severe

GVHR.[76–78] Similarly, specific immunity against critical infectious agents may be restored by addition of appropriate T-cell clones.[79]

In summary, the availability of PBSC has opened a broad spectrum of possibilities for allograft engineering. Designing an allograft tailored to the individual needs of the recipient by distinct selection of progenitor cells, GVL effector cells, and cells with specific anti-infectious activity appears to be feasible in the near future.

CONCLUSIONS

Transplantation of allogeneic peripheral blood stem cells is an attractive alternative to allogeneic BMT. Uncontrolled trials suggest that engraftment is faster than after allogeneic BMT, whereas incidence and severity of acute GVHR do not appear to be significantly different. Randomized studies are required to prove if allogeneic PBSCT is indeed superior to BMT in terms of donor convenience, engraftment, and leukaemia-free and overall survival. Such a trial is currently underway within the European Group for Blood and Marrow Transplantation

(EBMT). Since the first 100 patients have been accrued, an interim analysis is expected for early 1997. Regardless of the features of unmanipulated PBSC in comparison with marrow grafts, a major advantage of allogeneic PBSC over BM is their perfect suitability for graft engineering, such as T-cell depletion, ex vivo expansion, and generation of GVL effector cells.

If the main biological problems of allogeneic stem cell transplantation – namely GVHR, relapse and engraftment failure – could be overcome by using ex vivo manipulated PBSC, haplo-identical donors could also be considered for stem cell donation. Accordingly, a suitable stem cell graft would be available for almost every patient who needs it. On the other hand, the possibility of donating PBSC instead of BM and thus avoiding general anaesthesia and a surgical procedure should also facilitate the recruitment of unrelated stem cell donors. Furthermore, future improvements in stem cell mobilization procedures, for example by using additional cytokines or monoclonal antibodies against adhesion molecules,[80,81] may allow a sufficient progenitor cell number to be obtained by simple collection of 500 ml peripheral blood and thus eliminate the need for leukapheresis.

REFERENCES

1. Epstein RB, Graham TC, Buckner CD et al, Allogeneic marrow engraftment by cross circulation in lethally irradiated dogs. *Blood* 1966; **28:** 692–707.
2. Kessinger A, Armitage JO, Landmark JD, Weisenburger DD, Reconstitution of human hematopoietic function with autologous cryopreserved circulating stem cells. *Exp Hematol* 1986; **14:** 192–6.
3. Juttner CA, Blood stem cell transplants in acute leukemia. In: *Blood Stem Cell Transplants* (Gale RP, Juttner CA, Henon P, eds). Cambridge: Cambridge University Press, 1994: 101.
4. Kessinger A, Smith DM, Strandjord SE et al, Allogeneic transplantation of blood-derived, T cell-depleted hemopoietic stem cell after myeloablative treatment in a patient with acute lymphoblastic leukemia. *Bone Marrow Transplant* 1989; **4:** 643–6.
5. Sheridan WP, Begley CG, Juttner CA et al, Effect of peripheral-blood progenitor cells mobilized by filgrastim (G-CSF) on platelet recovery after high-dose chemotherapy. *Lancet* 1992; **339:**640–4.
6. Schmitz N, Linch DC, Dreger P et al, Randomised trial of filgrastim-mobilised peripheral blood progenitor cell transplantation versus autologous bone marrow transplantation in lymphoma patients. *Lancet* 1996; **347:** 353–7.
7. Dreger P, Grelle K, Eckstein V et al, Granulocyte-colony-stimulating factor induces increased serum levels of soluble interleukin-2 receptors preceding engraftment in autologous bone marrow transplantation. *Br J Haematol* 1993; **83:** 7–13.
8. Pan L, Delmonte J, Jalonen CK, Ferrara, JLM, Pretreatment of donor mice with granulocyte colony-stimulating factor polarizes donor T-lymphocytes toward type-2 cytokine production and reduces severity of experimental graft-versus-host disease. *Blood* 1995; **86:** 4422–9.
9. Stroncek DF, Clay ME, McCullough J, Experiences of normal individuals treated with granulocyte colony stimulating factor [Abstract]. *Blood* 1994; **84**(Suppl 1): 541a.
10. Bensinger WI, Buckner CD, Rowley S et al, Treatment of normal donors with recombinant growth factors for transplantation of allogeneic blood stem cells. *Bone Marrow Transplant* 1996; **17**(Suppl 2): S19–S21.
11. Grigg AP, Roberts AW, Raunow H et al, Optimizing dose and scheduling of filgrastim (granulocyte colony-stimulating factor) for mobilization and collection of peripheral blood progenitor cells in normal volunteers. *Blood* 1995; **86:** 4437–45.
12. Dreger P, Haferlach T, Eckstein V et al, G-CSF-mobilized peripheral blood progenitor cells for allogeneic transplantation: safety, kinetics of mobilization, and composition of the graft. *Br J Haematol* 1994; **87:** 609–13.
13. Höglund M, Smedmyr B, Simonsson B et al, Dose-dependent mobilisation of haematopoietic progenitor cells in healthy volunteers receiving glycosylated rHuG-CSF. *Bone Marrow Transplant* 1996; **18:** 19–27.
14. Azevedo WM, Aranha FJP, Gouvea JV et al, Allogeneic transplantation with blood stem cells

mobilized by rhG-CSF for hematological malignancies. *Bone Marrow Transplant* 1995; **16:** 647–53.

15. Anderlini P, Przepiorka D, Seong D et al, Transient neutropenia in normal donors after G-CSF mobilization and stem cell apheresis. *Br J Haematol* 1996; **94:** 155–8.

16. Caspar CB, Seger RA, Burger J, Gmür J, Effective stimulation of donors for granulocyte transfusions with recombinant methionyl granulocyte colony-stimulating factor. *Blood* 1993; **81:** 2866–71.

17. Russell NH, Hunter A, Rogers S et al, Peripheral blood stem cells as an alternative to marrow for allogeneic transplantation. *Lancet* 1993; **341:** 1482.

18. Körbling M, Huh YO, Durett A et al, Allogeneic blood stem cell transplantation: peripheralization and yield of donor-derived primitive hematopoietic progenitor cells (CD34$^+$ Thy-1) and lymphoid subsets, and possible predictors of engraftment and graft-versus-host disease. *Blood* 1995; **86:** 2842–8.

19. Matsunaga T, Sakamaki S, Kohgo Y et al, Recombinant human granulocyte colony-stimulating factor can mobilize sufficient amounts of peripheral blood stem cells in healthy volunteers for allogeneic transplantation. *Bone Marrow Transplant* 1993; **11:** 103–8.

20. Tjoennfjord GE, Steen R, Evensen SA et al, Characterization of CD34$^+$ peripheral blood cells from healthy adults mobilized by recombinant human granulocyte colony-stimulating factor. *Blood* 1994; **84:** 2795–801.

21. Chatta GS, Price TH, Allen RC, Dale DC, Effects of in vivo recombinant methionyl human granulocyte colony-stimulating factor on the neutrophil response and peripheral blood colony-forming cells in healthy young and elderly adult volunteers. *Blood* 1994; **84:** 2923–9.

22. Dreger P, Suttorp M, Haferlach T et al, Allogeneic G-CSF-mobilised peripheral blood progenitor cells for treatment of engraftment failure after bone marrow transplantation. *Blood* 1993; **81:** 1404–7.

23. Bensinger WI, Weaver CH, Appelbaum FR, Buckner CD, Transplantation of allogeneic peripheral blood stem cells mobilized by recombinant human granulocyte colony-stimulating factor (rh G-CSF). *Blood* 1995; **85:** 1655–8.

24. Sakamaki S, Matsunaga T, Hirayama Y et al, Haematological study of healthy volunteers 5 years after G-CSF. *Lancet* 1995; **346:** 1432–3.

25. Kawase Y, Akashi M, Ohtsu H et al, Effect of human recombinant granulocyte colony-stimulating factor on induction of myeloid leukemias by X-irradiation in mice. *Blood* 1993; **82:** 2163–8.

26. Imashuku S, Hibi S, Nakajima F et al, A review of 125 cases to determine the risk of myelodysplasia and leukemia in pediatric neutropenic patients after treatment with recombinant human granulocyte colony-stimulating factor. *Blood* 1994; **84:** 2380–1.

27. Kawakami M, Tsutsumi H, Kumakawa T et al, Levels of serum granulocyte colony-stimulating factor in patients with infections. *Blood* 1990; **76:** 1962–4.

28. Stroncek DF, Holland PV, Bartch G et al, Experiences of the first 493 unrelated marrow donors in the National Marrow Donor Program. *Blood* 1993; **81:** 1940–6.

29. Buckner CD, Petersen FB, Bolonese BA, Bone marrow donors. In: *Bone Marrow Transplantation* (Forman SJ, Blume KG, Thomas ED, eds). Boston: Blackwell Scientific Publications, 1994: 259.

30. Fritsch G, Fischmeister G, Haas OA et al, Peripheral blood hematopoietic progenitor cells of cytokine-stimulated healthy donors as an alternative for allogeneic transplantation. *Blood* 1994; **83:** 3420–1.

31. Lane TA, Law P, Maruyama M et al, Harvesting and enrichment of hematopoietic progenitor cells mobilized into the peripheral blood of normal donors by granulocyte–macrophage colony-stimulating factor (GM-CSF) or G-CSF: potential role in allogeneic marrow transplantation. *Blood* 1995; **85:** 275–82.

32. Aversa F, Tabilio A, Terenzi A et al, Successful engraftment of T-cell-depleted haploidentical 'three-loci' incompatible transplants in leukemia patients by addition of recombinant human granulocyte colony-stimulating factor-mobilized peripheral blood progenitor cells to bone marrow inoculum. *Blood* 1994; **84:** 3948–55.

33. Harada M, Nagafuji K, Fujisaki T et al, G-CSF-induced mobilization of peripheral blood stem cells from healthy adults for allogeneic transplantation. *J Hematother* 1996; **5:** 63–71.

34. Anderlini P, Przepiorka D, Huh Y et al, Duration of filgrastim mobilization and apheresis yield of CD34$^+$ progenitor cells and lymphoid subsets in normal donors for allogeneic transplantation. *Br J Haematol* 1996; **93:** 940–2.

35. Stroncek DF, Clay M, Jazcz W et al, Longer than 5 days of G-CSF mobilization of normal individuals results in lower CD34$^+$ counts [Abstract]. *Blood* 1994; **84**(Suppl 1): 541a.

36. Dreger P, Oberböster K, Schmitz N, PBPC grafts from healthy donors: analysis of CD34$^+$ and CD3$^+$ subpopulations. *Bone Marrow Transplant* 1996; **17**(Suppl 2): S22–S27.

37. Varas F, Bernard A, Bueren JA, Granulocyte colony-stimulating factor mobilizes into peripheral blood the complete clonal repertoire of hematopoietic precursors residing in the bone marrow of mice. *Blood* 1996; **88**: 2595–2601.

38. Molineux G, Pojda Z, Hampson IN et al, Transplantation potential of peripheral blood stem cells induced by granulocyte colony-stimulating factor. *Blood* 1990; **76**: 2153–8.

39. Baumann I, Testa NG, Lange C et al, Haemopoietic cells mobilised into the circulation by lenograstim as alternative to bone marrow for allogeneic transplants. *Lancet* 1993; **341**: 369.

40. Mackall CL, Granger L, Sheard MA et al, T-cell regeneration after bone marrow transplantation: Differential CD45 isoform expression on thymic-derived versus thymic-independent progeny. *Blood* 1993; **82**: 2585–94.

41. Ottinger HD, Beelen DW, Scheulen B et al, Improved immune reconstitution after allotransplantation of peripheral blood stem cells instead of bone marrow. *Blood* 1996; **88**: 2775–9.

42. Negrin RS, Kusnierz-Glaz C, Blume KG, Strober S, Enrichment of allogeneic CD34$^+$ cells and T cell depletion by Percoll density gradient centrifugation. *Bone Marrow Transplant* 1996; **17**(Suppl 2): S31–S33.

43. Krenger W, Snyder KM, Byon JHC et al, Polarized type 2 alloreactive CD4$^+$ and CD8$^+$ donor T cells fail to induce experimental acute graft-versus-host disease. *J Immunol* 1995; **155**: 585–93.

44. Glass B, Uharek L, Zeis M et al, Graft-versus-leukemia activity can be predicted by natural cytotoxicity against leukemia cells. *Br J Haematol* 1996; **93**: 412–20.

45. Weaver CH, Bensinger W, Longin K et al, Syngeneic transplantation with peripheral blood mononuclear cells collected after the administration of recombinant human granulocyte colony-stimulating factor. *Blood* 1993; **82**: 1981–4.

46. Dreger P, Haferlach T, Suttorp M et al, Rapid and sustained engraftment after syngeneic transplantation of G-CSF-mobilised peripheral blood progenitor cells [Abstract]. *Blood* 1993; **82**(Suppl 1): 630a.

47. Fefer A, Cheever MA, Thomas ED, Bone marrow transplantation for refractory acute leukemia in 34 patients with identical twins. *Blood* 1981; **57**: 421–30.

48. Schmitz N, Dreger P, Suttorp M et al, Primary transplantation of allogeneic peripheral blood progenitor cells mobilized by filgrastim (G-CSF). *Blood* 1995; **85**: 1666–72.

49. Körbling M, Przepiorka D, Engel H et al, Allogeneic blood stem cell transplantation for refractory leukemia and lymphoma: Potential advantage of blood over marrow allografts. *Blood* 1995; **85**: 1659–65.

50. Bensinger WI, Buckner CD, Storb R et al, Transplantation of allogeneic peripheral blood stem cells. *Bone Marrow Transplant* 1996; **17**(Suppl 2): S56–S57.

51. Bacigalupo A, Van Lint MT, Valbonesi M et al, Thiotepa/cyclophosphamide followed by granulocyte colony-stimulating factor mobilized allogeneic peripheral blood cells in adults with advanced leukemia. *Blood* 1996; **88**: 353–7.

52. Schmitz N, Bacigalupo A, Labopin M et al, Transplantation of peripheral blood progenitor cells from HLA-identical sibling donors: the EBMT experience. *Br J Haematol* 1996; **95**: 715–23.

53. Miflin G, Russel N, Hutchinson RM et al, Allogeneic peripheral blood stem cell transplantation for haematological malignancies – kinetics of engraftment and GvHD risk. *Bone Marrow Transplant* 1997; **19**: 9–13.

54. Bensinger WI, Clift R, Martin P et al, Allogeneic peripheral blood stem cell transplantation in patients with advanced hematologic malignancies: a retrospective comparison with marrow transplantation. *Blood* 1996; **88**: 2794–2800.

55. Molina L, Chabannon C, Viret F et al, Granulocyte colony-stimulating factor-mobilized allogeneic peripheral blood stem cells for rescue graft failure after allogeneic bone marrow transplantation in two patients with acute myeloblastic leukemia in first complete remission. *Blood* 1995; **85**: 1678–9.

56. Stachel D, Schmid I, Straka C et al, Allogeneic peripheral blood stem cell (PBSC) transplantation in two patients with graft failure. *Bone Marrow Transplant* 1995; **165**: 839–42.

57. Jansen J, Goselink HM, Veenhof WFJ et al, The impact of the composition of the bone marrow graft on engraftment and graft-versus-host disease. *Exp Hematol* 1983; **11**: 967–73.

58. Sosman JA, Oettel KR, Hank JA et al, Specific recognition of human leukemic cells by allogeneic T cell lines. *Transplantation* 1989; **48**: 486–90.

59. Elmaagacli AH, Beelen DW, Becks HW et al, Molecular studies of chimerism and minimal residual disease after allogeneic peripheral blood

progenitor cell or marrow transplantation [Abstract]. *Ann Hematol* 1996; **73**(Suppl 2): 84.

60. Zeis M, Uharek L, Glass B et al, Superior graft-vs-leukemia effects after transplantation of murine allogeneic peripheral blood progenitor cells (PBSC) as compared to bone marrow [Abstract]. *Blood* 1996; **88**(Suppl 1): 245a.

61. Giralt S, Escudier S, Kantarjian H et al, Preliminary results of treatment with filgrastim for relapse of leukemia and myelodysplasia after allogeneic bone marrow transplantation. *N Engl J Med* 1993; **329**: 757–61.

62. Alessandrino EP, Bernasconi P, Bonfichi M et al, Standard chemotherapy and donor peripheral blood stem cell (PBSC) infusion in early relapse after allo-BMT: preliminary results [Abstract]. *Bone Marrow Transplant* 1996; **17**(Suppl 1): S15.

63. Dreger P, Haferlach T, Winkemann T et al, Allogeneic peripheral blood progenitor cell infusion for treatment of relapse after allogeneic bone marrow transplantation [Abstract]. *Blood* 1995; **86**(Suppl 1): 292a.

64. Müller-Ruchholtz W, Wottge HU, Müller-Hermelink HK et al, Bone marrow transplantation across strong histocompatibility barriers by selective elimination of lymphoid cells in bone marrow. *Transplant Proc* 1976; **8**: 537–41.

65. Marmont AM, Horowitz MM, Gale RP et al, T-cell depletion of HLA-identical transplants in leukemia. *Blood* 1991; **78**: 2120–30.

66. Dreger P, Viehmann K, Steinmann J et al, G-CSF-mobilised peripheral blood progenitor cells for allogeneic transplantation: Comparison of T cell depletion strategies using different CD34$^+$ selection systems or CAMPATH-1. *Exp Hematol* 1995; **23**: 147–54.

67. Link H, Arseniev L, Bähre O et al, Transplantation of allogeneic CD34$^+$ blood cells. *Blood* 1996; **87**: 4903–9.

68. Finke J, Behringer D, Bertz H et al, Allogeneic peripheral blood stem cell transplantation with or without CD34$^+$ selection: rapid immune reconstitution and low incidence of GVHD [Abstract]. *Ann Hematol* 1996; **73**(Suppl 2): 165.

69. Bensinger WI, Buckner CD, Rowley S et al, Transplantation of allogeneic CD34$^+$ peripheral blood stem cells (PBSC) in patients with advanced hematologic malignancy. *Bone Marrow Transplant* 1996; **17**(Suppl 2): S38–S39.

70. Bensinger WI, Rowley S, Lilleby K et al, Reduction in graft-versus-host-disease (GVHD) after transplantation of CD34 selected, allogeneic peripheral blood stem cells (PBSC) in older

patients with advanced hematological malignancies [Abstract]. *Blood* 1996; **88**(Suppl 1): 421a.

71. Corringham RET, Ho AD, Rapid and sustained allogeneic transplantation using immunoselected CD34$^+$-selected peripheral blood progenitor cells mobilized by recombinant granulocyte and granulocyte–macrophage colony-stimulating factors. *Blood* 1995; **86**: 2052–4.

72. Kernan N, Collins NH, Juliano L et al, Clonable T lymphocytes in T cell-depleted bone marrow transplants correlate with development of graft-v-host disease. *Blood* 1986; **68**: 770–3.

73. Wieseneth M, Schreiner T, Friedrich W et al, Combination of CD34-selection and T-cell depletion as GVHD-prophylaxis in HLA-nonidentical blood progenitor cell transplantation [Abstract]. *Bone Marrow Transplant* 1996; **17**(Suppl 2): S70.

74. Handgretinger R, Lang P, Kuci S et al, Isolation and transplantation of highly purified autologous and allogeneic CD34$^+$ progenitors [Abstract]. *Blood* 1996; **88**(Suppl 1): 253a.

75. Martelli MF, Aversa F, Velardi A et al, New tools for crossing the HLA barrier: fludarabine and megadose stem cell transplants [Abstract]. *Blood* 1996; **88**(Suppl 1): 484a.

76. Barrett AJ, Mavroudis D, Molldrem J et al, Optimizing the dose and timing of lymphocyte add-back in T-cell depleted BMT between HLA-identical siblings [Abstract]. *Blood* 1996; **88**(Suppl 1): 460a.

77. Glass B, Uharek L, Zeis M et al, Graft-vs-leukemia (GVL) activity induced by MHC-mismatched activated natural killer cells given after bone marrow transplantation [Abstract]. *Blood* 1995; **86**(Suppl 1): 576a.

78. Uharek L, Sebens T, Zeis M et al, Leukemia-specific allogeneic T cell-lines for adoptive immunotherapy after allogeneic BMT in a murine model [Abstract]. *Blood* 1995; **86**(Suppl 1): 576a.

79. Rooney CM, Smith CA, Ng CY et al, Use of gene-modified virus-specific T lymphocytes to control Epstein–Barr-virus-related lymphoproliferation. *Lancet* 1995; **345**: 9–13.

80. Laterveer L, Lindley IJD, Heemskerk DPM et al, Rapid mobilization of hematopoietic progenitor cells in rhesus monkeys by a single intravenous injection of interleukin-8. *Blood* 1996; **87**: 781–8.

81. Papayannopoulou T, Nakamoto B, Peripheralization of hemopoietic progenitors in primates treated with anti-VLA4 integrin. *Proc Natl Acad Sci USA* 1993; **90**: 9374–8.

82. Russell JA, Luider J, Weaver M et al, Collection

of progenitor cells for allogeneic transplantation from peripheral blood of normal donors. *Bone Marrow Transplant* 1995; **15:** 111–15.

83. Rosenfeld C, Collins R, Pineiro L et al, Allogeneic blood cell transplantation without post-transplant colony-stimulation factors in patients with hematopoietic neoplasm: a phase II study. *J Clin Oncol* 1996; **14:** 1314–19.

84. Urbano-Ispizua A, Solano C, Brunet S et al, Allogeneic peripheral blood progenitor cell transplantation: analysis of short-term engraftment and acute GVHD incidence in 33 cases. *Bone Marrow Transplant* 1996; **18:** 35–40.

85. Martinez C, Urbano-Ispizua A, Mazzara R et al, Granulocyte colony-stimulating factor administration and peripheral blood progenitor cells collection in normal donors: analysis of leukapheresis-related side effects. *Blood* 1996; **87:** 4916–17.

11

Cord blood stem cell transplantation

Hal E Broxmeyer

CONTENTS • **Introduction** • **Characteristics of cord blood stem/progenitor cells** • **Cord blood banking** • **Clinical use of cord blood** • **Future uses of cord blood** • **Concluding remarks**

INTRODUCTION

There are many more patients in need of a stem cell transplant for reconstitution of a diseased hematopoietic system, or a hematopoietic system compromised by treatment, than can find a suitable stem cell donor. Stem cell transplants occur either in an autologous situation or in a situation in which allogeneic cells from family members or unrelated recipients are utilized. The major source of tissue for stem cell transplantation has been and currently continues to be from bone marrow, although stem cells mobilized from marrow to peripheral blood by use of growth factors and/or after the recovery phase from chemotherapy are increasingly utilized. To these tissue sources of clinically relevant stem cells have recently been added cells collected from the umbilical and placental blood of a newborn child.[1,2]

The author, having been a participant in identifying cord blood as a potential source of transplantable stem and progenitor cells,[1] and in translating this laboratory information into a clinically relevant effort,[2–4] has been extremely gratified to see the incredibly fast expansion of the use of cord blood transplantation for treatment of a growing number of blood and other

disorders, previously treated by bone marrow transplantation.

Most new and successful medical treatments involve a continuing interplay between laboratory and clinical efforts, and this has been and continues to be an important reason for the encouraging results obtained with clinical cord blood transplantation. It is appropriate to remember that the first cord blood transplant took place as recently as October 1988, the results of which were published in 1989,[2] the same year that the laboratory results suggesting the possibility for this were published.[1] The first few years saw only a few transplants with cord blood performed, and the vast majority of the first 40 or so transplants were done with either complete HLA-matched or one-antigen mismatched sibling cells for young recipients.[5] The first five and a total of seven of the first ten cord blood transplants were done with cells sent to the author's laboratory, where they were processed, assayed for progenitor cell content, cryopreserved and stored frozen until they were hand-delivered to the transplant site.[2–4] The first cord blood bank, which was in the author's laboratory, was soon followed by other banks for use either for storage of autologous and related cord bloods, or for storage of cord bloods for use in unrelated situations. It is the unrelated cord blood banking efforts[6,7] that have truly expanded the clinical utility of cord blood transplantation,[8,9] although it is the author's opinion that there is a place for unrelated as well as autologous/related cord blood banks. There was a healthy dose of scepticism after the first laboratory report[3,10] and the first clinical report,[3,11] and it is in large part through the establishment of the unrelated cord blood bank at the New York Blood Center[6–9] that we have been able to begin to answer some of the questions posed[12] regarding the broadness of applicability of cord blood as a source of transplantable cells.

This chapter will focus on:

- the characteristics of cord blood stem/ progenitor cells;
- cord blood banking;
- clinical use of cord blood;
- future uses of cord blood.

CHARACTERISTICS OF CORD BLOOD STEM/PROGENITOR CELLS

Cord blood is a rich source of immature subsets of hematopoietic progenitor cells, including those for the multipotential (CFU-GEMM), granulocyte–macrophage (CFU-GM), erythroid (BFU-E)[1,3,4,13] and megakaryocyte (CFU-MK, BFU-MK)[14,15] lineages. While these assays do not recognize the stem cell compartment subset that contains the long-term marrow repopulating cells, such assays were used to suggest that there would be enough cells in a single collection of cord blood to repopulate the hematopoietic system of myeloablated children and adults.[1,3,4,13] An example of the nucleated and progenitor cell content of single cord blood collections is shown in Table 11.1.

Stem and progenitor cells are considered to reside in a population of cells that express CD34 antigens, and this is also apparent for such cells from cord blood.[16–18] CD34 is a surface glycophosphoprotein,[19] and subsets of CD34+ cells can be subdivided based on levels of expression of CD34 and expression or lack of

expression of other antigens on the cell surface.[16–21] Other antigens useful for categorizing cord blood stem and progenitor cells include CD38,[17,22] thy-1[23] and c-kit.[24] The supravital dye rhodamine-123 has also been used to subset cord blood stem/progenitor cells.[25,26] Presently, the immature subsets of stem and progenitor cells in cord blood are believed to be present in the phenotypic subsets of CD34+++, CD34+CD38−, thy-1lo, and Rholo cell populations. Interestingly, mouse studies have suggested that the earliest subsets of murine stem cells with long-term marrow repopulating capacity may lack or express low levels of CD34 antigens.[27,28] It remains to be determined if some cord blood stem cell subsets are being missed because they express low levels or do not express CD34. This important question with obvious clinical relevance needs to be addressed in the near future.

The proliferative capacity of stem/progenitor cells from cord blood is extensive[16–18,29] and on the whole it is apparently greater than that of comparable subsets of cells obtained from adult bone marrow. While there are no in vitro assays yet available that identify the long-term marrow repopulating human stem cell, there are assays available for more mature cells that, through their proliferative and replating capacity in vitro and their engraftment in mice with severe combined immunodeficiency (SCID), are believed to reside in the stem cell compartment. These include the in vitro assays for subsets of CFU-GEMM,[30,31] as well as high-proliferative potential colony-forming cells (HPP-CFC)[18] and long-term culture-initiating cells (LTC-IC).[32–34] The frequency of these primitive cells in cord blood and their proliferative capacity is high. While it has not yet been proven that CFU-GEMM, HPP-CFC or LTC-IC contain long-term marrow repopulating subsets of stem cells, efforts with cells that repopulate SCID mice suggest that these cells may be more immature than those cells recognized by in vitro assessment.[35] These cells have been termed SCID repopulating cells (SRC). Human cord blood appears to have greater SCID marrow repopulating capacity than adult cells,[36–40] adding further evidence for the increased frequency and

Table 11.1 Characteristics of cord blood collections pre-freeze

Parameter	Mean ± 1SD
Blood collected (ml)	110 ± 48
Nucleated cells ($\times 10^6$)	1427 ± 1007
Progenitors (colonies, $\times 10^5$) in agar cultures	
CFU-GM (stimulated with GM-CSF)	2.43 ± 2.70
CFU-GM (stimulated with GM-CSF + SLF)	9.38 ± 9.79
Progenitors (colonies, $\times 10^5$) in methylcellulose cultures[a]	
CFU-GM (stimulated with Epo + IL-3 + SLF)	12.49 ± 23.64
BFU-E (stimulated with Epo + IL-3)	9.45 ± 9.94
CFU-GEMM (stimulated with Epo + IL-3 + SLF)	11.26 ± 12.77

The results shown are for 65 consecutive collections made with the intent that they might be used for sibling transplantation, and are adapted from a previous publication.[69] The progenitor cell assays were described elsewhere.[13]
[a] Epo = erythropoietin; SLF = stem cell factor.

proliferative capacity of cord blood versus marrow stem cells. A number of different SCID mice have been used that have demonstrated capacity for enhanced engraftment of human cells – these include mice containing human transgenes for granulocyte–macrophage colony stimulating factor (GM-CSF), interleukin (IL)-3 and steel factor (SLF = stem cell factor, *c-kit* ligand, mast cell growth factor),[38] and SCID mice that are of the non-obese diabetic genotypic.[38–40] In each case the repopulating capacity of cord blood seems to be greater than that of bone marrow.

Interestingly, immature subsets of cord blood progenitors are in a slow or non-cycling state;[41–44] however, they respond rapidly to stimulation by combinations of cytokines,[41–43] and their capacity to be expanded ex vivo is great.[13,16,17,34,42,43,45] Ex vivo expansion occurs in response to known cytokines as well as to as yet undefined growth factors in cord blood plasma.[45–47] It is clear that ex vivo expansion of cord blood cells will become a reality in the future, but presently this technology appears to be limited mainly by our inability to define an in vitro assay for the human long-term marrow repopulating stem cell. Thus, although a large number of reports have defined conditions for the extensive expansion of stem and progenitor cells from human cord blood, we have no way at present of determining if the earliest stem cells are expanded, or alternatively if they are maintained or decreased in numbers after ex vivo culture.

It is not known if there are stem cells in cord blood that are unique compared with stem cells in adult tissue with regard to greater proliferative and self-renewal capacity, or if merely the frequency of such cells in cord blood is greater. However, recent interest in telomere length[48] and telomerase activity[49] with regard to cell aging has suggested a possible molecular mechanism for the extensive proliferative capacity of immature cells. It has been noted that candidate human stem cells with a CD34$^+$CD38$^-$ phenotype purified from adult bone marrow have shorter telomeres than cells from fetal liver or cord blood.[48]

It is not apparent what characteristics of cord blood stem and progenitor cells are involved in their high-frequency presentation in the circulating blood of newborns, but this frequency is drastically decreased in the blood within 36 hours after the birth of a baby.[13] A gestational age-dependent decrease is also apparent, so that the frequency of progenitors is less at birth than at early gestation.[50] This heightens the need to collect as much cord blood as possible, without harm to the newborn, if it is anticipated that these cells are to be utilized for transplantation purposes. Analysis of progenitors from neonatal infants who are small and appropriate for gestational age suggests that cord blood collected from small newborns may be adequate for transplantation purposes in many cases.[51] The homing, migration and mobilization of stem cells during fetal development, at birth and in the adult are important topics, and are currently under intense investigation. While it has been reported that adherence molecules on CD34[+] cord blood and adult marrow are similar,[52] the activation state of these cell surface molecules may be of greater importance than their numbers on the cell surface.

CORD BLOOD BANKING

The future development of cord blood as a clinically useful source of transplantable stem cells is intimately related to the banking of these cells. To this end, the separation of cells, their cryopreservation and procedures for the establishment and regulation of cord blood banks are important areas of concern.

Our original report on cord blood progenitors noted a substantial loss of these cells with a number of different separation procedures.[1] This loss was subsequently substantiated by a number of other investigators.[53–56] Because it was not clear how many cord blood cells were needed for engrafting and hematopoietic repopulating capacity, we had originally suggested that cord blood should be frozen away without any maneuvers to separate the cells, and that upon use the cells should be thawed and infused without washing them.[1] We had

noted that even simple washing procedures would result in unacceptable losses of progenitors.[1] These suggestions led to the demonstration that cord blood could be successfully used as a clinical source of transplantable stem cells.[2–4,57,58] With the clinical procedure established, it became necessary to focus on ways to reduce the blood volume without significant loss of stem and progenitor cells, in order to address space concerns for cord blood banking, as well as concerns for removal of red cells prior to freezing and/or transplantation. A number of physical procedures for separating cord blood have been reported, including density cut on percol gradients, or separation with gelatin or starch.[59–65] While all of these procedures have apparently been of use in reducing volume of cord blood with minimal or no loss of progenitors, as assessed by in vitro culture, there is no one standard yet for separating cord blood cells. A simple procedure that has been used for a great number of the collections subsequently used for unrelated cord blood transplants originating from the New York Blood Center utilizes rouleaux formation induced by hydroxyethyl starch and centrifugation to reduce the bulk of erythrocytes and plasma, leading to a concentrated leukocyte preparation containing stem and progenitor cells.[65] Such separated cells have been used successful by us[66] and others.[65]

The freezing procedures vary, and here also there are no standard methods yet. Procedures utilize dimethyl sulfoxide as a cryopreservant, and range from timed freezing with a computerized machine to efforts in which cells are placed in styrofoam boxes, which are stored in −70°C freezers, where they are left to freeze overnight before being placed in liquid nitrogen.[1,13,65,68–70] Due to the large volume of samples processed and stored at the New York Blood Center, they have chosen to utilize a simplified freezing method that does not require a computerized timed freezing apparatus[6,7,65] for their cells to be used for transplantation.[8,9,66,67] The procedure they use for washing the thawed cells prior to use has also been reported.[65]

A concern of some has been how long one can store frozen cells and retrieve them in viable form. At present, the longest time period for which cord blood cells have been stored frozen prior to use and engraftment has been about three years. However, once cells have been frozen, they should theoretically remain in cryopreserved form for at least the lifetime of an individual, assuming there are no problems with the freezing, liquid nitrogen storage and thawing procedures. Bone marrow cells have been successfully used after storage in liquid nitrogen for up to eleven years.[71,72] We have found excellent recovery of viable nucleated cells and stem/progenitor cells with extensive proliferative capacity, as assessed by in vitro culture, after storage in liquid nitrogen for over ten years, even though relatively unsophisticated procedures were used to freeze the cells.[69] Our recoveries were based on calculations comparing the same pre-freeze and post-thaw samples in which culture conditions and cytokine combinations were the same at both these time assessments. Other studies have demonstrated the capacity to engraft SCID mice,[73] and to ex vivo expand progenitors[68,73] and transduce them to high efficiency,[68] after cryopreserved storage.

A number of reports have been published on procedures for the establishment of cord blood banks in the United States and Europe.[6,7,74–76] Guidelines for standards for cord blood collection, processing, testing, storage and transplantation are in the process of being evaluated. Examples of these are the combined efforts of the Foundation for Accreditation of Hematopoietic Cell Therapy (FAHCT), the International Society for Hematotherapy and Graft Engineering (ISHAGE), the American Society for Blood and Bone Marrow Transplantation (ASBMT), the Canadian Bone Marrow Transplant Group (CBMTG) and the American Association of Blood Banking (AABB). Additionally, the Federal Drug Administration (FDA) of the United States began addressing the issue of regulation of cord blood banking and transplantation. The FDA has voiced its opinion that such regulation should include an Establishment License Application (ELA), a Product License Application (PLA), and, because the stem cell product of cord blood cannot be assayed yet, an Investigational New Drug (IND) application. How stringent the regulatory controls will be here is not yet known, but the outcome will surely impact on the international collaboration for cord blood transplantation.

Presently, there are a number of private cord blood banks mainly interested in storing cryopreserved cord blood for autologous or family use, and there are a number of unrelated cord blood banks. Additionally, the National Heart Lung and Blood Institute (NHLBI) of the National Institutes of Health (NIH) in the United States has begun funding for three additional cord blood banks to store cells for unrelated use, as well for a number of cord blood transplantation centers. It is the desire of the NHLBI to use these banks and cord blood transplant centers to help determine the efficacy and broadness of applicability of cord blood transplantation in a controlled clinical trial setting.

An obvious advantage of banked cord blood is the potential for quick accessibility to matched or closely matched cells for patients in need of a stem cell transplant. The impact of racial genetic polymorphism on the probability of finding an HLA-matched donor[77] underscores the need for such a banking effort, since finding an HLA-matched bone marrow donor for certain racial groups is extremely difficult. However, this also means that numbers of samples of cord blood stored for these racial groups will have to be large. As the capacity to cross HLA-antigen barriers decreases, the number of samples that must be stored to meet transplantation needs also decreases. Most unrelated bone marrow transplants using less than complete HLA or one-antigen mismatched cells have resulted in high levels of graft versus host disease (GVHD). There is some accumulating clinical evidence that cord blood cells may elicit less GVHD than bone marrow in the context of sibling and unrelated donor cells for children, and possibly for adults.[2–5,8,9,57] If this holds up then we may need fewer HLA-typed cord bloods stored away than if cells were being stored that required more stringent HLA-matching.

CLINICAL USE OF CORD BLOOD

Since the first sibling transplant in October 1988, performed in Paris with cells from the author's cord blood bank, and the first unrelated transplant in August 1993, performed in Durham, North Carolina with cells from the New York Blood Center, there have been in the vicinity of 500 sibling plus unrelated cord blood transplants done. These have been for a variety of malignant and non-malignant disorders, some of which are listed in Table 11.2.[2–5,8,9,57,58,66,67,78–87] The results have thus far been encouraging for both sibling and unrelated transplants, with high engraftment rates, relatively low levels of GVHD, and no evidence so far that the low GVHD is associated with an enhanced rate of leukemic relapse. Thus, either the low GVHD is enough to mount a graft versus leukemia (GVL) effect or the cells mediating these effects are separable and differentially found in adult tissue, where GVHD and GVL have been closely linked, and in cord blood.

Not all clinical cord blood transplant results have been published. In order to organize information on those that had been done, an International Cord Blood Transplant Registry was formed, and the initial results of the first 44 sibling cord blood transplants were reported.[5] In that study, patients who had HLA-identical and one HLA-antigen disparate grafts had a probability of engraftment at 50 days after transplantation of 85%. No patient developed late graft failure. The probability of developing grade II–IV GVHD at 100 days was 3% and the probability of chronic GVHD at one year was 6%. With a medium follow-up of 1.6 years, the probability of survival for recipients of HLA-identical or one HLA-antigen disparate grafts was 72%. It should be noted that the first recipient of a cord blood transplant from his sister's cells[2] is alive and healthy more than eight years after the transplant and is cured of the hematological manifestations of Fanconi anemia.

The International Cord Blood Transplant Registry has not, for a variety of reasons, been able to keep up with the transplants done, especially for the unrelated situation. However, two recent reports[8,9] and meeting abstracts[66,67] have

Table 11.2 Examples of disorders for which cord blood transplantation has been utilized
Acute lymphoid leukemia – remission, relapse
Acute myeloid leukemia – remission, relapse
Chronic myeloid leukemia – accelerated/blastic
Juvenile chronic myeloid leukemia
Myelodysplastic syndrome
Neuroblastoma
Acute megakaryocytic thrombocytopenia
Severe combined immunodeficiency
Common variable immunodeficiency
Wiscott–Aldrich syndrome
X-linked lymphoproliferative disease
Hurler syndrome
Hunter syndrome
Fanconi anemia
Severe aplastic anemia
β-thalassemia
Sickle cell anemia
Lesch–Nyhan syndrome
Pure red cell aplasia
Osteopetrosis
Globoid cell leukodystrophy
Adrenoleukodystrophy
Gunther's disease – porphyrin accumulation
LAD syndrome – adhesive membrane glycoprotein deficiency
Kostmann's syndrome
Diamond–Blackfan syndrome

clearly demonstrated the feasibility of unrelated cord blood transplants.

In a one-center trial[8] where 25 consecutive patients received cord blood, 24 of the 25 donor–recipient pairs were discordant for one to three HLA antigens. Engraftment was noted in 23 of 25 patients (92%), acute GVHD grade level III occurred in 2 of 21 patients who could be evaluated (9.5%), and 2 of the patients manifested chronic GVHD. With a median follow-up of $12\frac{1}{2}$ months and a minimum follow-up of 100 days, the overall 100-day survival rate was 64% and the overall event-free survival was 48%. In another trial involving two centers,[9] 18 patients received either HLA-matched or one to three antigen disparate grafts. The probability of engraftment was 100%, with no graft failure evident at the time of the report. The probability of developing grade III–IV acute GVHD at 100 days was 11%. With a median follow-up of 6 months (range 1.6–17 months), the probability of survival at 6 months was 65%. Similar results were reported from our center.[66] The New York Blood Center, which supplied the frozen cells for most of the unrelated transplants mentioned above, was able to put together a preliminary evaluation of the first 243 transplants done in the first three years with cells from their cord blood bank.[67] It was noted that these transplants reflected over 2900 search requests and were performed in 59 transplant centers worldwide. Twenty-seven of 161 recipients died or relapsed within 30 days (16.7%), and 90.3% of the remaining, informative, patients engrafted with documented donor-type cells.

In all cases of sibling and unrelated cord blood transplants, time to neutrophil recovery was on the whole delayed somewhat, but time to platelet recovery was greatly delayed, compared with recovery from bone marrow transplantation. The reasons for this delay in platelet recovery are not known. Future efforts will address the ability of specific growth factors (e.g. thrombopoietin) or suppressors of negative regulation (e.g. lysophyline) to accelerate platelet recovery of recipients of cord blood transplants.

Most cord blood transplants have been done in children, although information is beginning to accumulate regarding the engrafting capability of cord blood for adults or large-sized recipients. Successes have been noted,[8,9,66,67,86] but it is too early to know the true engraftment efficiency in these patients. As more transplants are done, this information will become available. Certainly, large-sized cord blood collections will be helpful in these endeavors. Because of concerns for the newborn's safety, the question of how soon to clamp the cord

blood has been discussed.[88–91] Presently, there is no evidence that quick/early clamping for the cord blood collections has resulted in health problems for the newborns; however, until there are specific guidelines for this, we have felt it best to leave the decision of the time to clamping to the obstetrician.[89]

Interestingly, although GVHD has not been a problem in cord blood transplantation, which may in fact present less GVHD than with bone marrow, a concern originally voiced was that maternal cell contamination of the cord blood would be a problem. Initial efforts to detect maternal cells in cord blood were negative.[2–4] However, with more sensitive techniques it is apparent that maternal cell contamination does exist in cord blood collections.[92–96] The more sensitive techniques utilized include polymerase chain reaction (PCR) amplification of two minisatellite sequences,[92] fluorescence in situ hybridization using probes to the X and Y chromosomes,[93] an allele-specific PCR amplification,[94] locus-specific amplication of the non-inherited maternal HLA gene[95] and karyotyping of progenitor cell-derived colonies.[96] The detection of maternal cells in these cord blood collections by sensitive technologies raises the question of what, if any, effects the presence of these concentrations of maternal cells has on the reactivity of cord blood cell transplants for immune responses to the host. While investigators are currently aware that a close watch needs to be kept on correlating maternal cell contamination with GVHD, the presence of maternal cells has not engendered serious concerns at this time.

FUTURE USES OF CORD BLOOD

One potentially exciting use of cord blood is the correction of genetic disorders by gene transfer. Cord blood progenitors are efficiently transduced with new genetic material by both retroviral[97,98] and adeno-associated viral (AAV) vectors.[99] There has already been a beginning attempt to use cord blood for a gene therapy approach to treat a genetic disorder.[100] Cord blood was collected from three children who had been diagnosed in utero as being adenosine deaminase (ADA)-deficient patients with SCID. At birth, their cord blood was collected, and was subjected to column separation to enrich for CD34$^+$ cells. These cells were then placed into culture with growth factors for retroviral-mediated gene transduction with an *ADA* gene. The retroviral-mediated gene-manipulated CD34$^+$ cells were then returned to their respective autologous recipients. This clinical study was the first time that autologous transplantation was attempted, the first time that CD34$^+$ cord blood cells were used for transplantation and the first time that gene-transduced cord blood cells were transplanted. Although there is no evidence yet that this procedure has resulted in a therapeutic endpoint, it is clear that autologous transplantation is possible in a non-conditioned host if the timing is right, that CD34$^+$ cord blood cells can engraft and that some of the engrafted cells come from those that had been transduced with the *ADA* gene. This is an important start to other possible gene transfer/gene therapy scenarios with cord blood. A time can be envisioned when genetic defects can be corrected with gene transfer and autologous cord blood transplantation. Additionally, it may be possible to use such procedures to place genes for growth factors and/or growth factor receptors into cord blood cells to enhance specific types of hematopoietic cell growth. This of course would require that the gene expression be regulated, a possibility that awaits future technological advances.

CONCLUDING REMARKS

Results with cord blood have been very encouraging. From a time not so long ago when cord blood was considered mainly a discard material, to the present when in the vicinity of 500 cord blood transplants have been done in either a sibling or unrelated setting, the future looks bright for this newly emerged source of transplantable stem cells. As long as the basic laboratory and clinical studies are done carefully, we can be guaranteed that this exciting field will continue to progress. There are still a number of questions for which we would like answers. Among a plethora of questions are whether ex vivo expansion of cord blood long-term marrow repopulating stem cells can occur, whether adults can be routinely engrafted with cord blood, or if ex vivo expanded cells will be necessary to assure success with most cord blood transplants for adults. Also to be determined is whether gene transfer/gene therapy with cord blood stem cells will be feasible, and, if so, in what context. As soon as these questions have been answered, new ones to advance the field will no doubt take their place.

ACKNOWLEDGEMENTS

Thanks are due to Linda Cheung and Becki Miller for typing the manuscript. Some of the studies reported in this review were funded by US Public Health Service Grants R01 HL54037, R01 HL56416, T32 DK07519, and a project in P01 HL53586 from the National Institutes of Health to the author.

REFERENCES

1. Broxmeyer HE, Douglas GW, Hangoc G et al, Human umbilical cord blood as a potential source of transplantable hematopoietic stem/progenitor cells. *Proc Natl Acad Sci USA* 1989; **86:** 3828–32.
2. Gluckman E, Broxmeyer HE, Auerbach AD et al, Hematopoietic reconstitution in a patient with Fanconi anemia by means of umbilical-cord blood from an HLA-identical sibling. *N Engl J Med* 1989; **321:** 1174–8.
3. Broxmeyer HE, Gluckman E, Auerbach A et al, Human umbilical cord blood: a clinically useful source of transplantable hematopoietic stem/progenitor cells. *Int J Cell Cloning* 1990; **8:** 76–91.
4. Broxmeyer HE, Kurtzberg J, Gluckman E et al, Umbilical cord blood hematopoietic stem and repopulating cells in human clinical transplantation. *Blood Cells* 1991; **17:** 313–29.
5. Wagner JE, Kernan NA, Steinbuch M et al, Allogeneic sibling umbilical cord blood trans-

plantation in forty-four children with malignant and non-malignant disease. *Lancet* 1995; **346:** 214–19.

6. Rubinstein P, Rosenfield RE, Adamson JW, Stevens CE, Stored placental blood for unrelated bone marrow reconstitution. *Blood* 1993; **81:** 1679–90.

7. Rubinstein P, Taylor PE, Scaradavou A et al, Unrelated placental blood for bone marrow reconstitution: organization of the placental blood program. *Blood Cells* 1994; **20:** 587–600.

8. Kurtzberg J, Laughlin M, Graham ML et al, Placental blood as a source of hematopoietic stem cells for transplantation into unrelated recipients. *N Engl J Med* 1996; **335:** 157–201.

9. Wagner JE, Rosenthal J, Sweetman R et al, Successful transplantation of HLA-matched and HLA-mismatched umbilical cord blood from unrelated donors: Analysis of engraftment and acute graft-versus-host disease. *Blood* 1996; **88:** 795–802.

10. Linch DC, Brent L, Can cord blood be used? *Nature* 1989; **340:** 676.

11. Nathan DG, The beneficence of neonatal hematopoiesis [Editorial]. *N Engl J Med* 1989; **321:** 1190–1.

12. Broxmeyer HE, Questions to be answered regarding umbilical cord blood hematopoietic stem and progenitor cells and their use in transplantation. *Transfusion* 1995; **35:** 694–702.

13. Broxmeyer HE, Hangoc G, Cooper S et al, Growth characteristics and expansion of human umbilical cord blood and estimation of its potential for transplantation of adults. *Proc Natl Acad Sci USA* 1992; **89:** 4109–13.

14. Vainchenker W, Guichard J, Breton-Gorius J, Growth of human megakaryocyte colonies in culture from fetal, neonatal, and adult peripheral blood cells: ultrastructural analysis. *Blood Cells* 1979; **5:** 25–42.

15. Nishihira H, Toyoda Y, Miyazaki H et al, Growth of macroscopic human megakaryocyte colonies from cord blood in culture with recombinant human thrombopoietin (c-mpl ligand) and the effects of gestational age on frequency of colonies. *Br J Haematol* 1996; **92:** 23–8.

16. Lansdorp PM, Dragowska W, Mayani H, Ontogeny-related changes in proliferative potential of human hematopoietic cells. *J Exp Med* 1993; **178:** 787–91.

17. Cardoso AA, Li ML, Batard P et al, Release from quiescence of CD34$^+$CD38$^-$ human umbilical cord blood cells reveals their potentiality to engraft adults. *Proc Natl Acad Sci USA* 1993; **90:** 8707–11.

18. Lu L, Xiao M, Shen R-N et al, Enrichment, characterization and responsiveness of single primitive CD34^{+++} human umbilical cord blood hematopoietic progenitor with high proliferative and replating potential. *Blood* 1993; **81:** 41–8.

19. Krause DS, Fackler MJ, Civin CI, May WS, CD34: Structure, biology and clinical utility. *Blood* 1996; **87:** 1–13.

20. Knapp W, Strobl H, Scheinecker C et al, Molecular characterization of CD34$^+$ human hematopoietic progenitor cells. *Ann Hematol* 1995; **70:** 281–96.

21. Thoma SJ, Lamping CP, Ziegler BL, Phenotype analysis of hematopoietic CD34$^+$ cell populations derived from human umbilical cord blood using flow cytometry and cDNA-polymerase chain reaction. *Blood* 1994; **83:** 2103–14.

22. Hao QL, Shah AJ, Thiemann FT et al, A functional comparison of CD34$^+$CD38$^-$ cells in cord blood and bone marrow. *Blood* 1995; **86:** 3745–53.

23. Mayani H, Lansdorp PM, Thy-1 expression is linked to functional properties of primitive hematopoietic progenitor cells from human umbilical cord blood. *Blood* 1994; **83:** 2410–17.

24. Laver JH, Abboud MR, Kawashima I et al, Characterization of c-kit expression by primitive hematopoietic progenitors in umbilical cord blood. *Exp Hematol* 1995; **23:** 1515–19.

25. Traycoff CM, Abboud MR, Laver J et al, Evaluation of the in vitro behavior of phenotypically defined populations of umbilical cord blood hematopoietic progenitor cells. *Exp Hematol* 1994; **22:** 215–22.

26. Cicuttini FM, Welch KL, Boyd AW, The effect of cytokines in CD34$^+$ Rh-123^{high} and ^{low} progenitor cells from human umbilical cord blood. *Exp Hematol* 1994; **22:** 1244–51.

27. Cheng J, Baumhueter S, Thibodeaux H et al, Hematopoietic defects in mice lacking the sialomucin CD34. *Blood* 1996; **87:** 479–90.

28. Osawa M, Hanada KI, Hamada H, Nakauchi H, Long-term lymphohematopoietic reconstitution by a single CD34-low/negative hematopoietic stem cell. *Science* 1996; **273:** 242–5.

29. Hows JM, Bradley BA, Marsh JCW et al, Growth of human umbilical-cord blood in long term haematopoietic cultures. *Lancet* 1992; **340:** 73–6.

30. Carow C, Hangoc G, Cooper S et al, Mast cell

growth factor (c-kit ligand) supports the growth of human multipotential (CFU-GEMM) progenitor cells with a high replating potential. *Blood* 1991; **78:** 2216–21.

31. Carow CE, Hangoc G, Broxmeyer HE, Human multipotential progenitor cells (CFU-GEMM) have extensive replating capacity for secondary CFU-GEMM: An effect enhanced by cord blood plasma. *Blood* 1993; **81:** 942–9.

32. Pettengell R, Luft T, Henschier R et al, Direct comparison by limiting dilutions analysis of long-term culture-initiating cells in human bone marrow, umbilical cord blood, and blood stem cells. *Blood* 1994; **84:** 3653–9.

33. Hirao A, Kawano Y, Takaue Y et al, Engraftment potential of peripheral and cord blood stem cells evaluated by a long-term culture system. *Exp Hematol* 1994; **22:** 521–6.

34. Traycoff CM, Kosak ST, Grigsby S, Srour EF, Evaluation of ex vivo expansion potential of cord blood and bone marrow hematopoietic progenitor cells using cell tracking and limiting dilution analysis. *Blood* 1995; **85:** 2059–68.

35. Larochelle A, Vormoor J, Hanenberg H et al, Identification of primitive human hematopoietic cells capable of repopulating NOD/SCID mouse bone marrow: implications for gene therapy. *Nature Med* 1996; **2:** 1329–37.

36. Vormoor J, Lapidot T, Pflumio F et al, Immature human cord blood progenitors engraft and proliferate to high levels in immune-deficient SCID mice. *Blood* 1994; **83:** 2489–97.

37. Orazi A, Braun SE, Broxmeyer HE, Immunohistochemistry represents a useful tool to study human cell engraftment in SCID mice transplantation models. *Blood Cells* 1994; **20:** 323–30.

38. Bock TA, Orlic D, Dunbar CE et al, Improved engraftment of human hematopoietic cells in severe combined immunodeficient (SCID) mice carrying human cytokine transgenes. *J Exp Med* 1995; **182:** 2037–43.

39. Pflumio F, Izac B, Katz A et al, Phenotype and function of human hematopoietic cells engrafting immune-deficient CB17-severe combined immunodeficiency mice and nonobese diabetic–severe combined immunodeficiency mice after transplantation of human cord blood mononuclear cells. *Blood* 1996; **88:** 3731–40.

40. Lowry PA, Shultz LD, Greiner DL et al, Improved engraftment of human cord blood stem cells in NOD/LtSz-scid/scid mice after irradiation or multiple-day injections into unirradiated recipients. *Biol Blood Marrow Transplant* 1996; **2:** 15–23.

41. Lu L, Xiao M, Grigsby S et al, Comparative effects of suppressive cytokines on isolated single CD34^{+++} stem/progenitor cells from human bone marrow and umbilical cord blood plated with and without serum. *Exp Hematol* 1993; **21:** 1442–6.

42. Traycoff CM, Abboud MR, Laver J et al, Rapid exit from G_0/G_1 phases of cell cycle in response to stem cell factor confers on umbilical cord blood CD34$^+$ cells an enhanced ex vivo expansion potential. *Exp Hematol* 1994; **22:** 1264–72.

43. Moore MAS, Hopkins I, Ex vivo expansions of cord blood derived stem cells and progenitors. *Blood Cells* 1994; **20:** 468–81.

44. Leitner A, Strobl H, Fischmeister G et al, Lack of DNA synthesis among CD34$^+$ cells in cord blood and in cytokine mobilized blood. *Br J Haematol* 1996; **92:** 255–62.

45. Ruggieri L, Heimfeld S, Broxmeyer HE, Cytokine-dependent ex vivo expansion of early subsets of CD34$^+$ cord blood myeloid progenitors is enhanced by cord blood plasma, but expansion of the more mature subsets of progenitors is favored. *Blood Cells* 1994; **20:** 436–54.

46. Broxmeyer HE, Benninger L, Yip-Schneider M, Braun SE, A rapid proliferation assay for unknown co-stimulating factors in cord blood plasma possibly involved in enhancement of in vitro expansion and replating capacity of human hematopoietic stem/progenitor cells. *Blood Cells* 1994; **20:** 492–7.

47. Bertolini F, Lazzari L, Lauri E et al, Cord blood plasma-mediated ex vivo expansion of hematopoietic progenitor cells. *Bone Marrow Transplant* 1994; **14:** 347–53.

48. Vaziri H, Dragowska W, Allsopp RC et al, Evidence for a mitotic clock in human hematopoietic stem cells: loss of telomeric DNA with age. *Proc Natl Acad Sci USA* 1994; **91:** 9857–60.

49. Hiyama K, Hirai Y, Kyoizumi S et al, Activation of telomerase in human lymphocytes and hematopoietic progenitor cells. *J Immunol* 1995; **155:** 3711–15.

50. Clapp DW, Baley JE, Gerson SL, Gestational age-dependent changes in circulating hematopoietic stem cells in newborn infants. *J Lab Clin Med* 1989; **113:** 422–7.

51. Hiett AK, Britton KA, Hague NL et al, Comparative analysis of hematopoietic progen-

itor cells in human umbilical cord blood collections of small and appropriate for gestational age neonates. *Transfusion* 1995; **35:** 587–91.

52. Saeland S, Duvert V, Caux C et al, Distribution of surface-membrane molecules on bone marrow and cord blood CD34$^+$ hematopoietic cells. *Exp Hematol* 1992; **20:** 24–33.

53. Migliaccio G, Migliaccio AR, Druzin ML et al, Long-term generation of colony-forming cells in liquid culture of CD34$^+$ cord blood cells in the presence of recombinant human stem cell factor. *Blood* 1992; **79:** 2620–7.

54. Abboud M, Xu F, LaVia M, Laver J, Study of early hematopoietic precursors in human cord blood. *Exp Hematol* 1992; **20:** 1043–7.

55. Thierry D, Hervatin F, Traineau R et al, Hematopoietic progenitors cells in cord blood. *Bone Marrow Transplant* 1992; **9:** 101–4.

56. Falkenburg JHF, Van Luxemburg-Heijs SAP, Zijlmans JM et al, Separation, enrichment and characterization of human hematopoietic progenitor cells from umbilical cord blood. *Ann Hematol* 1993; **67:** 231–6.

57. Wagner JE, Broxmeyer HE, Byrd RL et al, Transplantation of umbilical cord blood after myeloblative therapy: analysis of engraftment. *Blood* 1992; **79:** 1874–81.

58. Kohli-Kumar M, Shahidi NT, Broxmeyer HE et al, Haematopoietic stem/progenitor cell transplant in Fanconi anemia using HLA-matched sibling umbilical cord blood cells. *Br J Haematol* 1993; **85:** 419–22.

59. Newton I, Charbord P, Schaal JP, Herve P, Toward cord blood banking: density-separation and cryopreservation of cord blood progenitors. *Exp Hematol* 1993; **21:** 671–4.

60. deWynter EA, Coutinho LH, Pei X et al, Comparison of purity and enrichment of CD34$^+$ cells from bone marrow, umbilical cord blood and peripheral blood (primed for apheresis) using five separation systems. *Stem Cells* 1995; **13:** 524–32.

61. Almici C, Carlo-Stella C, Mangoni L et al, Density separation of umbilical cord blood and recovery of hemopoietic progenitor cells: implications for cord blood banking. *Stem Cells* 1995; **13:** 533–40.

62. Yurasov SV, Flasshove M, Rafii S, Moore MAS, Density enrichment and characterization of hematopoietic progenitors and stem cells from umbilical cord blood. *Bone Marrow Transplant* 1996; **17:** 517–25.

63. Denning-Kendall P, Donaldson C, Nicol A et al, Optimal processing of human umbilical cord blood for clinical banking. *Exp Hematol* 1996; **24:** 1394–401.

64. Isoyama K, Yamada K, Hirota Y et al, Study of the collection and separation of umbilical cord blood for use in hematopoietic progenitor cell transplantation. *Int J Hematol* 1996; **63:** 95–102.

65. Rubinstein P, Dobrila L, Rosenfeld RE et al, Processing and cryopreservation of placental/umbilical cord blood for unrelated bone marrow reconstitution. *Proc Natl Acad Sci USA* 1995; **92:** 10 119–22.

66. Smith FO, Robertson KA, Lucas KG et al, Umbilical cord blood transplantation from HLA-mismatched unrelated donors: the Indiana University experience [Abstract]. *Blood* 1996; **88**(Suppl 1): 266a.

67. Rubinstein P, Carrier C, Adamson J et al, New York Blood Center's program for unrelated placental/umbilical cord blood (PCB) transplantation: 243 transplants in the first 3 years [Abstract]. *Blood* 1996; **88**(Suppl 1): 142a.

68. Lu L, Ge Y, Li Z-H et al, CD34^{+++} stem/progenitor cells purified from cryopreserved normal cord blood can be transduced with high efficiency by a retroviral vector and expanded ex vivo with stable integration and expression of Fanconi anemia complementation C gene. *Cell Transplant* 1995; **4:** 493–503.

69. Broxmeyer HE, Cooper S, High efficiency recovery of immature hematopoietic progenitor cells with extensive proliferative capacity from human cord blood cryopreserved for ten years. *Clin Exp Immunol* 1996; **107:** 45–53.

70. Li ZH, Broxmeyer HE, Lu L, Cryopreserved cord blood myeloid progenitor cells can serve as targets for retroviral-mediated gene transduction and gene-transduced progenitors can be cryopreserved and recovered. *Leukemia* 1995; **9:** S12–S16.

71. Aird W, Labopin M, Gorin NC, Antin JH, Long-term cryopreservation of human stem cells. *Bone Marrow Transplant* 1992; **9:** 487–90.

72. Attarian H, Feng Z, Buckner CD et al, Long-term cryopreservation of bone marrow for autologous transplantation. *Bone Marrow Transplant* 1996; **17:** 425–30.

73. DiGiusto DL, Lee R, Moon J et al, Hematopoietic potential of cryopreserved and ex vivo manipulated umbilical cord blood progenitor cells evaluated in vitro and in vivo. *Blood* 1996; **87:** 1261–71.

74. McCullough J, Clay ME, Fautsch S et al,

Proposed policies and procedures for the establishment of a cord blood bank. *Blood Cells* 1994; **20:** 609–26.

75. Gluckman E, European Organization for Cord Blood Banking. *Blood Cells* 1994; **20:** 601–8.

76. Fisher CA, Establishment of cord blood banks for use in stem cell transplantation: Commentary. *Curr Probl Obstet Gynecol Fertil* 1996; **19:** 55–8.

77. Beatty PG, Mori M, Milford E, Impact of racial genetic polymorphism on the probability of finding an HLA-matched donor. *Transplantation* 1995; **60:** 778–83.

78. Bogdanic V, Nemet D, Kastelan A et al, Umbilical cord blood transplantation in a patient with Philadelphia chromosome-positive chronic myeloid leukemia. *Transplantation* 1993; **56:** 477–9.

79. Vilmer E, Sterkers G, Rahimy C et al, HLA-mismatched cord-blood transplantation in a patient with advanced leukemia. *Transplantation* 1992; **53:** 1155–7.

80. Vowels MR, Lam-Po-Tang R, Berdoukas V et al, Brief report: correction of X-linked lymphoproliferative disease by transplantation of cord-blood stem cells. *N Engl J Med* 1993; **329:** 1623–5.

81. Pahwa RN, Fleischer A, Than S, Good RA, Successful hematopoietic reconstitution with transplantation of erythrocyte-depleted allogeneic human umbilical cord blood cells in a child with leukemia. *Proc Natl Acad Sci USA* 1994; **91:** 4485–8.

82. Issaragrisil S, Visuthisakchai S, Suvatte V et al, Brief report: transplantation of cord-blood stem cells into a patient with severe thalassemia. *N Engl J Med* 1995; **332:** 367–9.

83. Brichard B, Vermylen C, Ninane J et al, Transplantation of umbilical cord blood in a refractory lymphoma. *Pediatr Hematol Oncol* 1995; **12:** 79–81.

84. Zix-Kieffer I, Langer B, Eyer D et al, Successful cord blood stem cell transplantation for congenital erythropoietic porphyria (Gunther's disease). *Bone Marrow Transplant* 1996; **18:** 217–20.

85. Stary J, Bartunkova J, Kobylka P et al, Successful HLA-identical sibling cord blood transplantation in a 6-year-old boy with leukocyte adhesion deficiency syndrome. *Bone Marrow Transplant* 1996; **18:** 249–52.

86. Laporte JP, Gorin NC, Rubinstein P et al, Cord-blood transplantation from an unrelated donor in an adult with chronic myelogenous leukemia. *N Engl J Med* 1996; **335:** 167–70.

87. Brichard B, Vermylen C, Ninane J, Cornu G, Persistence of fetal hemoglobin production after successful transplantation of cord blood stem cells in a patient with sickle cell anemia. *J Pediatrics* 1996; **128:** 241–3.

88. Ende N, Questions to be answered about umbilical cord blood [Letter to the Editor]. *Transfusion* 1996; **36:** 288–9.

89. Wagner JE, Broxmeyer HE, Questions to be answered about umbilical cord blood [Response to Letter to the Editor]. *Transfusion* 1996; **36:** 289–90.

90. Sirchia G, Rebulla P, Lecchi L, More on the safety of cord blood collection [Letter to the Editor]. *Transfusion* 1996; **36:** 937–8.

91. Bertolini F, Battaglia M, DeIulio C et al, Placental blood collection: effects on newborns [Letter to the Editor]. *Blood* 1995; **85:** 3361–2.

92. Socie G, Gluckman E, Carosella E et al, Search for maternal cells in human umbilical cord blood by polymerase chain reaction amplification of two minisatellite sequences. *Blood* 1994; **83:** 340–4.

93. Hall JM, Lingenfelter P, Adams SL et al, Detection of maternal cells in human umbilical cord blood using fluorescence in situ hybridization. *Blood* 1995; **86:** 2829–32.

94. Petit T, Gluckman E, Carosella E et al, A highly sensitive polymerase chain reaction method reveals the ubiquitous presence of maternal cells in human umbilical cord blood. *Exp Hematol* 1995; **23:** 1601–5.

95. Scaradavou A, Carrier C, Mollen N et al, Detection of maternal DNA in placental/umbilical cord blood by locus-specific amplification of the noninherited maternal HLA gene. *Blood* 1996; **88:** 1494–500.

96. Almici C, Carlo-Stella C, Rizzoli V, Wagner JE, Detection of maternal progenitor cells in human umbilical cord blood by single-colony karyotyping [Letter to the Editor]. *Blood* 1996; **88:** 1520–1.

97. Moritz T, Keller DC, Williams DA, Human cord blood cells as targets for gene transfer: potential use in genetic therapies of severe combined immunodeficiency disease. *J Exp Med* 1993; **178:** 529–36.

98. Lu L, Xiao M, Clapp DW, Li Z-H, Broxmeyer HE, High efficiency retroviral-mediated gene transduction into single isolated immature and replatable $CD34^{+++}$ hematopoietic stem/progenitor cells from human umbilical cord blood. *J Exp Med* 1993; **178:** 2089–96.

99. Zhou SZ, Cooper S, Kang LY et al, Adeno-associated virus 2-mediated high efficiency gene transfer into immature and mature subsets of hematopoietic progenitor cells in human umbilical cord blood. *J Exp Med* 1994; **179:** 1867–75.

100. Kohn DB, Weinberg KI, Nolta JA et al, Engraftment of gene-modified umbilical cord blood cells in neonates with adenosine deaminase deficiency. *Nature Med* 1995; **10:** 1–7.

12

Gene therapy

John M Cunningham, Stephen M Jane and Helen E Heslop

CONTENTS • **Introduction** • **Delivery systems** • **Gene transfer to hematopoietic progenitors** • **Gene therapy for single-gene defects** • **Modification of T lymphocytes** • **Gene transfer to modify malignant cells** • **Conclusions**

INTRODUCTION

Hematopoietic stem cell (HSC) transplantation with genetically modified cells offers the potential to treat many congenital disorders where allogeneic bone-marrow transplantation (BMT) is the only current curative therapy. However, problems in obtaining long-term stable expression of transferred genes in human hematopoietic cells have delayed the use of HSC transplantation as a vehicle for gene therapy apart from a few selected diseases where low-level transfer may produce therapeutic benefit. A more common use of gene transfer in clinical hematology over the past few years has been to answer biological questions about BMT and to develop novel therapies for cancer. Transfer of marker genes has provided important information on the biology of reconstitution and the origin of relapse after autologous transplantation. Gene transfer may also be used as a means of modifying T cells either to abrogate adverse effects of alloreactivity or to enhance activity of antileukemic effectors. In this chapter, we will review delivery systems for gene transfer into marrow-derived cells, as well as strategies to optimize gene transfer and select transduced cells. We will then review the results of clinical studies involving gene transfer for marking or therapeutic intent and discuss potential future applications.

DELIVERY SYSTEMS

A requirement for gene therapy is an efficient delivery system to transfer the gene of interest to the target cell. An ideal vector for the gene delivery would be selectively targeted to the desired cell, have a high efficiency of transduction and result in long-term expression of the transferred gene. None of the currently available vectors meets these specifications, and all have varying limitations. Gene correction by homologous recombination would be the preferred delivery in diseases where complex regulation is required. However, this technique is probably some years from clinical application. Current methods for gene delivery use recombinant viruses or physical methods[1,2] to introduce genetic material into non-homologous sites. The utility of any gene transfer system depends on six parameters:

(i) a high frequency of infection of the target cells;

(ii) efficient integration (if long-term expression of the transgene is required);

(iii) a selective advantage over non-transduced cells;

(iv) adequate transgene expression for reversal of the disease phenotype;

(v) stable regulatable expression in the desired cell type;

(vi) a genetically neutral event.

The biology and problems identified with the commonly used systems in hematopoiesis are discussed below.

Retroviral vectors

Retroviruses, particularly the Moloney murine leukemia virus (MoMuLV),[2] have been used extensively as a gene-delivery system. More recently, studies exploring the usefulness of recombinant Friend virus,[3] myeloproliferative sarcoma virus[4] and lentiviruses (such as HIV),[5] amongst others, have shown promise. Viral particles contain two single-stranded RNA molecules and the enzyme reverse transcriptase. Transcription results in production of duplex DNA, with subsequent genomic integration in mitotic cells. The proviral DNA serves as a template for virus production, since it encodes all sequences necessary for particle formation and productive infection. The wild-type retrovirus consists of two long terminal repeats (LTR), which are responsible for transcriptional control, polyadenylation, replication and integration (Figure 12.1A), and three structural genes: *gag*, which encodes structural proteins and confers high packaging efficiency; *pol*, which codes for replicative polymerases and integrase; and *env*, which codes for envelope proteins. In addition, a 350-nucleotide packaging signal (ψ) is required for retroviral encapsidation.[2]

Gene transfer requires a replication-defective virus, since there exists a risk of insertional mutagenesis with the wild-type retrovirus. This is achieved by replacing the *gag*, *pol* and *env* genes with the desired therapeutic genes, together with any necessary regulatory elements (Figure 12.1B).[2] Replication-defective viral vectors infect a target cell and integrate the therapeutic gene into the host genome, but lack the ability to reinfect. Murine fibroblast packaging cell lines provide structural genes in *trans* to package the recombinant virus, which is subsequently secreted into the culture medium (Figure 12.1B). To improve the safety of viral vectors, clinical-grade packaging cell lines have been refined such that three separate recombination events are required to produce a replication-competent retrovirus.[6] High-titer supernatants (10^6–10^7 particles/ml), optimal for HSC transduction, are thus produced.

The host range of MoMuLV viruses is determined by the gp70 envelope protein. Two major gp70 polypeptides have been used: ecotropic, which infects murine cells only, and amphotropic, which have a broader range that includes human cells. Interaction of these molecules with their cognate cellular receptors, transmembrane polypeptides that are normally involved in ion transport,[7,8] is associated with internalization. However, the poor transduction efficiency of human HSC and the limited number of amphotropic receptors on the stem cell surface[9] have prompted studies to improve specific viral targeting. Several approaches are presently being assessed:

(i) pseudotyping the virus, with VSV-G protein,[10] or a ligand for a cell surface receptor (e.g. erythropoietin or kit);[11]

(ii) changing the viral envelope, to the gibbon ape leukemia virus envelope for example;[12] or

(iii) transient expression of a retroviral receptor on the surface of non-permissive cells.[13]

In addition, these manipulations may allow concentration of the retrovirus (e.g. VSV-G).

Once in the cell, mitosis is required for efficient retroviral integration. Thus hematopoietic progenitors provide a good target for viral infection and integration. In contrast, most HSC are quiescent. This problem has been addressed by the use of cytokines, adhesion molecules and bone-marrow stroma to induce stem cell cycling. However, despite murine HSC transduction efficiencies of 20–50%, non-human pri-

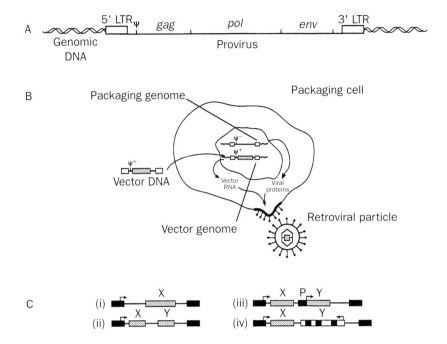

Figure 12.1 Recombinant retrovirus production.

(A) Integrated proviral genome. The virus is divided into regions consisting of (i) 5′ and 3′ LTR, which contain promoter, enhancer and polyadenylation sequences as well as inverted repeats; (ii) a packaging signal (ψ); three structural genes *gag*, *pol* and *env* which are required in *trans* for replication and packaging.

(B) Production of helper-free retroviral particles. A retroviral vector is introduced by transfection into the packaging cell line. This vector is capable of being packaged, but lacks the structural proteins necessary for infectious particle formation. This packaging genome provides these proteins, *gag*, *pol* and *env* in *trans*. Retroviral RNA transcripts complex with these proteins to form infectious particles. Supernatant from these cells thus contains replication-defective retroviruses that are free of wild-type virus, termed 'helper-free'.

(C) Basic types of recombinant retroviral vector: (i) simple type used in marking studies where a single gene X is regulated by the LTR; (ii) retroviral vector containing two genes each regulated by the LTR, in which viral transcripts are spliced prior to translation to give two transcripts X and Y; a similar construct in which splicing is prevented is termed a 'polycistronic vector'; (iii) a dual promoter construct in which the Y gene is driven by an external promoter and the X gene is regulated by the LTR; (iv) a construct where regulatory sequences of the genomic structure of one gene (Y) are used; this design has been used for β-globin constructs to prevent inappropriate splicing of intronic variants during the viral life cycle. (Adapted from reference 21.)

mate[14] and human studies[15] are disappointing, with transduction efficiencies of 1–10%.

Retroviruses accommodate 8–9 kb of exogenous DNA, gene expression being dependent on the regulatory sequences present in the viral construct.[2] Several possibilities exist, as illustrated in Figure 12.1C, including regulation of a single exogenous gene by the LTR, or expression of two genes using splicing or polycistronic variants where one gene is regulated by the LTR and one by an exogenous promoter.

For example, the recent identification of the elements required for high-level expression from the CD34 promoter suggests a possible mechanism of hematopoietic progenitor-specific expression.[16] Alternatively, LTR-driven expression of two genes can be achieved by the placement of an internal ribosomal re-entry site (IRES) between the two genes.[17] Several factors may affect the level of expression of the transgene, including the effects of the flanking viral sequences required for transduction and the stability of the viral transcript. The use of recombinases to inactivate or remove these flanking sequences,[18] introduction of hepatitis viral elements that ensure transcript stability,[19] and modification of LTR sequences to enhance expression are some of the possible approaches being explored.[20]

In summary, the advantages of recombinant retroviral particles include homogeneity of vector particles in the supernatant, the high titer and the lack of helper virus contamination. Problems of retroviral vector usage still exist, such as low hematopoietic stem cell transduction efficiency, lack of sufficient expression of the therapeutic gene and inconsistent long-term expression. This is exemplified by experience with globin-based vectors (see below).

Adeno-associated viruses

The non-pathogenic, defective parvovirus, adeno-associated virus (AAV), is a single-stranded DNA virus with a broad host range.[21] The 4.7-kb genome is bordered by inverted terminal repeat (ITR) sequences of 145 nucleotides (Figure 12.2). Two sets of structural genes, *rep* and *cap*, provide replicative and capsid proteins respectively. In addition, *rep* is required for site-specific integration of the virus into human chromosome 19, with consequent establishment of a latent state.[22] AAV is a dependovirus requiring a DNA helper virus, adenovirus or herpes simplex, for viral reactivation and packaging.

The ability of recombinant AAV (rAAV) to infect cells was first demonstrated by replacing the *cap* genes with a selectable marker.[23]

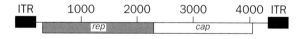

Figure 12.2 Wild-type adeno-associated virus genome. The virus is flanked by ITR (inverted terminal repeats), which are single-stranded hairpin structures. These are all that is required for recombinant vector production. The structural *rep* and *cap* genes are regulated by internal promoters.

Transduction efficiencies of 80% were observed in tissue culture. Subsequent experiments replaced all sequences between the AAV ITR with exogenous DNA, the ITR being necessary for integration, replication and packaging signals.[24] The construct is cotransfected with a second plasmid expressing the *rep* and *cap* genes and live adenovirus into a permissive cell line. This procedure permits up to 5 kb of DNA to be packaged without AAV helper contamination. Adenoviral contamination is excluded by differential heat inactivation. Initial titers of 10^4–10^5 particles were obtained with this system, and subsequent refinement resulted in titers exceeding 10^9 infectious particles/ml. Ongoing development of efficient packaging cell lines, similar to those developed for retroviruses, should make this approach less cumbersome.[25]

The efficacy of rAAV to transduce and integrate into the genome with consequent transgene expression was demonstrated in numerous tissue culture cells.[26,27] In addition, rAAV integrates into mitotic and quiescent cells, thus increasing its target range.[28] Initial experiments suggested that a similar result was possible with primary cells, including bone marrow and cord blood hematopoietic progenitors.[29–31] These cells showed high levels of expression of the transgene after 14–21 days in culture, suggesting that AAV vectors may be useful for hematopoietic stem cell targeted gene transfer. Unlike wild-type AAV, the recombinant form of the virus appears to integrate randomly as 3–5 tandemly arranged copies.[30] However, subsequent studies suggest that rAAV exists predominantly as an episomal genome for several days to weeks after infection.[13] Integration events are rare, and appear to depend on vector design, the presence of *rep* and the viral titer. Thus this viral system has the advantages of lack of pathogenicity, the ability to transduce and integrate into quiescent hematopoietic stem cells,[30] and an apparent lack of interference from flanking viral sequences. However, significant disadvantages, including the lack of an efficient packaging system, the relatively small amount of DNA that can be packaged and the low efficiency of viral integration, have limited its use.

Other viruses

The development of recombinant herpes simplex and adenoviral vectors has focussed on their utility in pulmonary, hepatic and CNS gene therapy.[21] Extensive reviews of their biology have been published elsewhere.[32] They are attractive in view of the large amount of DNA that can be packaged, and their ability to infect non-dividing and dividing cells. In contrast to the systems described above, they are limited by their inability to integrate efficiently into recipient cell nuclear DNA. However, the recent demonstration of the ability of adenovirus to infect hematopoietic progenitors,[33] the utilization of adenoviral vectors for transient expression of ecotropic viral receptors on non-permissive human hematopoietic cells, and the short-term expression of cytokines and costimulatory molecules in primary leukemic cells to induce immune stimulation suggest that these vectors may be valuable in hematopoietic cell-directed gene therapy. Similarly, a disabled single-cycle herpes simplex virus can transduce hematopoietic progenitors or leukemic blasts efficiencies of 80–100%.[34] While expression is transient, this vector may be useful for applications where short-term expression is adequate. Several other viral vector systems are currently in the early stages of development. These include the spumavirus human foamy virus, other parvoviruses and the hepatitis viruses.[35] However, efficient packaging systems, host range and integration efficiency still require determination.

GENE TRANSFER TO HEMATOPOIETIC PROGENITORS

The genetic modification of hematopoietic progenitor cells could theoretically correct many single-gene defects of marrow-derived cells. The advantages of using hematopoietic progenitors as targets for gene transfer include easy procurement and manipulation ex vivo and the possibility of gene transfer to multiple cell lineages. The major disadvantages are that transduction efficiency with current vectors is low, and the biology of the true hematopoietic stem cell is not yet well defined. Clinical studies have therefore been confined to situations where low-efficiency transduction may produce therapeutic benefit (such as ADA deficiency) or where useful information may be obtained (such as in marking studies).

Gene-marking studies in autologous HSC transplantation

Since 1991, studies using this approach have been undertaken in a variety of malignancies where autologous HSC transplantation may be part of the therapy, including acute myeloid leukemia (AML), neuroblastoma, chronic myeloid leukemia (CML), acute lymphoblastic leukemia (ALL), lymphoma, multiple myeloma and breast cancer (Table 12.1). In these studies, HSC have been marked with retroviral vectors encoding the neomycin resistance gene. This marker gene can subsequently be detected in transduced cells: either phenotypically because it confers resistance to the neomycin analogue G418, or genotypically by PCR.

The first marking study was undertaken at St Jude Children's Research Hospital between September 1991 and March 1993 in patients with AML or neuroblastoma receiving autologous transplantation. Marrow mononuclear cells were marked in a simple 6-hour transduction protocol in the absence of growth factors. Twelve patients were enrolled on the AML study and follow-up ranges from 47 to 63 months. In three of four patients who have relapsed, the marker gene was definitively shown in leukemia cells that had a collateral leukemia-specific marker,[36] while the fourth patient was uninformative.

In the neuroblastoma study, five of nine patients have relapsed, and gene-marked neuroblastoma cells, co-expressing the neuroblastoma-specific antigen GD2 together with the transferred marker gene, were detected in four cases.[37,38] In one of these patients, marked neuroblastoma cells were detected in an extramedullary relapse in the liver.[37] Similarly marked malignant cells co-expressing the t(9;22)

Table 12.1 Marking studies in autologous BMT

Institution	Disease	Study question
St Jude Children's Research Hospital	Acute myeloid leukemia	Source of relapse
	Neuroblastoma	Efficacy of purging
	Pediatric solid tumors	Reconstitution: blood versus marrow
		Reconstitution: unmanipulated versus cytokine-expanded CD34 cells
MD Anderson Cancer Center	Chronic myeloid leukemia	Source of relapse
	Chronic lymphoid leukemia	Efficacy of purging
	Lymphoma	Reconstitution: blood versus marrow
National Institutes of Health	Breast cancer	Reconstitution: blood versus marrow
	Multiple myeloma	
University of Indiana	Acute lymphoid leukemia	Source of relapse
	Acute myeloid leukemia	
Fred Hutchinson Cancer Institute	Lymphoma	Cytokine-mobilized peripheral blood supplementation
	Solid tumors	of marrow grafts
University of Southern California	Lymphoma	Source of relapse
	Breast cancer	Reconstitution: blood versus marrow
Karolinska Institute	Multiple myeloma	Source of relapse
University of Minnesota	Chronic myeloid leukemia	Contribution of CD34 DR⁻ population
University of Toronto	Multiple myeloma	Gene transfer in long-term bone-marrow culture

and *neo* transcripts were found in two patients with CML at relapse.[39] These data show that marrow harvested in apparent clinical remission in these three malignancies may contain residual tumorigenic cells that can contribute to a subsequent relapse. In contrast, marked cells have not been found in adult patients relapsing after autografts for ALL.[40] However, only around 10% of the marrow was marked in this study, and gene transfer to normal cells was very low. In the National Institutes of Health (NIH) study, transplantation was undertaken using CD34-selected HSC from blood and marrow. Two patients with breast cancer have relapsed, and the marker gene was not found.[15] This may reflect a lower efficiency of marking of breast cancer cells, or CD34 selection may reduce contamination with malignant cells. Alternatively, relapse in this disease may occur predominantly from residual disease in the patient. No patient has yet relapsed in the myeloma studies.

In second-generation studies, two genetically distinct marker genes are being used to compare either marrow purging versus no purging, or two different purging techniques. The two vectors used in these studies, G1N and LNL6, differ in 3′ non-coding sequence, so primers can be designed that will result in amplification of fragments of different sizes. Fifteen patients have been transplanted in an AML study that compares two purging techniques,[41] but only two patients have relapsed and no information is yet available on the efficacy of purging.

These studies also allowed assessment of the efficiency of gene transfer to normal progenitors. In the St Jude studies, the marker gene has continued to be detected and expressed for up to five years in both marrow clonogenic cells and their mature progeny, including peripheral blood T and B cells and neutrophils.[42,43] It is interesting that the level of transfer was highest in marrow clonogenic hemopoietic progenitors and about 1 log lower in peripheral blood.[42,44] In peripheral blood cells, expression was higher in myeloid cells than in T lymphocytes, with the lowest level of transfer in B lymphocytes. These observations suggest that autologous marrow makes a substantial contribution to long-term reconstitution following autologous transplantation. Similar results were seen in the MD Anderson study,[39] where cells were also transduced in a short incubation in the absence of growth factors. In the NIH study, CD34 cells were transduced in a 72-hour culture with the growth factors IL-3, IL-6 and stem cell factor. Although this technique produces high-efficiency transfer in clonogenic assays and murine reconstitution models, levels of gene transfer in hematopoietic cells post transplant has been lower than in the St Jude and MD Anderson studies.[15] This may reflect the different patient population, or alternatively may show that culture with growth factors commits transduced cells to differentiation. The highest levels of gene transfer have been observed by the Toronto group, who are transducing marrow cells in long-term bone-marrow culture,[45,46] based on studies in a canine model that have shown high levels of long-term transfer.[47] In the clinical study in myeloma patients, in situ PCR studies have shown that up to 10% of peripheral blood cells contain the marker gene.[46]

Marking studies to compare different sources of hematopoietic stem cells

Double marking techniques can also be used to compare long-term reconstitution from different sources of HSC. The availability of multiple sources of HSC, such as umbilical cord blood and peripheral blood progenitor cells, has led to debate over the optimal source of HSC for transplantation and gene therapy applications. Currently available in vitro and xenograft models provide only a surrogate analysis of the behavior of HSC following clinical transplantation. The use of two distinguishable retroviral markers allows intrapatient comparison of the short- and long-term reconstituting capacity of different populations of HSC. In the NIH study, CD34-selected cells from blood or marrow of patients receiving HSC transplant were randomized to marking with two distinguishable retroviral vectors. Although the levels of transfer detected in vivo were low, the contribution from the marker gene derived from the blood stem cells has been detected for up to 18 months.[15] In a marrow purging study in patients with AML,[41] the double marking component has allowed comparison of reconstitution of normal progenitors after the two purging procedures. In peripheral blood, the signal from the 4-hydroperoxycyclophosphamide (4HC)-purged fraction has been consistently stronger and longer-lived than that from the IL-2-purged fraction, implying that the 4HC-purged fraction is making a greater contribution to hematopoietic reconstitution.[44] This strategy may also be used to compare the reconstitution of different subsets of HSC or differentially treated aliquots. For example, we plan to compare the contribution of different CD34 subsets to short- and long-term reconstitution[43] and to compare the reconstitution of unmanipulated and ex vivo expanded progenitors.[48]

Drug resistance genes

The low efficiency of current gene-transfer techniques into hematopoietic progenitor cells necessitates an ability to select in vivo for the transduced cell population. The neomycin resistance gene, used to select retroviral producer clones, is unsuitable for in vivo selection. Thus genes involved in the metabolism of several cytotoxic agents have become attractive candidates for in vivo hematopoietic stem cell selection/protection.[49,50] These dominant selectable markers allow dose escalation of chemotherapeutic regimens by protecting normal progenitors from the toxic effects of these compounds, forming the basis of several recently approved clinical trials. Other selectable markers include surface antigens such as CD24[51,52] or a truncated version of the nerve growth factor receptor.[53]

The dihydrofolate reductase gene (DHFR), which is involved in methotrexate (MTX) metabolism, was the first gene evaluated for its potential use as a dominant selectable marker. Mice transplanted with marrow previously transduced with a DHFR-containing retrovirus were protected from subsequent MTX-induced myelosuppression.[49] Subsequent studies suggested that this gene protects committed progenitors but not HSC.[33] However, more recent studies demonstrate that the combination of MTX and an inhibitor of thymidine rescue (e.g. dipyridamole) bypasses this effect and permits stem cell selection.[54]

The multidrug resistance-1 gene (*MDR-1*), which is involved in the efflux of several naturally occurring cytotoxic agents such as the vinca alkaloids, Taxol and anthracycline-based compounds, has been evaluated in murine and human studies. *MDR-1*-transduced marrow when transplanted into mice protected them from the effects of Taxol.[50] Recently, the work of Pastan and colleagues suggested that a bicistronic vector (see Figure 12.1C), containing an *MDR-1* gene and a therapeutic glucocerebrosidase gene, allows high-level coexpression of both transcripts in tissue culture, and selection of transduced cells.[55] Studies of human hematopoietic progenitors have confirmed the results seen in mice, but with a lower transduction efficiency.[56] Clinical trials now underway will help to validate this selection strategy.

GENE THERAPY FOR SINGLE-GENE DEFECTS

A number of monogenic diseases resulting from single-gene defects can be treated by allogeneic BMT and are candidates for correction by modified hematopoietic progenitors. To illustrate some of the issues with gene therapy for such disorders, we will discuss gene transfer for adenosine deaminase deficiency, hemoglobinopathies and metabolic storage disorders.

Adenosine deaminase deficiency

In adenosine deaminase (ADA) deficiency, accumulation of toxic metabolites in T cells results in one form of severe combined immunodeficiency. This disease is a good model for gene therapy since the gene is not subject to complex regulation and clinical benefit may occur with correction of only a small number of T cells. Furthermore, there should be a growth advantage for transduced cells. Three clinical protocols have evaluated transfer of ADA into peripheral blood lymphocytes, bone marrow and umbilical cord blood cells that have been transduced ex vivo and returned to the patients.[57–59] In all these studies, there has been an increase in numbers of circulating T cells and ADA levels in conjunction with reconstitution of immune function.[57–59] As all the children continue to receive treatment with polyethylene glycol (PEG) ADA, these results must be interpreted with caution. Nevertheless, the observation that the percentage of ADA-transduced T cells increases by 1–2 logs when PEG ADA is tapered[60] suggests that the transduced cells may have a selective advantage that will allow them to contribute to long-term reversal of phenotype.

Hemoglobinopathies

The challenges of the hemoglobinopathies mirror those of many gene defects that may be amenable to HSC-targeted gene therapy. Therapy is limited and non-curative, with the exception of allogeneic BMT, which is an option in only a minority of patients.[61,62] Gene therapy for these diseases requires replacement of the defective β-globin gene: with a functional β-globin gene in β-thalassemia, while a regulatable γ-globin gene is preferable in sickle cell disease. Significant amelioration of the disease phenotype requires at least 20% expression of a transduced γ- or β-globin gene relative to the endogenous levels.[61] To achieve this goal, we must first understand the normal regulation of the human β-globin genes,[63] develop more efficient gene-delivery systems, and ensure that the expression of the transduced gene is both tissue-specific and maintained at high levels by erythroid progenitors.

The genes of the β-globin locus (ε, ^{G}γ, ^{A}γ, δ, β), are coordinately regulated at the level of gene transcription.[63] Studies in transgenic mice have shown that both gene-proximal promoters and enhancers as well as a far-upstream 15-kb dominant regulatory region termed the locus control region (LCR) are required for high-level expression. Prior to identification of the LCR, retroviral vectors containing genomic fragments of the β- or γ-genes demonstrated the feasibility of gene transfer of globin sequences, albeit with low levels of gene expression.[64–67] Identification of the LCR and its addition to these constructs resulted in high-level expression in tissue culture cells.[68] However, inability to manufacture high-titer unrearranged producer cell lines and poor expression of these contructs in primary cells (<1%) has provided significant obstacles to their clinical applicability. More recently, constructs containing LCR elements and a human β-globin gene altered to reduce recombination were reported to induce transgene expression of up to 70% in MEL cells and relatively high expression in mice.[69] Although encouraging, these results require confirmation in non-human primate models.

Owing to the difficulties of viral preparation and transgene expression, rAAV has been proposed as an alternative vector system. The major potential advantage of AAV is its ability to stably integrate in a relatively site-specific manner in quiescent cells. Early experiments yielded transgene expression levels 40–110% of the endogenous gene in K562 erythroleukemia cells.[26] Genomic analysis revealed a randomly integrated single copy of unrearranged provirus per cell. These encouraging results have led several laboratories to investigate the expression of similar constructs in erythroid progenitors.[29] A construct containing a truncated LCR coupled to the ^{A}γ gene (v432^{A}γ) without a selectable marker has given high-level expression in human BFUe.[70] However, poor efficiency of viral integration both in primary cell culture and in primate studies suggest that further work is necessary prior to the availability of a clinical-grade vector. More recently, an increased rate of integration has been observed with high-titer preparations and the addition of ancillary globin elements to the construct that interact with the nuclear scaffold, suggesting that this approach warrants further study.[71]

In general, further advancement in gene transfer to correct hemoglobinopathies requires improved vector technology, a broader understanding of the role of the *cis-* and *trans-*acting elements in globin gene regulation, and improved stem cell transduction. An alternative approach presently being pursued is the correction of the mutation by gene conversion utilizing an RNA–DNA oligonucleotide. Specific conversion was observed in lymphoblastoid cell lines from patients with sickle cell disease. Further studies are required to assess the validity of this approach in primary cells.[72]

Metabolic storage diseases

Gene therapy for metabolic storage diseases has been the focus of much interest. Similar problems related to stem cell transduction and long-term expression that were described for the hemoglobinopathies have been encountered.[73] Gaucher disease is the most prevalent autosomal recessive lysosomal storage disease. It is due to glucocerebrosidase deficiency, which predominantly affects macrophage metabolism. Although recombinant enzyme replacement is available, a less expensive form of therapy is required.[74] Correction of this enzyme deficiency by gene transfer has been demonstrated in skin fibroblasts, human lymphoblastoid cell lines and bone-marrow culture.[73,75] Long-term reconstitution, and expression in most cases, was achieved in mice with hematopoietic stem cells containing glucocerebrosidase-expressing retroviral constructs.[73] In addition, expression in both circulating macrophage and CNS microglia was documented, which is a prerequisite for successful therapy of most metabolic storage diseases.[76] Similar results have also been reported from studies of human in vitro cell culture.[77] Clinical trials using this construct are due to begin soon. Further studies, including the use of variant retroviral backbones, bicistronic vectors incorporating dominant selectable markers such as MDR, alternate HSC sources and the AAV system, are being pursued in order to achieve optimal transgene expression.[27,52]

Other single-gene-defect syndromes, including the other lipidoses, mucopolysaccharidoses, chronic granulomatous disease, inborn errors of metabolism and leukocyte adhesion abnormalities, have been corrected, at least in part, in tissue culture cell lines or in murine models.[27,73] Of particular note is the correction of a subset of Fanconi anemia phenotypes by both retroviral and AAV vectors containing a correct copy of the defective DNA repair enzymes.[78] This is particularly important in view of the high risk of both regimen-related toxicity and graft-versus-host disease when allogeneic BMT is undertaken in such patients.

MODIFICATION OF T LYMPHOCYTES

Over the past few years, adoptive transfer studies in allogeneic BMT recipients have shown that donor T cells can be effective in the therapy of relapsed malignancy or viral infection following BMT.[79–81] Although such adoptive immunotherapy approaches have produced clinical benefit, they are complicated by the frequent development of graft-versus-host disease (GVHD). Several gene-transfer studies in allogeneic BMT (Table 12.2) are providing a means of monitoring such approaches, ablating allogeneic T cells in the event of GVHD or conferring novel recognition properties.

Gene transfer to evaluate adoptive transfer strategies

Gene marking is being used in an adoptive transfer study to determine if donor-derived Epstein–Barr virus (EBV)-specific cytotoxic T lymphocytes (CTL) provide effective prophylaxis for EBV lymphomas that arise after BMT. The pathogenesis of EBV lymphoproliferation is outgrowth of EBV-infected B cells that express a number of EBV-encoded antigens and are highly immunogenic. Normally, outgrowth is prevented by EBV-specific CTL[82] and will occur only in severely immunosuppressed individuals such as patients receiving T-cell-depleted allogeneic bone marrow from HLA-mismatched or HLA-matched unrelated donors.[83] The frequency of EBV-specific CTL precursors (CTLp) in seropositive individuals is

Table 12.2 Gene-transfer studies in allogeneic BMT

Institution	Target cell (gene)	Study question
St Jude Children's Research Hospital	EBV-specific CTL (*neo*)	Persistence and safety of adoptively transferred cells
HMS Raffaele, Milan, Italy	Donor T cells (*Tk/NGFR*)	Feasibility of suicide gene strategy
Fred Hutchinson Cancer Institute	CD8$^+$ HIV-specific CTL (*Tk/hygromycin*)	Persistence and safety of adoptively transferred cells Feasibility of suicide gene strategy
University of Arkansas	Donor T cells (*Tk/neo*)	Feasibility of suicide gene strategy
Laboratoire d'Histocompatibilité et Therapeutique Immuno-Moléculaire, Besançon, France	Donor T cells (*Tk/neo*)	Feasibility of suicide gene strategy

CTL = cytotoxic T lymphocytes; *Tk* = thymidine kinase; *NGFR* = nerve growth factor receptor.

high, and donor-derived peripheral blood leukocytes[81,84] are effective therapy for this complication. However, the frequency of alloreactive CTLp is also high, resulting in a significant risk of severe GVHD. In addition, treatment of established disease can lead to toxicity from inflammatory responses to virus-infected cells.[81,85]

Patients at high risk of developing EBV lymphoproliferation after receiving T-cell-depleted BMT from HLA-mismatched family members or unrelated donors are eligible to receive donor-derived, EBV-specific CTL as prophylaxis for EBV-associated lymphoma, from day 45 post-BMT.[86] To allow tracking of infused cells and to determine if they produced adverse effects, CTL were marked with the *neo*R gene. Thirty-three patients have received CTL lines on the prophylaxis component of this study and no immediate adverse effects from infusion have been seen. In particular, there was no induction of GVHD. The marker gene was detected by PCR for up to 16 weeks in unmanipulated peripheral blood mononuclear cells and for over 36 months in EBV-specific CTL lines regenerated from patients following treatment with gene-marked CTL.[87] We also have evidence for efficacy in that, of the 33 patients receiving prophylactic CTL, six had developed greatly elevated titers of EBV DNA prior to administration of CTL – a result strongly predictive of the onset of lymphoma.[88] In all six patients, titers rapidly returned to baseline within 2–4 weeks of CTL infusion.[85] Moreover, in two patients who received CTL therapeutically rather than prophylactically, there was a dramatic therapeutic response to CTL infusion.[89] In one of these patients, the marking component of the study allowed us to show by in situ hybridization and semiquantitative PCR that the infused cells had selectively accumulated and expanded at disease sites.[85] However, while prophylactic CTL did not produce any adverse effects, the patient who received therapeutic CTL for bulky established disease developed initial tumor swelling and respiratory obstruction prior to response. This patient illustrates that, even when alloreactivity is absent, it is possible to get morbidity from tissue inflammation during therapy of bulky disease.

Gene transfer to confer drug sensitivity

Infusing donor-derived T cells following BMT can lead to GVHD initiated by alloreactive T cells. Even if CTL clones are used, cross-reaction with MHC polymorphisms may cause GVHD in an allogeneic setting.[90] In addition, as discussed above, therapy of established disease with T cells can result in tissue damage from inflammatory reactions. Transduction of T cells with a 'suicide gene' so that cell death may be induced if adverse effects occur is one solution to this problem.[53,91] The vector most commonly used encodes the thymidine kinase gene (*Th*), which renders host cells sensitive to the cytotoxic effects of nucleotide analogues such as ganciclovir. For this approach to be successful, it is necessary that all cells contain the suicide gene and that expression is maintained in vivo. To achieve this, suicide gene constructs have included a selectable marker such as *neo*[91] or a cell-surface marker.[53]

Suicide genes are currently being evaluated in a number of clinical trials of adoptive immunotherapy post-transplant. Bonini and colleagues, who are using donor T cells to treat relapse or EBV lymphoma following BMT,[92] transfect lymphocytes, after a brief 24–48-hour primary stimulation with antigen, with a construct containing a suicide gene and a truncated version of the low-molecular-weight nerve growth factor gene to serve as a selectable marker. Eight patients have been treated, and in three patients who developed GVHD, signs and symptoms resolved after ganciclovir therapy.[92] Riddell and colleagues have administered *gag*-specific CTL transduced with a construct encoding *Tk* and the hygromycin resistance gene to HIV-infected patients receiving allogeneic BMT for lymphoma.[93] In this study, five of six patients developed CTL responses specific for the transgene, which destroyed the infused cells. One patient in the Italian study also developed *Tk*-specific CTL, so this approach may be limited by the immunogenicity of the transgene.

Gene transfer to modulate T-cell function

The antitumor activity of T cells may also be enhanced by increasing the levels of cytotoxic cytokines they produce at local tumor sites or by transducing them with appropriate antigen-specific T-cell receptors to confer novel tumor-recognition properties. Many tumors express surface antigens that may be recognized by specific antibodies. If a cytotoxic T cell is transduced with a construct encoding a chimeric gene that contains a single-chain variable-region antibody linked with the γ or ζ chain of the immunoglobulin receptor or the T-cell receptor, then that CTL will recognize the tumor cell via the chimeric receptor. On binding to a tumor-specific antigen on the tumor cell surface, the effector function of these modified CTL could be triggered. Unlike conventional CTL, which recognize antigen in the context of one MHC polymorphism, these modified lymphocytes would recognize a tumor-specific antigen in an MHC-unrestricted fashion. This approach has also shown promise when non-T-cell immune effectors are modified with such receptors.[94] If CTL targeted to leukemic cells could be generated, their administration post BMT may produce a graft-versus-leukemia (GVL) effect without GVHD.

GENE TRANSFER TO MODIFY MALIGNANT CELLS

Gene transfer may be used to modify tumor cells in an attempt to increase immunogenicity (Figure 12.3). With increasing knowledge of the requirements for antigen presentation and for co-stimulation in induction of CTL responses, investigators have evaluated the effect of transducing tumor cells with cytokine genes, co-stimulatory molecules or allogeneic MHC molecules.[95] In a number of different murine models, administration of transduced tumor cells has led to the recruitment of immune system effector cells and tumor rejection. For example, in a murine leukemia model, the B7-1 molecule was transduced into a *bcr–abl*-transformed subline of the 32Dc13 myeloid cell line

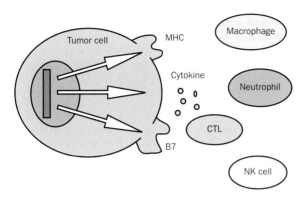

Figure 12.3 Increasing immunogenicity of tumors. This figure illustrates how transfection of a tumor cell with an MHC molecule, a cytokine gene, or a co-stimulatory molecule results in recruitment of immune system effectors. All these effects may induce rejection of tumor locally, and some of these effectors will also eradicate distant tumor deposits. CTL=cytotoxic T lymphocyte.

that is normally lethal.[96] If the line was transduced with B7-1, it remained lethal in nude mice, but caused only a transient leukemia in immunocompetent syngeneic mice, who subsequently developed protective immunity to rechallenge. Optimum benefit may be obtained when tumor cells are transduced with combinations of molecules affecting different phases of the immune reponse.[97] As of September 1997, over 50 clinical studies were evaluating this tumor vaccine approach. Initial results of these studies suggest that both IL-2-transduced neu-

roblastoma cells and GM-CSF-transduced melanoma cells produce immunomodulatory effects.[98]

CONCLUSIONS

Gene transfer will have a significant impact on hematopoietic stem cell transplantation in several ways. First, it may provide alternate therapies for genetic disorders due to single-gene defects currently treated by allogeneic BMT. For therapy of most single-gene defects to be effective, better delivery systems are required, as well as more precise knowledge of the optimal conditions for hematopoietic stem cell transduction. For patients with leukemia who will still require allogeneic BMT, genetic modification of infused T cells may provide a means of ablating alloreactive T cells and preventing GVHD. Finally, gene transfer to antigen-specific CTL may allow separation of GVHD and GVL effects, with enhancement of anti-leukemia effects.

ACKNOWLEDGEMENTS

This work was supported in part by NIH Cancer Center Support CORE Grant P30, HL55703, CA 61384, HL53749, the Assisi Foundation of Memphis, the NHMRC, and the American Lebanese Syrian Associated Charities (ALSAC). JMC is a scholar of the American Society of Hematology.

REFERENCES

1. Crystal RG, Transfer of genes to humans: early lessons and obstacles to success. *Science* 1995; **270:** 404–10.
2. Miller AD, Retroviral vectors. *Curr Top Microbiol Immunol* 1992; **158:** 1–24.
3. Clapp DW, Freie B, Srour E et al, Myeloproliferative sarcoma virus directed expression of beta-galactosidase following retroviral transduction of murine hemopoietic cells. *Exp Hematol* 1995; **23:** 630–8.
4. Baum C, Eckert HG, Stocking C, Ostertag W, Activity of Friend mink cell focus-forming retrovirus during myelo-erythroid hematopoiesis. *Exp Hematol* 1996; **24:** 364–70.
5. Naldini L, Blomer U, Gallay P et al, In vivo gene delivery and stable transduction of nondividing cells by a lentiviral vector. *Science* 1996; **272:** 263–7.
6. Danos O, Mulligan RC, Safe and effective generation of recombinant retroviruses with ampho-

tropic and ecotropic host ranges. *Proc Natl Acad Sci USA* 1988; **85:** 6460–4.

7. Miller DG, Edwards RH, Miller AD, Cloning of the cellular receptor for amphotropic murine retroviruses reveals homology to that for gibbon ape leukemia virus. *Proc Natl Acad Sci USA* 1994; **91:** 78–82.

8. Albritton LM, Tseng L, Scadden D, Cunningham JM, A putative murine ecotropic retrovirus receptor gene encodes a multiple membrane-spanning protein and confers susceptibility to viral infection. *Cell* 1989; **57:** 659–66.

9. Orlic D, Girard LJ, Jordan CT et al, The level of mRNA encoding the amphotropic retroviral receptor in mouse and human hematopoietic stem cells is low and correlates with the efficiency of retrovirus transduction. *Proc Natl Acad Sci USA* 1996; **93:** 11 097–102.

10. Yee JK, Miyanohara A, LaPorte P et al, A general method for the generation of high titer, pantropic retroviral vectors: highly efficient infection of primary hepatocytes. *Proc Natl Acad Sci USA* 1994; **91:** 9564–8.

11. Kasahara N, Dozy AM, Kan YW, Tissue-specific targeting of retroviral vectors through ligand-receptor interactions. *Science* 1994; **266:** 1373–6.

12. Porter CD, Collins MK, Tailor CS et al, Comparison of efficiency of human gene therapy target cells via four different retroviral receptors. *Human Gene Ther* 1996; **7:** 913–19.

13. Bertran J, Miller JL, Yang Y et al, Recombinant adeno-associated virus-mediated high-efficiency, transient expression of the murine cationic amino acid transporter (ecotropic retroviral receptor) permits stable transduction of human HeLa cells by ecotropic retroviral receptors. *J Virol* 1996; **70:** 6759–66.

14. Bodine DM, Moritz T, Donahue RE et al, Long-term in vivo expression of a murine adenosine deaminase gene in rhesus monkey hematopoietic cells of multiple lineages after retroviral mediated gene transfer into CD34$^+$ bone marrow cells. *Blood* 1993; **82:** 1975–80.

15. Dunbar CE, Cottler–Fox M, O'Shaunessy JA et al, Retrovirally marked CD34-enriched peripheral blood and marrow cells contribute to long term engraftment after autologous transplantation. *Blood* 1995; **85:** 3048–57.

16. May G, Enver T, Targeting gene expression to haemopoietic stem cells: chromatin-dependent upstream element mediates cell type-specific expression of the stem cell antigen CD34. *EMBO J* 1995; **14:** 564–74.

17. Sokolic RA, Sekhsaria S, Sugimoto Y et al, A bicistronic retroviral vector containing a picornavirus internal ribosome entry site allows for correction of X-linked CGD by selection for *MDR1* expression. *Blood* 1996; **87:** 42–50.

18. Russ AP, Friedel C, Grez M, von Melchner H, Self-deleting retrovirus vectors for gene therapy. *J Virol* 1996; **70:** 4927–32.

19. Huang ZM, Yen TSB, Role of hepatitis B virus posttranscriptional regulatory element in export of intronless transcripts. *Mol Cell Biol* 1995; **15:** 3864–9.

20. Challita PM, Skelton D, el-Khoueiry A et al, Multiple modifications in *cis* elements of the long terminal repeat of retroviral vectors lead to increased expression and decreased DNA methylation in embryonic carcinoma cells. *J Virol* 1995; **69:** 748–55.

21. Nienhuis AW, Walsh CE, Liu J, Young NS, Viruses as therapeutic gene transfer vectors. In: *Viruses and Bone Marrow; Basic Research and Clinical Practice* (Young NS, ed). New York: Marcel Dekker, 1993: 353–414.

22. Samulski RJ, Zhu X, Xiao X et al, Targeted integration of adeno-associated virus (AAV) into chromosome 19. *EMBO J* 1991; **10:** 3941–50.

23. Hermonat P, Muzyczka N, Use of adeno-associated virus as a mammalian DNA cloning vector: transduction of neomycin resistance into mammalian tissue culture cells. *Proc Natl Acad Sci USA* 1984; **81:** 6466–70.

24. Samulski RJ, Chang LS, Shenk T, Helper-free stocks of recombinant adeno-associated viruses: normal integration does not require viral gene expression. *J Virol* 1989; **63:** 3822–8.

25. Tamayose K, Hirai Y, Shimada T, A new strategy for preparation of high-titer recombinant adeoo-associated virus vectors by using packaging cell lines and sulfonated cellulose column chromatography. *Hum Gene Ther* 1996; **7:** 507–13.

26. Walsh CE, Liu JM, Xiao X et al, Regulated high level expression of a human gamma-globin gene introduced into erythroid cells by an adeno-associated virus vector. *Proc Natl Acad Sci USA* 1992; **89:** 7257–61.

27. Wei FF, Wei F, Samulski RJ, Barranger JA, Expression of the human glucocerebridase and arylsulfatase genes in murine and patient primary fibroblasts transduced by an adeno-associated virus vector. *Gene Ther* 1994; **1:** 261–8.

28. Russell DW, Miller AD, Alexander IE, Adeno associated virus vectors preferentially transduce cells in S phase. *Proc Natl Acad Sci USA* 1994; **91:**

8915–20.

29. Zhou SZ, Li O, Stamatoyannopoulos G, Srivastava A, Adeno-associated virus 2-mediated gene transfer in murine hematopoietic progenitor cells. *Exp Hematol* 1993; **21:** 928–33.

30. Goodman S, Xiao X, Donahue RE et al, Recombinant adeno-associated virus-mediated gene transfer into hematopoietic progenitor cells. *Blood* 1994; **84:** 1492–500.

31. Zhou SZ, Cooper S, Kang LY et al, Adeno-associated virus 2-mediated high efficiency gene transfer into immature and mature subsets of hematopoietic progenitor cells in human umbilical cord blood. *J Exp Med* 1994; **179:** 1867–75.

32. Wilson JM, Adenoviruses as gene delivery vehicles. *N Engl J Med* 1996; **334:** 1185–7.

33. Neering SJ, Hardy SF, Minamoto D et al, Transduction of primitive human hematopoietic cells with recombinant adenovirus vectors. *Blood* 1996; **88:** 1147–55.

34. Dilloo D, Rill D, Entwistle C et al, A novel herpes vector for the high efficiency transduction of normal and malignant human hemopoietic cells. *Blood* 1997; **89:** 119–27.

35. Russell DW, Miller AD, Foamy virus vectors. *J Virol* 1996; **70:** 217–22.

36. Brenner MK, Rill DR, Moen RC et al, Gene-marking to trace origin of relapse after autologous bone marrow transplantation. *Lancet* 1993; **341:** 85–6.

37. Rill DR, Santana VM, Roberts WM et al, Direct demonstration that autologous bone marrow transplantation for solid tumors can return a multiplicity of tumorigenic cells. *Blood* 1994; **84:** 380–3.

38. Brenner M, Heslop HE, Rill D et al, Transfer of marker genes into hemopoietic progenitor cells. *Cytokines Mol Ther* 1996; **2:** 193–200.

39. Deisseroth AB, Zu Z, Claxton D et al, Genetic marking shows that Ph$^+$ cells present in autologous transplants of chronic myelogenous leukemia (CML) contribute to relapse after autologous bone marrow in CML. *Blood* 1994; **83:** 3068–76.

40. Cornetta K, Srour EF, Moore A et al, Retroviral gene transfer in autologous bone marrow transplantation for adult acute leukemia. *Hum Gene Ther* 1996; **7:** 1323–9.

41. Brenner MK, Krance R, Heslop HE et al, Assessment of the efficacy of purging by using gene marked autologous marrow transplantation for children with AML in first complete remission. *Hum Gene Ther* 1994; **5:** 481–99.

42. Brenner MK, Rill DR, Holladay MS et al, Gene marking to determine whether autologous marrow infusion restores long-term haemopoiesis in cancer patients. *Lancet* 1993; **342:** 1134–7.

43. Heslop HE, Rooney CM, Brenner MK, Gene-marking and haemopoietic stem-cell transplantation. *Blood Rev* 1995; **9:** 220–5.

44. Brenner MK, Gene marking. *Hum Gene Ther* 1996; **7:** 1927–36.

45. Stewart AK, Dube ID, Kamel-Reid S, Keating A, A Phase 1 study of autologous bone marrow transplantation with stem cell gene marking in multiple myeloma. *Hum Gene Ther* 1995; **6:** 107–10.

46. Stewart AK, Nanji S, Krygsman P et al, Engraftment of gene marked long term bone marrow culture (LTMC) cells in myeloma patients [Abstract]. *Blood* 1996; **88** (Suppl 1): 270a.

47. Bienzle D, Abrams-Ogg ACG, Kruth SA et al, Gene transfer into hematopoietic stem cells: long-term maintenance of in vitro activated progenitors without marrow ablation. *Proc Natl Acad Sci USA* 1994; **91:** 350–4.

48. Heslop HE, Brenner MK, Krance RA et al, Use of double marking with retroviral vectors to determine rate of reconstitution of untreated and cytokine expanded CD34$^+$ selected marrow cells in patients undergoing autologous bone marrow transplantation. *Hum Gene Ther* 1996; **7:** 655–67.

49. Williams DA, Hsieh K, DeSilva A, Mulligan RC, Protection of bone marrow transplant recipients from lethal doses of methotrexate by the generation of methotrexate-resistant bone marrow. *J Exp Med* 1987; **166:** 210.

50. Sorrentino BP, Brandt SJ, Bodine D et al, Selection of drug-resistant bone marrow cells in vivo after retroviral transfer of human *MDR1*. *Science* 1992; **257:** 99–103.

51. Pawliuk R, Kay R, Lansdorp P, Humphries RK, Selection of retrovirally transduced hematopoietic progenitor cells using CD24 as a marker of gene transfer. *Blood* 1994; **84:** 2868–77.

52. Medlin JA, Migita M, Pawliuk R et al, A bicistronic therapeutic retroviral vector enables sorting of transduced CD34$^+$ cells and corrects the enzyme deficiency in cells from Gaucher patients. *Blood* 1994; **84:** 1754–62.

53. Mavilio F, Ferrari G, Rossini S et al, Peripheral blood lymphocytes as target cells of retroviral vector-mediated gene transfer. *Blood* 1994; **83:** 1988–97.

54. Allay JA, Spencer HT, Wilkinson SL et al, In vivo

selection of DHFR-modified murine hemopoietic progenitors by combined therapy with trimetrexate and thymidine transport inhibitors [Abstract]. *Blood* 1997; **88** (Suppl 1): 645a.

55. Aran JM, Gottesman MM, Pastan I, Drug-selected coexpression of human glucocerebrosidase and P-glycoprotein using a bicistronic vector. *Proc Natl Acad Sci USA* 1994; **91**: 3176–80.

56. Ward M, Richardson C, Pioli P et al, Transfer and expression of the human multiple drug resistance gene in human CD34[+] cells. *Blood* 1994; **84**: 1408–14.

57. Bordignon C, Notarangelo LD, Nobili N et al, Gene therapy in peripheral blood lymphocytes and bone marrow for ADA-immunodeficient patients. *Science* 1995; **270**: 470–5.

58. Blaese RM, Culver KW, Miller AD et al, T lymphocyte-directed gene therapy for ADA-SCID: initial trial results after 4 years. *Science* 1995; **270**: 475–80.

59. Kohn DB, Weinberg KI, Nolta JA et al. Engraftment of gene-modified umbilical cord blood in neonates with adenosine deaminase deficiency *Nature Med* 1995; **1**: 1017–23.

60. Kohn DB, Weinberg KI, Lenarsky C et al, Selective accumulation of ADA gene-transduced T lymphocytes upon PEG-ADA dosage reduction after gene therapy with transduced CD34[+] umbilical cord blood cells [Abstract]. *Blood* 1995; **86**(Suppl 1): 295a.

61. McDonagh K, Nienhuis AW, The thalassemias. In: *Hematology of Infancy and Childhood* (Nathan DG, Oski FA, eds). Philadelphia: WB Saunders 1992: 783–879.

62. Lucarelli G, Galimberti M, Polchi P et al, Marrow transplantation in patients with advanced thalassemia. *N Engl J Med* 1987; **316**: 1050–6.

63. Stamatoyannopoulos G, Nienhuis AW (eds), Hemoglobin switching. In: *The Molecular Basis of Blood Diseases*. Philadelphia: WB Saunders, 1994 107–56.

64. Cone RD, Weber-Benarous A, Baorto D, Mulligan RC, Regulated expression of a complete human β-globin gene encoded by a transmissible retrovirus vector. *Mol Cell Biol* 1987; **7**: 887–97.

65. Karlsson S, Papayannopoulos T, Schweiger SG et al, Retroviral-mediated transfer of genomic globin genes leads to regulated production of RNA and protein. *Proc Natl Acad Sci USA* 1987; **84**: 2411–15.

66. Dzierzak EA, Papayannopoulou T, Mulligan RC, Lineage-specific expression of a human beta-globin gene in murine bone marrow transplant recipients reconstituted with retrovirus-transduced stem cells. *Nature* 1988; **331**: 35–41.

67. Bender MA, Gelinas RE, Miller AD, A majority of mice show long-term expression of a human β-globin gene after retrovirus transfer into hematopoietic stem cells. *Mol Cell Biol* 1989; **9**: 1426–34.

68. Novak U, Harris EAS, Forrester W et al, High-level β-globin expression after retroviral transfer of locus activation region-containing human β-globin gene derivatives into murine erythroleukemia cells. *Proc Natl Acad Sci USA* 1990; **87**: 3386–90.

69. Plavec I, Papayannopoulou T, Maury C, Meyer F, A human β-globin gene fused to the human β-globin locus control region is expressed at high levels in erythroid cells of mice engrafted with retrovirus-transduced hematopoietic stem cells. *Blood* 1993; **81**: 1384–92.

70. Miller JL, Donahue RE, Seller SE et al, Recombinant adeno-associated virus (rAAV)-mediated expression of a human gamma-globin gene in human progenitor-derived erythroid cells. *Proc Natl Acad Sci USA* 1994; **91**: 10 183–7.

71. Hargrove P, Vanin EF, Nienhuis AW, High level globin gene expression mediated by a recombinant adeno-associated virus genome which contains the 3′ gamma globin gene regulatory element and integrates as tandem copies in erythroid cells. *Blood* 1997; **89**: 2167–75.

72. Cole-Strauss A, Yoon K, Xiang Y et al, Correction of the mutation responsible for sickle cell anemia by an RNA–DNA oligonucleotide. *Science* 1996; **273**: 1386–9.

73. Karlsson S. Treatment of genetic defects in hematopoietic cell function by gene transfer. *Blood* 1991; **78**: 2481–92.

74. Beutler E, Gaucher disease as a paradigm of current issues regarding single gene mutations of humans. *Proc Natl Acad Sci USA* 1993; **90**: 5384–90.

75. Correll PH, Fink JK, Brady RO et al, Production of human glucocerebrosidase in mice after retroviral gene transfer into multipotential hematopoietic progenitor cells. *Proc Natl Acad Sci USA* 1989; **86**: 8912–16.

76. Krall WJ, Challita PM, Perlmutter LS et al, Cells expressing human glucocerebrosidase from a retroviral vector repopulate macrophages and central nervous system microglia after murine bone marrow transplantation. *Blood* 1994; **83**: 2737–48.

77. Xu L, Stahl SK, Dave HP, Schiffmann R et al, Correction of the enzyme deficiency in hematopoietic cells of Gaucher patients using a clincally acceptable retroviral supernatant transduction protocol. *Exp Hematol* 1994; **22:** 223–30.

78. Walsh CE, Grompe M, Vanin E et al, A functionally active retrovirus vector for gene therapy in Fanconi anemia group C. *Blood* 1994; **84:** 453–9.

79. Kolb H, Schattenberg A, Goldman JM et al, Graft-versus-leukemia effect of donor lymphocyte infusions in marrow grafted patients. *Blood* 1995; **86:** 2041–50.

80. Slavin S, Naparstek E, Nagler A et al, Allogeneic cell therapy with donor peripheral blood cells and recombinant human interleukin-2 to treat leukemia relapse after allogeneic bone marrow transplantation. *Blood* 1996; **87:** 2195–204.

81. Papadopoulos EB, Ladanyi M, Emanuel D et al, Infusions of donor leukocytes to treat Epstein–Barr virus-associated lymphoproliferative disorders after allogeneic bone marrow transplantation. *N Engl J Med* 1994; **330:** 1185–91.

82. Rickinson AB, Lee SP, Steven NM, Cytotoxic T lymphocyte responses to Epstein–Barr virus. *Curr Opin Immunol* 1996; **8:** 492–7.

83. O'Reilly RJ, Lacerda JF, Lucas KG et al (eds), Adoptive cell therapy with donor lymphocytes for EBV-associated lymphomas developing after allogeneic marrow transplants. In: *Important Advances in Oncology.* Philadelphia: Lippincott-Raven, 1996: 149–66.

84. Heslop HE, Brenner MK, Rooney CM, Donor T cells to treat EBV-associated lymphoma. *N Engl J Med* 1994; **331:** 679–80.

85. Heslop HE, Rooney CM, Adoptive immunotherapy of EBV lymphoproliferative diseases. *Immunol Rev* 1997; **157:** 217–22.

86. Heslop HE, Brenner MK, Rooney CM et al, Administration of neomycin-resistance-gene-marked EBV-specific cytotoxic T lymphocytes to recipients of mismatched-related or phenotypically similar unrelated donor marrow grafts. *Hum Gene Ther* 1994; **5:** 381–97.

87. Heslop HE, Ng CYC, Li C et al, Long-term restoration of immunity against Epstein–Barr virus infection by adoptive transfer of gene-modified virus-specific T lymphocytes. *Nature*

88. Rooney CM, Loftin SK, Holladay MS et al, Early identification of Epstein–Barr virus-associated post-transplant lymphoproliferative disease. *Br J Haematol* 1995; **89:** 98–103.

89. Rooney CM, Smith CA, Ng C et al, Use of gene-modified virus-specific T lymphocytes to control Epstein–Barr virus-related lymphoproliferation. *Lancet* 1995; **345:** 9–13.

90. Burrows SR, Khanna R, Burrows JM, Moss DJ, An alloresponse in humans is dominated by cytotoxic T lymphocytes (CTL) cross-reactive with a single Epstein–Barr virus CTL epitope: implications for graft-versus-host disease. *J Exp Med* 1994; **179:** 1155–61.

91. Tiberghien P, Reynolds CW, Keller J et al, Ganciclovir treatment of herpes simplex thymidine kinase-transduced primary T lymphocytes: an approach for specific in vivo donor T-cell depletion after bone marrow transplantation? *Blood* 1994; **84:** 1333–41.

92. Bonini C, Ferrari G, Verzeletti S et al, HSV-TK gene transfer into donor lymphocytes for control of allogeneic graft versus leukemia. *Science* 1997; **276:** 1719–24.

93. Riddell SR, Elliot M, Lewinsohn DA et al, T-cell mediated rejection of gene-modified HIV-specific cytotoxic T lymphocytes in HIV-infected patients. *Nature Med* 1996; **2:** 216–23.

94. Hege KM, Cooke KS, Finer MH et al, Systemic T cell-independent tumor immunity after transplantation of universal receptor-modified bone marrow into SCID mice. *J Exp Med* 1996; **184:** 2261–9.

95. Pardoll DM, Paracrine cytokine adjuvants in cancer chemotherapy. *Annu Rev Immunol* 1995; **13:** 399–415.

96. Matulonis UA, Dosiou C, Lamont C et al, Role of B7-1 in mediating an immune response to myeloid leukemia cells. *Blood* 1995; **85:** 2507–15.

97. Dilloo D, Bacon K, Holden W et al, Combined chemokine and cytokine gene transfer enhances antitumor immunity. *Nature Med* 1996; **2:** 1090–5.

98. Dranoff G, Granulocyte–macrophage colony stimulating factor based tumor vaccines [Abstract]. *Biol Blood Marrow Transplant* 1996; **2:** 158.

Med 1996; **2:** 551–5.

Index